Essential Forensic Medicine

Essentials of Forensic Science

Titles in the series

Essential Forensic Medicine

Edited by

Peter Vanezis
Emeritus Professor of Forensic Medical Sciences, Queen Mary University of London

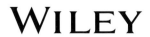

Registered Offices
John Wiley & Sons, Inc., 111 River Street, Hoboken, NJ 07030, USA
John Wiley & Sons Ltd, The Atrium, Southern Gate, Chichester, West Sussex, PO19 8SQ, UK

Editorial Office
The Atrium, Southern Gate, Chichester, West Sussex, PO19 8SQ, UK

For details of our global editorial offices, customer services, and more information about Wiley products visit us at www.wiley.com.

Wiley also publishes its books in a variety of electronic formats and by print-on-demand. Some content that appears in standard print versions of this book may not be available in other formats.

Library of Congress Cataloging-in-Publication Data

Names: Vanezis, Peter, author.
Title: Essential forensic medicine / Peter Vanezis.
Description: First edition. | Hoboken, NJ : Wiley, [2020]. | Series:
    Essentials of forensic science | Includes bibliographical references and
    index. |
Identifiers: LCCN 2019016116 (print) | LCCN 2019017012 (ebook) | ISBN
    9781119186885 (Adobe PDF) | ISBN 9781119186892 (ePub) | ISBN 9780470748633
    (paperback)
Subjects: | MESH: Forensic Medicine–methods | Wounds and Injuries–pathology
Classification: LCC RA1151 (ebook) | LCC RA1151 (print) | NLM W 700 | DDC
    614/.1–dc23
LC record available at https://lccn.loc.gov/2019016116

Cover image: Courtesy of Peter Vanezis
Cover design: Wiley

Set in 10.5/13pts Times Ten by SPi Global, Pondicherry, India
Printed and bound in Singapore by Markono Print Media Pte Ltd

10 9 8 7 6 5 4 3 2 1

Contents

5 The Medico-legal Autopsy   55
Peter Vanezis

6 Interpretation of Injuries: General Principles, Classification, and Age Estimation   73
Peter Vanezis

12 Sexual Offences   199
Philip Beh

13 Paediatric Forensic Medicine   213
Philip Beh and Peter Vanezis

14 Sudden Natural Death   233
Peter Vanezis

15 Heat, Cold, and Electricity   245
Peter Vanezis

16 Diagnosing Death and Changes after Death   261
Peter Vanezis

17   Identification: General Principles, including Anthropology, Fingerprints, and the Investigation of Mass Deaths   285

Peter Vanezis

23   Forensic Toxicology: Clinico-pathological Aspects and Medico-legal Issues   383
Nadia Porpiglia, Chiara Laposata, and Franco Tagliaro

24   Illicit Drug Use   405
Giovanni Serpelloni and Claudia Rimondo

List of Contributors

Dr Philip Beh - Consulting Editor
Associate Professor, Department of Pathology,
Li Ka Shing Faculty of Medicine, University of
Hong Kong, Hong Kong, PR China

Dr Mahomed Dada
Consultant Histopathologist, Histopathology
Department, West Suffolk Hospital NHS
Foundation Trust, Bury St. Edmunds, UK

Dr Vivek Khosla
Consultant Forensic Psychiatrist and
Associate Medical Director (Adult), Oxford
Clinic Medium Secure Unit, Littlemore
Mental Health Centre, Oxford Health NHS
Foundation Trust, Oxford, UK

Dr Chiara Laposata
Medical Specialist in Legal Medicine, Unit of
Forensic Medicine, Department of Diagnostics
and Public Health, University of Verona,
Verona, Italy

Dr Phil Marsden
Consultant Forensic Odontologist, London, UK

Dr Nadia Porpiglia
Post-doctoral Researcher in Forensic
Toxicology, Unit of Forensic Medicine,
Department of Diagnostics and Public
Health, University of Verona, Verona, Italy

Dr Claudia Rimondo
Senior consultant on substance of abuse and
addictions, Department of Diagnostic and Public
Health, University of Verona, Verona, Italy
Assistant at the European Chemicals Agency

Dr Giovanni Serpelloni
Director of UOC Addiction Department,
Verona, Italy

Professor Denise Syndercombe Court
Professor of Forensic Genetics, Department
of Analytical, Environmental and Forensic
Sciences, King's College London, London, UK

Professor Franco Tagliaro
Professor and Head of Unit of Forensic
Medicine, Department of Diagnostics and
Public Health, University of Verona, Verona,
Italy

Dr Orlando Trujillo-Bueno
Oxford Health NHS Foundation Trust,
Oxford, UK

Professor Peter Vanezis OBE
Professor Emeritus of Forensic Medical
Sciences Queen Mary, University of
London, UK

Series Foreword

Essentials of Forensic Science

The world of forensic science is changing at pace in terms of the provision of quality forensic science services, the development of technologies and knowledge, and the interpretation of analytical and other data as it is applied to evidence types presented in our court rooms. Practising forensic scientists are constantly striving to deliver the very best for the judicial process. As such, they need a reliable, valid, and robust scientific basis to underpin the evidence they present in our courts in the service of justice.

It is hoped that this book series will provide a resource by which such validated scientific underpinning can be articulated to both students and practitioners of forensic science alike.

Professor Niamh Nic Daéid, FRSE
Leverhulme Research Centre for Forensic Science
University of Dundee
Series Editor
2019

Preface

There are numerous excellent forensic medical texts available that fulfil the needs of the various professional forensic medicine or science experts in their day-to-day work. Whilst naturally experts will be drawn to texts in their own sub-specialty, the expectation of those wishing to have a wide understanding of the various disciplines is better suited to a more broad-based text. Such individuals fall into main two groups: undergraduate and postgraduate students with a science or medical background, and forensic professionals who wish to widen their knowledge base and enhance their career opportunities.

This text provides essential knowledge in the different areas of the forensic medical sciences to both these groups and is particularly useful for all students taking post-graduate examinations and diplomas up to Masters level.

The text is not designed to be exhaustive and the reader is encouraged and guided towards further reading to supplement their study material when preparing for examinations.

I hope very much that that you find this book a useful companion and would very much appreciate your critical feedback to assist us for future editions.

Peter Vanezis

Acknowledgements

I would firstly like to thank my Consulting Editor Philip Beh for his invaluable advice and contribution to the text, particularly with regard to clinical forensic topics. I would also like to thank all contributors, Mahomed Dada, Vivek Khosla, Chiara Laposata, Philip Marsden, Nadia Porpiglia, Claudia Rimondo, Denise-Syndercome-Court, Giovanni Serpelloni, Franco Tagliaro and Orlando Trujillo-Bueno,

My thanks go to all the staff at Wiley for their assistance with the book through its long gestation period and they include, Vinodhini Mathiyalagan, Nicky McGirr, Elsie Merlin, Lesley Montford, Emma Strickland, Audrie Tan, Mounisamy Thilagavathy, and many others in their team.

I lastly wish to express my gratitute for the permissions granted from various individuals and organisations for many of the illustrations used in the book.

Peter Vanezis

1

The Legal System, Courts, and Witnesses

Peter Vanezis

Queen Mary University of London, London, UK

1.1   Introduction

Forensic medicine in its broadest sense is that branch of medicine which is involved with legal matters and proceedings. The term 'forensic' is derived from the Latin *forensis*, meaning 'the forum'.[1] Forensic practitioners work within the legal system of their area of practice and occasionally may be required to provide reports and give evidence in jurisdictions beyond their own. It is outside the scope of this text to describe in detail different legal systems and here only a brief description of the different main legal systems is given.

There are a number of legal systems and many countries have a mixture of different systems that has ultimately resulted from cultural, religious, and other influences in the development of each particular nation. The main legal systems include common law, Roman law (civil law), religious law and a mixed system. Furthermore, in the European Union (EU) the Court of Justice takes an approach mixing civil law (based on the treaties) with an attachment to the importance of case law.

---

[1] In ancient Rome the forum was a market place where people gathered not just to buy things, but also to conduct all kinds of business, including that of public affairs. The meaning of 'forensic' later came to be restricted to refer to the courts of law. The word entered English usage in 1659.

Essential Forensic Medicine, First Edition. Edited by Peter Vanezis.
© 2020 John Wiley & Sons Ltd. Published 2020 by John Wiley & Sons Ltd.

1.1.1 Common law

Common law developed in England, was influenced by the Norman conquest, which introduced legal concepts from Norman law, and was later inherited by the Commonwealth of Nations and adopted by almost every former colony of the British Empire.

Common law has its source in decisions on cases made by judges. The doctrine of precedent is the main difference from codified law systems. A precedent is a legal case establishing a principle or rule that a court or other judicial body may utilise when deciding subsequent cases with similar issues or facts. Alongside this system of law, there is a legislature that passes new laws and statutes, and the relationships between statutes and judicial decisions can be complex.

The court's role is to apply and develop common law. Statute law, which is created by Parliament, takes precedence over common law and is the supreme legal authority in the United Kingdom (UK). Membership of the EU has meant that European law takes precedence over British Acts of Parliament.

1.1.2 Civil law (Roman law)

Civil law is the most widespread system of law around the world and is sometimes known as *continental European law*. Scots law is a mixed system based on Roman and continental law with elements of common law dating back to the Middle Ages.

The authoritative source of civil law is based on codifications in a constitution or statute passed by legislature (rather than judicial precedents, as in common law).

Historically, the Code of Hammurabi in Babylon c. 1790 BCE is recognised as the first codification (Hooker 1996). The main origin of civil law, however, is from the Roman Empire, the *Corpus Juris Civilis* issued by the Emperor Justinian c. 529 CE. In addition, civil law in its development was also partly influenced by religious laws such as Canon law and Islamic law (Kunkel 1966).

1.2 British courts

There are three court system structures in the UK governed by three different legal systems: England and Wales (English law), Scotland (Scots law), and Northern Ireland (Northern Ireland law).

1.3 The Supreme court of the United Kingdom

The United Kingdom Supreme Court was established by the Ministry of Justice in October 2009 following the passing of the Constitutional Reform Act 2005. Twelve professional judges who are members of the House of Lords carry out its judicial functions. It has assumed the jurisdiction of the Appellate Committee of the House of Lords and the devolution jurisdiction of the Judicial Committee of the Privy Council. It is therefore the final and highest court of appeal for all UK civil cases, and criminal cases from England, Wales, and Northern Ireland. It hears appeals on arguable points of law of general public importance and concentrates on cases of the greatest public and constitutional importance. It also maintains and develops the role of the highest court in the UK as a leader in the common law world.

The Supreme Court cannot consider a case unless a relevant order has been made in a lower court. The courts from which appeals are heard in the UK include:

- *England and Wales*: the Court of Appeal, Civil Division; the Court of Appeal, Criminal Division; the High Court in some limited cases
- *Scotland*: the Court of Session
- *Northern Ireland*: the Court of Appeal in Northern Ireland; the High Court in some limited cases.

Most courts in England and Wales are the responsibility of the Ministry of Justice and Her Majesty's Courts and Tribunals Service (HMCTS 2011), an agency of the Ministry of Justice, for their administration.

The HMCT was created on 1 April 2011 and brings together Her Majesty's Courts Service and the Tribunals Service into one integrated agency providing support for the administration of justice of the criminal, civil, and family courts and tribunals in England and Wales and non-devolved tribunals in Scotland and Northern Ireland. It uniquely operates as a partnership between the Lord Chancellor, the Lord Chief Justice, and the Senior President of Tribunals.

1.4 English and Welsh courts

1.4.1 Court of Appeal

This court consists of two divisions, the Criminal Division and the Civil Division. Decisions of the Court of Appeal may be appealed to the Supreme Court. The Civil Division hears appeals concerning civil law and family justice from the High Court, from tribunals, and certain cases from county courts. The Criminal Division of the Court of Appeal hears appeals from the Crown Court.

1.4.2 High Court

The High Court consists of three divisions, the Chancery Division, the Family Division and the Queen's Bench Division. Decisions of this court may be appealed to the Civil Division of the Court of Appeal.

1.4.3 County Courts

These courts deal with all except the most complicated and most simple civil cases (including most matters under the value of £5000). Decisions in county courts may be appealed to the appropriate division of the High Court.

1.4.4 Crown Court

The Crown Court deals with indictable criminal cases that have been transferred from the Magistrates' Courts, including serious criminal cases (such as murder, rape, and robbery). Cases are sent for sentencing and appeals. Cases are heard by a judge and a jury. Decisions by the Crown Court may be appealed to the Criminal Division of the Court of Appeal.

1.4.5   Magistrates' Courts

These courts deal with summary criminal cases and committals to the Crown Court, with simple civil cases, including family proceedings courts and youth courts, and with licencing of betting, gaming, and liquor. Cases are normally heard by three magistrates or by a district judge, without a jury. Criminal decisions may be appealed to the Crown Court and civil decisions to the county courts.

1.4.6   Tribunals

The Tribunal Service makes decisions on matters of asylum, immigration, criminal injuries, employment, compensation, social security, education, child support, pensions, tax, and lands. Decisions may be appealed to the appropriate division of the High Court.

The structure of the court system in England, Wales, and Northern Ireland is shown in Figure 1.1.

1.5   Scottish Courts

In Scotland, the Superior Courts consist of the Court of Session and the High Court of Justiciary. The Supreme Court of the United Kingdom (described above) hears appeals from the Inner House of the Court of Session.

1.5.1   The court of session

The supreme civil court in Scotland sits in an appeal capacity and also as a civil court dealing with disputes between people or organisations. It consists of the Inner House and Outer House. The Inner House deals mainly with appeals. Appeals are heard from the Outer House, from the Sheriff Court, and from certain tribunals and other bodies. Decisions may be appealed to the Supreme Court. The Outer House hears cases at first instance on a wide range of civil matters. Decisions of the Outer House may be appealed to the Inner House.

1.5.2   The High Court of Justiciary

The High Court of Justiciary deals with criminal appeals and serious criminal cases. Decisions may be appealed to the Privy Council (functions have been taken over by the Supreme Court).

1.5.3   The Sheriff Court

Most cases are heard before a judge called a sheriff. The work of the Sheriff Courts can be divided into three main categories: civil, criminal and commissary. They deal with more serious cases than Justice of the Peace Courts.

1.5.4   Justice of the Peace Courts

From 10 March 2008 the Scottish Court Service is responsible for the administration of the former District Courts – now Justice of the Peace Courts (JP Courts).

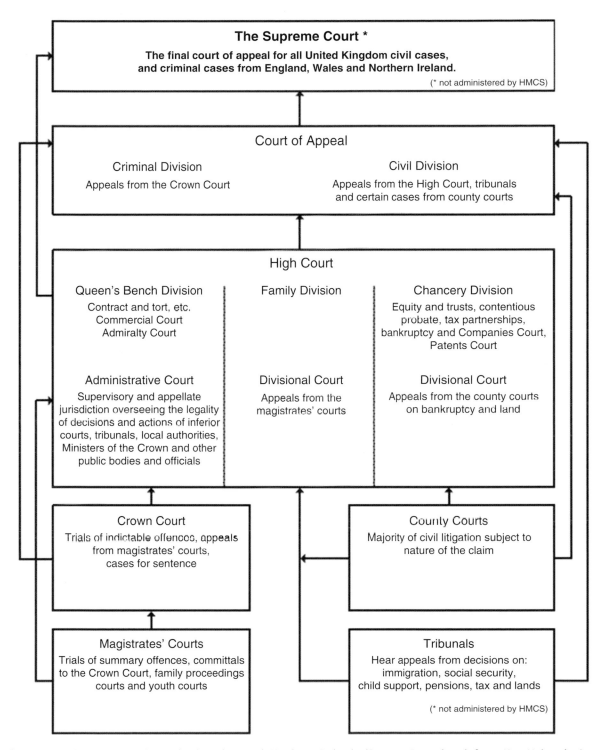

Figure 1.1 Court system in England, Wales, and Northern Ireland. (Source: Reproduced from Her Majesty's Court Service – Structure of HMCS https://webarchive.nationalarchives.gov.uk/aboutus/structure/index.htm.)

1.6   Northern Ireland Courts

Northern Ireland's legal system is similar to that in England and Wales. The Lord Chancellor is responsible for court administration through the Northern Ireland Court Service. The Northern Ireland Office deals with policy and legislation concerning criminal law, the police, and the prison system.

The court system is similar to English courts, with a few modifications, and includes: The Court of Appeal, the High Court (three divisions as in England: Queen's Bench, Family and Chancery), the Crown Court, county courts and magistrates' courts.

1.7   Other courts

There are many other courts in existence. The following is not an exhaustive list.

1.7.1   The Court of Justice of the European Union

A case may be referred to the Court of Justice of the European Union (CJEU), based in Luxembourg. This may happen if European legislation has not been implemented properly by a national government, if there is confusion over its interpretation, or if it has been ignored. The case is then sent back to the national court to make a decision based on the ruling of the CJEU.

1.7.2   The European Court of Human Rights

The European Court of Human Rights, based in Strasbourg, deals with cases in which a person thinks their human rights have been contravened and for which there is no legal remedy within the national legal system.

1.7.3   Court martial (military court)

The Armed Forces Act 2006 established the Court Martial as a permanent standing court, effective from 1 November 2009. The Court Martial may try any offence against service law, which includes all criminal offences under the law of England and Wales. The procedure is broadly similar to that of the Crown Court in England and Wales. It is presided over by a Judge Advocate, and there is a jury (known as a 'board') of between three and seven officers.

1.7.4   International Courts

International courts are set up either between nations through treaties or by international organisations such as the United Nations (UN) and also include international tribunals established for specific purposes.

The *International Criminal Court (ICC)* governed by the Rome Statute (a multilateral treaty), is the first permanent, treaty-based court and was established to help end impunity for the perpetrators of the most serious crimes of concern to the international community. The ICC is an independent international organisation and is not part of the UN system. Its seat is at The Hague in the Netherlands. The international community has long aspired to the creation of a permanent international court and in the twentieth century it reached consensus on definitions of genocide, crimes against humanity, and war crimes. The Nuremberg and Tokyo trials addressed war crimes, crimes against peace, and crimes against humanity committed during the Second World War. In the 1990s, after the end of the Cold War, tribunals like the International Criminal Tribunal for the former Yugoslavia and for Rwanda were the result of a consensus that impunity is unacceptable. However, because they were established to try crimes committed only within a specific time-frame and during a specific conflict, there was general agreement that an independent, permanent criminal court was needed. On 17 July 1998, the international community reached a historic milestone when 120 states adopted the Rome Statute, the legal basis for establishing the permanent ICC, which entered into force on 1 July 2002 after ratification by 60 countries.

The *International Court of Justice (ICJ)* is the principal judicial organ of the UN. It was established in June 1945 by the UN and began work in April 1946. It is based in The Hague (Netherlands). The Court's role is to settle, in accordance with international law, legal disputes submitted to it by states and to give advisory opinions on legal questions referred to it by authorised UN organs and specialised agencies. Fifteen judges, who are elected for a term of nine years by the UN General Assembly and the Security Council of the UN, comprise the court. It is assisted by a Registry, its administrative organ, and the official languages are English and French.

1.7.5 Coroner Courts

Coroner courts are covered in Chapter 2.

1.8 Types of witnesses and evidence

1.8.1 Ordinary witness

An ordinary witness is anyone who can give a first-hand factual account of what they have seen or otherwise experienced in some way, e.g. an eyewitness in a road traffic collision. Any person may be called upon in such a capacity to give evidence.

1.8.2 Professional witness versus the expert witness

The terms professional witness and expert witness are often used synonymously although in the UK the distinction is made where a witness gives evidence in relation to a case in which they may be involved in a professional capacity, e.g. a casualty doctor who has treated the victim of an assault. The doctor will be requested to provide a statement for the court giving a factual account of what injuries they found and how they were investigated and treated. An opinion in relation to the causation of the injuries may be requested if the court agrees and if it is likely that the causation is not contentious, although opinions derived from the facts of a case are the province of expert witness testimony. It would be a common occurrence for a medical expert in the same case to give opinion based on the evidence of the treating doctor. The Faculty of Forensic and Legal Medicine clarified the position in relation to forensic physicians (FPs) acting as professional witnesses as opposed to expert witnesses, stating that FPs document the clinical findings and may include a limited opinion with respect to the significance of the examination findings, e.g. causation of a bruise (Academic Committee of the Faculty of Forensic and Legal Medicine, UK 2008). Although it is expected that all FPs should have had training in how to produce a factual statement, and have ongoing support with writing statements from an experienced FP, the author of a professional statement is merely a witness of fact and does not have to have any experience or expertise with regard to the interpretation of the clinical findings. However, the courts will often need expert interpretation of the medical evidence and this task will fall to an expert witness. The Crown Prosecution Service, alluding to the investigation of rape cases, makes the point that investigating officers and rape specialist prosecutors need to be aware that many FPs, whilst competent to carry out the examination and collect samples, lack the experience and expertise to provide expert opinion (Crown Prosecution Service 2011). This results in professional rather than expert status and may apply particularly where police forces have outsourced services. In these circumstances consideration should always be given to instructing an expert to provide an opinion on the FP's findings.

1.8.3   Expert evidence

An expert witness may give evidence on both fact and opinion or on opinion alone. With respect to criminal proceedings in England and Wales, and following a number of concerns about forensic medical and scientific expert evidence that have resulted in a number of miscarriages of justice, the Law Commission recently published a report that has been presented to Parliament recommending a number of changes (The Law Commission 2011). One of the key recommendations of the report is that there should be a statutory admissibility test which would provide that an expert's opinion evidence is admissible in criminal proceedings only if it is sufficiently reliable to be admitted.

Four requirements have developed at common law in relation to the admissibility of expert evidence in criminal cases.

Assistance

For expert opinion evidence to be admissible it must be able to provide the court with information which is likely to be outside a judge or jury's knowledge and experience, but it must also be evidence which gives the court the help it needs in forming its conclusions.

Relevant expertise

To demonstrate expertise in a particular area, it is essential to furnish the judge or jury with the necessary scientific criteria for testing the accuracy of expert conclusions so as to enable the judge or jury to form their own independent judgement as to the accuracy of their conclusions (Davie v Magistrates of Edinburgh 1953).

The expert usually has academic qualification and experience within their field of expertise. However, expertise can be gained through experience alone, e.g. a police officer may be an accident investigator, or a charity worker with drug abusers may give opinion on the amount of drugs for personal use. An expert may therefore qualify as such through study, training or experience in a particular area (Keane 2000).

Federal rule 702 (Federal Rules of Evidence USA 2006) deals with conditions under which testimony by experts can be given and states, '*If scientific, technical, or other specialized knowledge will assist the trier of fact to understand the evidence or to determine a fact in issue, a witness qualified as an expert by knowledge, skill, experience, training, or education, may testify thereto in the form of an opinion or otherwise, if (1) the testimony is based upon sufficient facts or data, (2) the testimony is the product of reliable principles and methods, and (3) the witness has applied the principles and methods reliably to the facts of the case*'.

Impartiality

The expert must be able to provide impartial, objective evidence on the matters within their field of expertise.

The Civil Procedure Rules (2011) state that (i) it is the duty of experts to help the court on matters within their expertise and (ii) this duty overrides any obligation to the person from whom experts have received instructions or by whom they are paid.

Criminal Procedure Rules (2010) state that (i) an expert must help the court to achieve the overriding objective by giving objective, unbiased opinion on matters within his/her expertise, (ii) this duty overrides any obligation to the person from whom he/she receives instructions or by whom he/she is paid, and (iii) this duty includes an obligation to inform all parties and the court if the expert's opinion changes from that contained in a report served as evidence or given in a statement.

Evidential reliability

Courts in the USA and elsewhere have developed through common law from 'general acceptance' to 'reliability'.

The Frye test (Frye v 1923). In this case the appellant (defendant), was convicted of the crime of murder in the second degree. The case is based on the admissibility of the polygraph (lie detector test).[2] It followed from this judgement that scientific evidence presented to the court must be interpreted by the court as 'generally accepted' by a meaningful segment of the associated scientific community'. This applies to procedures, principles or techniques that may be presented in the proceedings of a court case.

In R v Bonython (1984), King CJ explained the court's approach as follows: 'Before admitting the opinion of a witness into evidence as expert testimony, the judge must consider and decide two questions.

The first is whether the subject matter of the opinion falls within the class of subjects upon which expert testimony is permissible. This first question may be divided into two parts: (i) whether the subject matter of the opinion is such that a person without instruction or experience in the area of knowledge or human experience would be able to form a sound judgement on the matter without the assistance of witnesses possessing special knowledge or experience in the area [common knowledge rule – see below] and (ii) whether the subject matter of the opinion forms part of a body of knowledge or experience which is sufficiently organised or recognised to be accepted as a reliable body of knowledge or experience, a special acquaintance with which of the witness would render his opinion of assistance to the court'.

The second question is whether the witness has acquired by study or experience sufficient knowledge of the subject to render his opinion of value in resolving the issue before the court.

Frye was followed in England in R v Gilfoyle (2001), though it had been superseded by Daubert (Daubert v Merrell Dow Pharmaceuticals Inc. 1993).[3] The Court of Appeal in Dallagher (2002) stated that the approach in English law followed Daubert, although they referred to the pre-2000, 702 amendment.

---

[2] The Appeal Court judges stated 'We think the systolic blood pressure deception test has not yet gained such standing and scientific recognition among physiological and psychological authorities as would justify the courts in admitting expert testimony deduced from the discovery, development, and experiments thus far made'.

[3] Jason Daubert and Eric Schuller had been born with serious birth defects. They and their parents sued Merrell Dow Pharmaceuticals Inc., a subsidiary of Dow Chemical Company, in a California state court, claiming that the drug Bendectin had caused the birth defects.

In the USA the conservative approach in Frye has now been replaced in most states by the case of Daubert, which provides a less conservative approach to admissibility and recognises validity and reliability. 'Daubert hearings' are voir dires to assess whether the expert evidence can be subject to falsifiability, refutability or testability taking into account methodology (including peer review and publication, known or potential error rate, and existence and maintenance of standards), and furthermore, whether the technique has gained general acceptance within the scientific community.

1.8.4   Common knowledge rule

The common knowledge rule bars the admission of expert evidence on matters that can be decide by the court based on its own common sense and everyday experience, and without the assistance of expert knowledge. The purpose of this rule is to preserve the integrity of the decision-making process of the tribunal of fact. It is not designed to filter out inaccurate, invalid or inexpert evidence. Therefore, the common knowledge rule operates to exclude opinion evidence even if the evidence is extremely reliable. Such evidence would include expert evidence on intoxication and intent, character, credit, and credibility Furthermore, evidence from psychiatrists and psychologists is not admissible to prove the veracity of the accused's evidence or the credibility of witness accounts. The case of R v Turner (1975) stands as the main authority for the common knowledge rule at common law.[4] The case of R v Chard (1972) is also of relevance in relation to intention.[5]

1.8.5   Basis rule

The basis rule requires the underpinning of an expert's opinion to be proven by admissible evidence, failing which the expert's opinion is either inadmissible or carries much-reduced weight. The conceptual principle underlying the basis rule is that if an expert is to render the assistance for which his/her evidence is adduced, he/she must furnish the trier of fact with criteria enabling evaluation of the validity of the expert's conclusions. In other words, to state explicitly the facts or assumptions upon which his/her opinion is based.

In England at common law a liberal attitude is taken on the use of hearsay evidence by an expert. This approach is rooted in pragmatism rather than conceptual coherence. The concern is the virtual impossibility of strict compliance with the hearsay rule and the potential for excluding much highly useful and highly reliable opinion evidence. As the English courts said in another case (Borowski v Quayle 1966) 'no one professional man can know from personal observation more than a minute fraction of the data which he must every day treat as working truths'.

---

[4] The defendant was charged with murdering his girlfriend and raised the defence of provocation. He alleged that he had committed the crime in a fit of blind rage when she confessed that she had been unfaithful to him. The defence sought to adduce expert testimony for three purposes: first, to establish that the defendant lacked intent, second, to establish that the defendant was of a nature to be easily provoked, and, third, to bolster the defendant's credibility. The trial judge refused to accept a psychiatrist's report on these issues and since the defendant in *Turner* was not suffering from any mental illness, the Court of Appeal was of the view that the jury did not *need* expert assistance on the issue because the way he was likely to react to his girlfriend's distressing news was a matter well within ordinary human experience.

[5] A is charged with murder. Defence counsel desired to question a prison doctor on the supposed inability of A to form any intent to kill or to do grievous bodily harm, but the judge refused to admit the evidence and this was upheld on appeal. Roskill LJ '... it seems to this Court abundantly plain, on first principles of the admissibility of expert evidence, that it is not permissible to call a witness, whatever his personal experience, merely to tell the jury how he thinks an accused man's mind – assumedly a normal mind – operated at the time of the alleged crime with reference to the crucial question of what that man's intention was'.

1.8.6 Ultimate issue rule

The general rule was that a witness, whether an expert or ordinary witness, may not give evidence about a matter that is an 'ultimate issue' in the case, as this would usurp the function of the judge or jury. This rule has now been abandoned in civil cases and effectively in criminal cases (Civil Evidence Act 1972). The important feature in each such case is that the jury are reminded that it is their assessment of the totality of the evidence that matters and that they are not bound to accept the expert's opinion (R v Stockwell 1993).

References

Academic Committee of the Faculty of Forensic and Legal Medicine (2008) Forensic physicians as witnesses in criminal proceedings.

Borowski v Quayle (1966) VR 382 at 386–387.

Civil Evidence Act 1972, S3 (1).

Civil Procedure Rules 2011. Part 35.3, updated 4 August 2011.

Constitutional Reform Act 2005.

Criminal Procedure Rules 2010, r.33.2.

Crown Prosecution Service (2011). A Protocol between the Police and Crown Prosecution Service in the investigation and prosecution of allegations of rape. http://www.cps.gov.uk/publications/agencies/rape_protocol.html (accessed November 2011).

Dallagher (2002) EWCA Crim 1903, [2003] 1 Cr App R 12 at [29].

Daubert v Merrell Dow Pharmaceuticals Inc. (1993) 509 US 579, 589.

Davie v Magistrates of Edinburgh (1953) S.C. 34.

Federal Rules of Evidence (2006) US Government Printing Office, Washington, 1 December 2006.

Frye v US (1923) Frye v. United States 54 App. D. C. 46, 293 F. 1013, No. 3968 Court of Appeals of District of Columbia.

Her Majesty's Courts and Tribunals Service (2011) www.justice.gov.uk/about/hmcts/index.htm (accessed November 2011).

Hooker, R. (ed.) (1996). *Mesopotamia: The Code of Hammurabi* (trans. L.W. King). Washington State University.

Keane, C. (2000). *The Modern Law of Evidence*, 5e, 503–504. Butterworths.

Kunkel, W. (1966). *An Introduction to Roman Legal and Constitutional History* (translated into English by Kelly JM). Oxford.

R v Bonython (1984) 38 SASR 45.

R v Chard (1972) 56 Cr. App. R. 268.

R v Gilfoyle (No.2) (2001) Cr. App. R 5.

R -v- Stockwell (1993) 97 Cr App R 260.

R v. Turner (1975) 1 QB 834.

The Law Commission (2011) Expert evidence in criminal proceedings in England and Wales. (Law COM No 325) 21st March 2011, HC 829 London. The Stationery Office.

2
Investigation of the Deceased and Their Lawful Disposal

Peter Vanezis
Queen Mary University of London, London, UK

2.1 Introduction

There are a number of different medico-legal systems throughout the world concerned with the proper certification of dead persons and their disposal according to national legal requirements and local customs. In the UK and in the vast majority of its former Empire, the coroner system, mostly modified to meet local needs, is still in place. In the USA the coroner system also remains operative in some states such as California, alongside other states which operate a medical examiner system. Countries of mainland Europe and many of its former colonies employ an examining magistrate to investigate deaths and in Scotland the procurator fiscal system is not that dissimilar to the rest of Europe, although it also has many similarities with the rest of the UK.

This chapter is based on the coroner system although some brief reference is made to other systems of death investigation.

2.2 Certification of details of death by the Registrar of births and deaths and lawful disposal of the body

In order to enable a deceased person to be lawfully disposed of, a number of procedures are essential (the following description applies to the coroner system as it currently operates in England, Wales and Northern Ireland, although with some modifications, the fundamental underlying principles of the other systems are similar).

Essential Forensic Medicine, First Edition. Edited by Peter Vanezis.
© 2020 John Wiley & Sons Ltd. Published 2020 by John Wiley & Sons Ltd.

2.3 Death certificate

Regulations have existed since the latter part of the nineteenth century (Births and Deaths Registration Act 1874) to prevent concealment of a crime and to obtain information about the cause of death for statistical purposes. The disposal of a body must be lawful and the Births and Deaths Registration Act 1926 s.1 stipulates that 'The body of a deceased person may not be disposed of before a certificate of the Registrar (of Deaths) or an order of the coroner has been delivered to the person effecting the disposal'. Furthermore, if the body is to be taken out of England, an 'Out of England Order' is needed from a coroner prior to its removal (s3).

2.4 When may a doctor issue a death certificate?

A person may issue a death certificate if they are a registered medical practitioner. Furthermore, there is a statutory duty on a medical practitioner to issue a medical certificate of the cause of death (MCCD) if he/she attended the deceased during their last illness; in practice usually within 14 days of death (s.22(1) of the Births and Deaths Registration Act (1953)). If these conditions are satisfied then the doctor is obliged to issue a certificate, even if the cause is unknown or unnatural. The registrar will then notify the coroner or the procurator fiscal (Scotland only). Usually, however, the doctor notifies the coroner or procurator fiscal and withholds the certificate. Where there are no grounds for reporting a death to the coroner or procurator fiscal, a death certificate is issued, except where a post-mortem is requested on the grounds of clinical interest and not to ascertain the nature of the illness.

2.5 The form of the certificate in England and Wales

The MCCD (Figure 2.1a and b) comprises a main part, a counterfoil for doctor's retention and a notice to the informant (usually a relative). The main part of the certificate requests the doctor to fill in details of the deceased, whether the cause of death takes into account findings at autopsy (if one was performed), and the cause of death. There is also provision to state whether more information may become available at a later date, usually after further investigations.

  The cause of death is divided into parts I and II. Great care should be exercised in filling in a cause of death so that somewhere in part I the disease or condition leading to death is entered. To enter the mode rather than the cause and its underlying condition is not acceptable. In addition, when one is entering the underlying condition, in many instances a terminal complication or outcome is necessary, particularly when dealing with a chronic illness.

2.6 Legal procedures in the coroner system

The office of coroner has its origin in Saxon times: an official with such a name was in existence during the reign of King Alfred (871–910 CE). However, the official mention of the coroner that we recognise today was in 1194 in the reign of Richard I. It seems that the reason for the revival of the office was initially financial. The coroner had a number of duties but one of the prime reasons for introduction of the office was to keep a check on the corruption of sheriffs of the counties, who were the main executors of the law at that time. The main purpose of the medieval coroner as the office developed was to keep all records of events leading to court cases, including all violent deaths.

(a)

MED.A 22 007539

BIRTHS AND DEATHS REGISTRATION ACT 1953
(Form prescribed by the Registration of Births and Deaths Regulations 1987)

MEDICAL CERTIFICATE OF CAUSE OF DEATH

• For use only by a Registered Medical Practitioner WHO HAS BEEN IN ATTENDANCE during the deceased's last illness, and to be delivered by him forthwith to the Registrar of Births and Deaths.

MED.A 22 007539

Registrar to enter No. of Death Entry

MED.A 22 007539

(Form prescribed by the Registration of Births and Deaths Regulations 1987)

COUNTERFOIL

For use of Medical Practitioner, who should complete in all cases.

Name of deceased

Date of death

Age

Place of death

Last seen alive by me

Post-mortem/* Coroner   1   2   3   4

Whether seen after death*   a   b   c

Cause of death:

I   (a)

     (b)

     (c)

II

Employment?   ☐ *Please tick where applicable*

B. Further information offered?

Signature

Date

Ring appropriate digit(s) and letter.

Name of deceased

Date of death as stated to me .... day of .... Age as stated to me

Place of death

Last seen alive by me .... day of

1 The certified cause of death takes account of information obtained from post-mortem.
2 Information from post-mortem may be available later.
3 Post-mortem not being held.
4 I have reported this death to the Coroner for further action.
   [See overleaf]

Please ring appropriate digit(s) and letter

a Seen after death by me.
b Seen after death by another medical practitioner but not by me.
c Not seen after death by a medical practitioner.

CAUSE OF DEATH

The condition thought to be the 'Underlying Cause of Death' should appear in the lowest completed line of Part I.

These particulars not to be entered in death register

Approximate interval between onset and death

I (a) Disease or condition directly leading to death †

(b) Other disease or condition, if any, leading to I(a)

(c) Other disease or condition, if any, leading to I(b)

II Other significant conditions CONTRIBUTING TO THE DEATH but not related to the disease or condition causing it

The death might have been due to or contributed to by the employment followed at some time by the deceased.   ☐ Please tick where applicable

†This does not mean the mode of dying, such as heart failure, asphyxia, asthenia, etc.: it means the disease, injury, or complication which caused death.

I hereby certify that I was in medical attendance during the above named deceased's last illness, and that the particulars and cause of death above written are true to the best of my knowledge and belief.

Signature ....   Qualifications as registered by General Medical Council

Residence ....   Date

For deaths in hospital: Please give the name of the consultant responsible for the above-named as a patient

NOTICE TO INFORMANT

I hereby give notice that I have this day signed a medical certificate of cause of death of

Signature

Date

This notice is to be delivered by the informant to the registrar of births and deaths for the sub-district in which the death occurred.

The certifying medical practitioner must give this notice to the person who is qualified and liable to act as informant for the registration of death (see list overleaf). Where the informant intends giving information for the registration outside of the area where the death occurred, this notice may be handed to the informant's agent.

DUTIES OF INFORMANT

Failure to deliver this notice to the registrar renders the informant liable to prosecution. The death cannot be registered until the medical certificate has reached the registrar

When the death is registered the informant must be prepared to give to the registrar the following particulars relating to the deceased:

1. The date and place of death.
2. The full name and surname (and the maiden surname if the deceased was a woman who had married).
3. The date and place of birth.
4. The occupation (and if the deceased was a married woman or a widow the name and occupation of her husband).
5. The usual address.
6. Whether the deceased was in receipt of a pension or allowance from public funds.
7. If the deceased was married, the date of birth of the surviving widow or widower.

THE DECEASED'S MEDICAL CARD SHOULD BE DELIVERED TO THE REGISTRAR

(b)

PERSONS QUALIFIED AND LIABLE TO ACT AS INFORMANTS

The following persons are designated by the Births and Deaths Registration Act 1953 as qualified to give information concerning a death; in order of preference they are:

DEATHS IN HOUSES AND PUBLIC INSTITUTIONS

(1) A relative of the deceased, present at the death.

(2) A relative of the deceased, in attendance during the last illness.

(3) A relative of the deceased, residing or being in the sub-district where the death occurred.

(4) A person present at the death.

(5) The occupier* if he knew of the happening of the death.

(6) Any inmate if he knew of the happening of the death.

(7) The person causing the disposal of the body.

DEATHS NOT IN HOUSES OR DEAD BODIES FOUND

(1) Any relative of the deceased having knowledge of any of the particulars required to be registered.

(2) Any person present at the death.

(3) Any person who found the body.

(4) Any person in charge of the body.

(5) The person causing the disposal of the body.

*"Occupier" in relation to a public institution includes the governor, keeper, master, matron, superintendent, or other chief resident officer.

Complete where applicable

A

I have reported this death to the Coroner for further action.

Initials of certifying medical practitioner.

B

I may be in a position later to give, on application by the Registrar General, additional information as to the cause of death for the purpose of more precise statistical classification.

Initials of certifying medical practitioner.

The death should be referred to the coroner if.

• the cause of death is unknown
• the deceased was not seen by the certifying doctor *either* after death *or* within the 14 days before death
• the death was violent or unnatural or was suspicious
• the death may be due to an accident (whenever it occurred)
• the death may be due to self-neglect or neglect by others

• the death may be due to an industrial disease or related to the deceased's employment
• the death may be due to an abortion
• the death occurred during an operation or before recovery from the effects of an anaesthetic
• the death may be a suicide
• the death occurred during or shortly after detention in police or prison custody

LIST OF SOME OF THE CATEGORIES OF DEATH WHICH MAY BE OF INDUSTRIAL ORIGIN

MALIGNANT DISEASES	Causes include	INFECTIOUS DISEASES	Causes include
(a) Skin	– radiation and sunlight – pitch or tar – mineral oils	(a) Anthrax	– imported bone, bonemeal hide or fur
(b) Nasal	– wood or leather work – nickel	(b) Brucellosis	– farming or veterinary
(c) Lung	– asbestos – chromates – nickel – radiation	(c) Tuberculosis	– contact at work
		(d) Leptospirosis	– farming, sewer or under-ground workers
(d) Pleura and peritoneum	– asbestos	(e) Tetanus	– farming or gardening
(e) Urinary tract	– benzidine – dyestuff manufacture – rubber manufacture	(f) Rabies	– animal handling
(f) Liver	– PVC manufacture	(g) Viral hepatitis	– contact at work
(g) Bone	– radiation	CHRONIC LUNG DISEASES	
(h) Lymphatics and haematopoietic	– radiation – benzene	(a) Occupational asthma	– sensitising agent at work
POISONING		(b) Allergic alveolitis	– farming
(a) Metals	e.g. arsenic, cadmium, lead	(c) Pneumoconiosis	– mining and quarrying – potteries – asbestos
(b) Chemicals	e.g. chlorine, benzene	(d) Chronic bronchitis and emphysema	– underground coal mining
(c) Solvents	e.g. trichlorethylene		

NOTE:—The Practitioner, on signing the certificate, should complete, sign and date the Notice to the Informant, which should be detached and handed to the informant. Where the informant intends giving information for the registration outside of the area where the death occurred, the notice may be handed to the informant's agent. The Practitioner should then, without delay, deliver the certificate itself to the Registrar of Births and Deaths for the sub-district in which the death occurred. Envelopes for enclosing the certificates are supplied by the Registrar.

Figure 2.1 Medical certificate of the cause of death (MCCD) used in the UK apart from Scotland: (a) side 1 and (b) side 2. (Source: http://www.certificatestemplatesfree.com/death-certificate-uk-1735.html.)

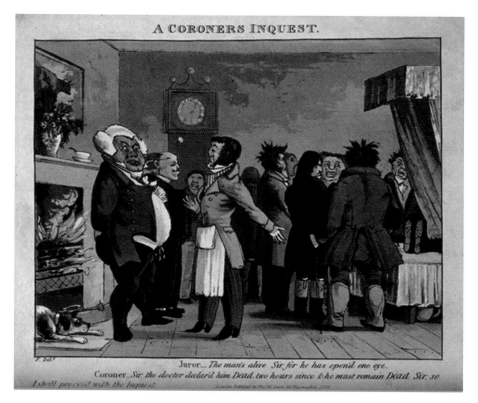

Figure 2.2   A juror protesting that the subject of a coroner's inquest is alive; showing the danger of blind faith in doctors. (Source: Coloured aquatint by F. (published by Thos. McLean, London [26 Haymarket] 1826.) Wellcome Library, London, Iconographic Collections.)

Until the end of the nineteenth century, inquests were held in public houses and inns, mainly because of their large size and for convenience. The coroner would also take a leading role in the investigation, regularly visiting the scene of discovery of a body together with his jurors (Figure 2.2).

Over the years the coroner has gradually lessened his considerable power. Since the Coroners Act 1887, coroners have been concerned with determining the circumstances and actual medical causes of sudden, violent, and unnatural deaths as categorised below. The coroner also has the vestigial but important other function of investigating treasure trove, which does not concern us here.

There have been a number of attempts to reform and improve the coroner system to satisfy the requirement of society for a relevant, transparent, and efficient death investigation system. In 1935 a Committee of Enquiry under the chairmanship of Lord Wright enquired into the law and practice relating to coroners, although few of their recommendations were implemented. A further extensive enquiry carried out in 1971 was the Brodrick Report. Many of the recommendations of this far-reaching enquiry have now been implemented, including the abolition of a coroner's power to commit a person for trial on a charge of criminally causing a death (Criminal Law Act 1977), the abolition of the need for the coroner to view a body before inquest (Coroners Act 1980), the acceptance of written instead of oral evidence at inquest (Coroner's Rules 1980), the referral of criminally caused deaths to the then Director of Public Prosecution (now the

Crown Prosecution Service) (Coroner's Rules 1977), and the power to dispense with a jury in several types of inquest (Criminal Law Act 1977). Both the Wright Committee (Report of the Departmental Committee on Coroners 1936) and the Report on the Committee of Death Certification and Coroners (1971) chaired by Brodrick re-affirmed confidence in the office of the coroner. The Coroners Act (1988) made a number of modifications to the previous Acts, including the new regulation that a person shall not be qualified to be appointed as coroner unless he/ she is a barrister, solicitor or legally qualified medical practitioner of not less than five years' standing in their profession.

A number of events over the last few years have highlighted some serious failings of death certification and the coroner system. In particular, the murders committed by Harold Shipman of his patients, a doctor in general practice in Hyde, Cheshire, made it clear that the current system did not provide adequate protection against malpractice. This led to a lengthy judicial inquiry by Dame Janet Smith comprising six reports, with the third report dealing specifically with death certification and investigation of deaths by coroners (The Shipman Inquiry 2003) Other enquiries also reinforced the need for reform of the system.

The Government acknowledged that there was a need for radical reform of the system (Death Certification and Investigation in England, Wales and Northern Ireland 2003) and this resulted in the Coroners and Justice Act 2009, which, although enacted, has yet to be fully implemented. The new Act provides for the creation of a new Chief Coroner post for England and Wales to lead the jurisdiction and for local medical examiners to oversee a new death certification scheme applicable equally to burial and cremation cases. On 22 May 2012 the first Chief Coroner of England and Wales was announced. He had overseen the implementation of the new provisions of the 2009 Act on 25 July 2013 (Coroners Society England and Wales (2013).

The numbers of cases reported to coroners and their management under the 2009 Act are summarised below (Ministry of Justice 2015).

– Over the last decade, the number of registered deaths in England and Wales has decreased from 512 993 in 2005 to 500 122 in 2014. Of these, 223 841 deaths were reported to coroners in 2014, a decrease of 4143 (2%) from 2013, reflecting in part the fall in the number of registered deaths from 2013 to 2014 (down 1%).
– Just under half (45%) of all registered deaths were reported to coroners in 2014, the same level as seen in 2013. Over the last 10 years this proportion has been relatively consistent, within the range of 45–47%.
– The number of inquests opened in 2014 reduced by 14% to 25 889, which coincided with the Coroners and Justice Act 2009 coming into effect in July 2013. This means coroners can now conduct a brief investigation prior to deciding whether an inquest should take place.
– Post-mortem examinations were ordered by coroners in 40% of all cases reported to them in 2014, down by one percentage point since 2013 and consistent with the long-term downward trend. Since 1995, the proportion of post-mortems ordered has decreased by 21 percentage points, from 61 to 40%.
– In 2014, the proportion of post-mortems conducted in inquest cases was 76%, down eight percentage points on 2013. Following the implementation of the Coroners and Justice Act 2009 in July 2013, coroners are allowed to hold post-mortems as part of a brief investigation before deciding if an inquest needs to be opened, which may account for the drop in the figures.

- Despite a fall of 8% in the total number of conclusions recorded (in part due to the fall in the number of deaths reported to coroners), the number of suicide conclusions in 2014 has increased by almost 3% from 2013 and has been steadily rising since 2007.
- Just three of the ten possible inquest conclusion short forms account for almost 62% of all conclusions recorded (accident and misadventure 27%, unclassified 18%, and natural causes 17%).
- Between 2010 and 2013, 'natural causes' was the most commonly used inquest conclusion, but compared with 2013, the number of natural causes fell by 45% in 2014. This may partly be due to the decrease in the number of cases reported to coroners, but may also be due to the Coroners and Justice Act 2009 coming into effect in July 2013. This means that coroners can now issue a death certificate without holding an inquest when it is known that a death has occurred naturally.
- The estimated average time taken to process an inquest in 2014 (from the date the death was reported until the conclusion of the inquest, where the death occurred in England and Wales) was 28 weeks, with a minimum of 3 weeks and maximum 53 weeks across coroner areas.

2.6.1   Notification of cases to the coroner

Any member of the public may notify a death to the coroner, although the vast majority of deaths (around 90%) are reported by doctors and 10% by registrars of births, deaths, and marriages. There is nevertheless currently no statutory duty on doctors to report deaths, whereas registrars are governed by The Registration of Births and Deaths Regulations (1987) which require referral to the coroner of certain types of death.

All deaths which require to be notified by all the above fall into the following categories:

- deaths resulting from different types of physical injury, whether due to accident, self-harm or homicide
- other types of unnatural deaths, including from poisoning, the effects of heat or cold, drowning, asphyxia, etc.
- death related to a medical procedure or treatment, lack of medical care or adverse reaction to a procedure or medication as opposed to the disease per se
- fatal outcome was unexpected for the injury/disease
- injury or disease received in the course of employment or industrial poisoning
- any death of a person detained in a prison or in military detention, in police custody, or related to police confrontation, e.g. in a riot or demonstration (This category includes a person dying in a special hospital or under statutory mental health powers, or resident in a bail or asylum hostel.)
- where the cause of death is unknown
- where the deceased was not attended by a registered medical practitioner during his/her last illness
- where the cause of death has not been certified by a doctor who saw the deceased after death or within the 14 days before death
- deaths in children where the cause of death is unexpected, including cases where it is uncertain whether a newborn infant was stillborn or had a separate existence (Throughout the UK, stillbirths must be registered by law. The Still-birth Definition Act (1992) states, 'any "child" expelled or issued forth from its mother after the 24th week of pregnancy that did not breathe or show any other signs of life should be registered as a stillbirth'. In England and Wales, this must be

done within 42 days and a Stillbirth Certificate is issued to the parent(s). In Scotland, this must be done within 21 days.)

– any death which is the subject of significant unresolved concern or suspicion as to its cause or circumstances on the part of any family member, or any member of the public, or any health-care, funeral services or other professional with knowledge of the death.

In addition, the registrar is under a statutory duty (see above) to report to the coroner any deaths which are brought to his/her attention and had not previously been reported. These include:

– deaths in which the registrar may have a continuing concern
– deaths where the registrar has been unable to obtain delivery of a completed certificate of the cause of death
– where it appears to the registrar that the cause of death is unnatural, or caused by violence or neglect or by abortion or to have been attended by suspicious circumstances.

Once a death has been referred to the coroner, the coroner, or more usually the coroner's officer, may wish to discuss the case further with the doctor and relatives, and a decision may be made that the death was due to natural causes. In such circumstance the coroner will issue a Pink (or peach-coloured) Form A, which is a notification to the registrar to enable the death to be registered. If the cause of death is uncertain or unknown the coroner may order a post-mortem examination. If the cause of death after the examination is natural and there is no reason to think that the death was unnatural, the coroner will issue a Pink Form B for the registrar and no inquest will be held.

Post-mortem examinations under the 2009 Act replace the old S19 and S20 of the 1988 Act.

– The person carrying out a post-mortem must be a 'suitable practitioner', which could be of a type designated by the Chief Coroner.
– Post-mortem examination is carried out to enable the senior coroner to determine whether a duty to investigate arises.
– The distinction between post-mortems and 'special examinations' is removed, allowing the senior coroner to determine the kind of examination he/she would like the practitioner to make.

2.7 Deaths abroad

Deaths in England and Wales *must* be reported to the Registrar of Deaths. Deaths abroad may be registered – it is a voluntary system. The law requires coroners to treat bodies lying in their jurisdiction but who died outside England and Wales in the same way as those who died in the UK. There are statutory exceptions for visiting forces and diplomats.

2.8 Inquests

Conclusions were recorded for 29 153 inquests in 2014, down by 2426 (8%) from 2013, reversing the continuing upward trend seen since 1996. The conclusions recorded in 2014 may relate to cases opened in 2014 or earlier years. Almost all inquests have a conclusion recorded (98%) and this has remained at the same level since 2012.

Inquests are held on unnatural deaths and others where the coroner feels an enquiry would be beneficial. An inquest is held into every death in prison. An inquest may also be held with respect to bodies brought into England. There are, however, some exceptions where an inquest is not held, such as for diplomats and visiting forces.

The procedure is inquisitorial rather than adversarial and its purpose is a fact-finding inquisition and not a trial which is conducted on behalf of the sovereign.

Furthermore, the hearsay rules do not apply and the coroner will select the witnesses.

In a coroner's court there are no 'parties' but there are 'interested persons' (rule 20). Advocates may represent interested persons, but no-one may address the coroner or the jury on the facts. The coroner may allow evidence to be documentary which in his opinion is unlikely to be disputed, unless a person who in the opinion of the coroner objects to the documentary evidence being admitted.

2.8.1   Scope of the inquest

The scope of the inquest is to answer the following four essential questions:

- *who* deceased was
- *where* they met their death
- *when* death occurred
- *how* the person died (i.e. by what means) but *not why* they died (the reason behind their death).

The Human Rights Act (1988) and Article 2 ECHR (1950) has widened the scope of some inquests. Deaths 'in the care of the state' include deaths in National Health Service (NHS) hospitals and in custody. The inquest must then investigate 'by what means and in what circumstances' the deceased came by his/her death.

A coroner (or jury where there is one) must not frame a conclusion in such a way as to appear to decide any question of criminal liability on the part of a named person, or civil liability, e.g. negligence, in contrast with law before 1977. Indeed in the Coroners Rules 1984, rule 22, provision is made against self-incrimination. The rule states that, '(1) No witness at an inquest shall be obliged to answer any question tending to incriminate himself and, (2) Where it appears to the coroner that a witness has been asked such a question, the coroner shall inform the witness that he may refuse to answer'.

2.8.2   Inquest conclusions

The answer to 'how the person came by their death' is known as the conclusion. Sometimes the short labels that we are familiar with hearing are appropriate and the coroner will use one of them. However, he can also make up his own label or write a narrative of the facts of the case.

When there is a jury at the inquest, the coroner will make the decision about which conclusions are reasonable in law. He would not, for example, leave the jury the option of choosing 'natural causes' if that was clearly wrong. The jury will then choose between the conclusions they have been left. The jury also make the findings of fact.

The whole of the Inquisition (the form completed by the coroner at the end of an inquest) is the conclusion (verdict, before the 2009 Act) and provides additionally for a short narrative of the time, place, and circumstances of the death. Inquest conclusions must not identify someone as having criminal liability nor may they appear to determine civil liability.

Possible short-form conclusions of the inquest include:

- natural causes
- accident or misadventure
- he/she killed him/herself
- unlawful or lawful killing
- industrial disease
- open (where there is insufficient evidence for any other conclusion)
- narrative.

As a result of the development of case law in response to the enactment of the Human Rights Act, coroners increasingly now return a narrative conclusion when this seems more helpful. This is a short paragraph describing the circumstances of the death.

2.9 Registration of death

The informant attends the registrar's office and gives details of the deceased to be entered on the register and to hand the registrar the MCCD and other documents (medical card, passport, pension books, etc.). The registrar will then issue a certificate for disposal and a Certificate of Registration of Death. This will be needed by the executor or administrator when sorting out the person's affairs.

2.10 Burial

The Certificate for Disposal is delivered to funeral director for burial to proceed. The person responsible is the executor or, if deceased is intestate, the next of kin. If no relatives can be found, then the local authority has an obligation to organise and dispose of the body.

After burial, notification of disposal is sent to the registrar.

2.11 Cremation

2.11.1 Introduction

Dr William Price from Llantrisant in South Wales (1800–1893) was regarded as an eccentric doctor who achieved notoriety for his support of Welsh nationalism, Chartism, and his involvement with the Neo-Druidic religious movement (Figure 2.3). He has been recognised as one of the most significant figures in nineteenth century Welsh history, as well as being one of the most unusual in Victorian Britain. He is recognised as the pioneer of cremation in the UK. His first child was born in 1883 and died only five months later, in January 1884. Believing that it was wrong to bury a corpse, thereby polluting the earth, Price decided to cremate his son's body, an act which at the time was taboo, although across the country there were already several proponents of it as a form of corpse disposal. He performed the funeral in the early evening of Sunday 13 January 1884, upon the summit of a hill to one side of Llantrisant. He was arrested for what

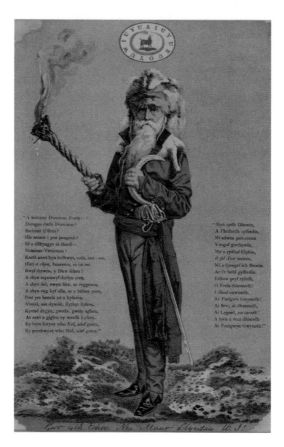

Figure 2.3 Dr William Price. (Source: A lithograph portrait from the Welsh Portrait Collection at the National Library of Wales (unknown artist c. 1870).)

was believed to be the illegal disposal of a corpse, and the body of his son, which had not yet been engulfed by the flames, was removed from the pyre.

From an autopsy carried out by a local doctor, it was concluded that the child had died of natural causes and had not been murdered. Price was therefore not charged with infanticide, but was instead tried in a Cardiff courtroom for performing cremation rather than burial, which the police believed to be illegal. Price argued that while the law did not state that cremation was legal, it also did not state that it was illegal. The judge, Mr Justice Stephen, agreed and Price was freed. The case set a precedent which, together with the activities of the newly founded Cremation Society of Great Britain, led to the first Act of Parliament concerning cremation, which was the Cardiff Corporation Act (1894). Section 71 of this Act empowered the Corporation to establish a crematorium in its cemetery. Between then and 1902, four other similar local Acts were passed. In 1902, Parliament passed the Cremation Act (1902), the first general Cremation Act. It repealed all the previously passed local Acts. Since then Parliament has passed one other Cremation Act (1952). Both general Acts are still in force, although they have been amended. In addition, Parliament has approved a set of Cremation Regulations, made under section 7 of the Cremation Act 1902. These were replaced successively up to 2008, and the Cremation Regulations 2008 are currently in force in England and Wales.

Similar provisions for cremation also apply in Scotland and Northern Ireland through local regulations.

2.11.2 The current cremation procedure

Before any cremation can take place there are a series of forms that have to be completed, which are laid down in the Cremation Regulations 2008 and came into effect on 1 January 2009. They modernise and consolidate all previous regulations, replacing the Cremation Regulations 1930 as amended.

- *Form Cremation 1 – Application for cremation of remains of deceased person (replacing Form A)*: The applicant for cremation should usually be a near relative or an executor. Part 5 of the form deals with the applicant's right to inspect the medical forms (forms Cremation 4 and Cremation 5) before the medical referee authorises cremation. In certain circumstances, the death may need to be referred to a coroner. The coroner may then require a post-mortem examination to be held or an inquest to be opened. In these circumstances there is no right of inspection, as there are no medical forms to inspect and the death is being fully investigated. If the applicant's inspection of the forms raises a possibility that the cause of death was not natural, the medical referee may consider that the case should be referred to a coroner for further consideration.
- *Form Cremation 2 – Application for cremation of body parts (replacing Form AA):* Should be completed by a near relative or an executor. If it is more appropriate for the form to be completed by someone acting on behalf of the next of kin (perhaps the bereavement officer at the hospital) then an explanation for this should be given on the form.
- *Form Cremation 3 – Application for cremation of stillborn baby:* May be completed by one of the parents but may also be completed by the bereavement officer at the hospital.
- *Form Cremation 4 – Medical certificate (replacing Form B):* To be completed by a doctor who can certify the cause of death. It contains the most detailed information about the circumstances surrounding the death. The doctor will need to give information as to whether any hazardous implant has been removed and whether the death has been discussed with a coroner.
- *Form Cremation 5 – Confirmatory medical certificate (replacing Form C):* Regulation 17 of the Cremation Regulations 2008 requires the confirmatory medical certificate to be completed by a registered medical practitioner of at least 5 years' standing.[1]
- *Form Cremation 6 – Certificate of coroner (replacing Form E)*
- *Form Cremation 7 – Certificate following anatomical examination (replacing Form H)*
- *Form Cremation 8 – Certificate releasing body parts for cremation (replacing Form DD)*
- *Form Cremation 9 – Certificate of stillbirth*: This form should be linked with form Cremation 3 and the appropriate registration document. The form may be completed by a registered midwife as well as by a fully registered medical practitioner.
- *Form Cremation 10 – Authorisation of cremation of deceased person by medical referee (replacing Form F)*

---

[1] An overseas doctor who has a primary European qualification in an EEA member state will be eligible to sign form Cremation 5 provided he or she has been registered for 5 years and holds a licence to practise (European Qualifications (Health and Social Care Professions) Regulations 2007 [Regulation 31]).

– *Form Cremation 11 – Certificate after post-mortem examination (replacing Form D):* Cremation authorities will need to be satisfied that all the relevant provisions of the Human Tissue Act 2004 are met. These include any necessary consent from the applicant or other family member for the post-mortem examination to take place, that the post-mortem is made by a pathologist under the authority of a licence issued for that purpose by the Human Tissue Authority, and that the place where the post-mortem is to take place is also duly licenced.
– *Form Cremation 12 – Authorisation of cremation of body parts by medical referee (replacing Form FF)*
– *Form Cremation 13 – Authorisation of cremation of remains of stillborn child by medical referee.*

2.12   The Human Tissue Act 2004 and Human Tissue (Scotland) Act 2006

Investigation of deaths reported to the coroner as well as clinical non-coroner autopsies are subject to the Human Tissue Act 2004, which took effect in England, Wales, and Northern Ireland from April 2006. (Human Tissue Act legislation followed in Scotland in 2006.) Pathologists retaining tissue for further investigation are required to notify the coroner with what has been retained and state how long it is intended to retain the tissue and be aware of what arrangements have been made for its disposal depending on the wishes of the next of kin. The Human Tissue Authority (HTA), established on 1 April 2005 under the Human Tissue Act, extends to England, Wales, and Northern Ireland. The HTA is an executive non-departmental public body sponsored by the Department of Health and is the regulatory body responsible for providing a legal framework, issuing codes of practice, providing guidance, licencing, and inspection of relevant organisations.

The Authority's Chair and 11 members are appointed by the Secretary of State for Health. The Chair and eight of the members are lay and the remaining six are professionals drawn from some of the groups with a direct interest in the application of the Human Tissue Act.

The Human Tissue Act makes consent the fundamental principle underpinning the lawful storage and use of tissues and organs from the living, and the removal, storage, and use of material from the bodies of deceased persons. The Human Tissue Act identifies a number of activities for which a licence must be sought from the HTA:

– The storage of human bodies for anatomical examination and related research.
– The carrying out of a post-mortem examination, including the removal and storage of human tissue.
– The removal and storage of tissue from the body of a deceased person for scheduled purposes (except transplantation), e.g. research.
– The storage of human tissue or cells for human application.
– The storage and use of human bodies or parts for public display.

Offences under the new legislation relate to the removal, storage or use of human tissue for scheduled purposes without appropriate consent and for engagement in licensable activities without an appropriate licence. The Human Tissue Act makes it an offence to have human tissue, which includes hair, nail, and gametes in this context, with the intention of its DNA being analysed without the consent of the individual from whom the tissue came or of those close to them if they have died.

Purposes generally requiring consent where the tissue is from the living or the deceased include:

– anatomical examinations – requires witnessed consent in writing before death
– determining the cause of death – except where a post-mortem is ordered by a coroner
– establishing after a person's death the efficacy of any drug or other treatment administered to them, e.g. hospital post-mortem
– obtaining scientific or medical information about a living or deceased person which may be relevant to any other person (including a future person), e.g. genetic information
– public display – requires witnessed consent in writing before death
– research in connection with disorders or the functioning of the human body
– transplantation – includes all bodily material, such as blood, bone marrow, skin, tissues, and organs.

2.12.1 Existing holdings

Consent is not required for the use of tissue from the living or the deceased held in storage before 1 September 2006 for any scheduled purpose. This includes the use of existing tissue samples for DNA analysis. Use of existing holdings of human tissue for research requires a favourable ethical opinion from an appropriate Research Ethics Committee (REC) and for the tissue samples to be anonymised.

2.13 Exhumation is discussed in detail in Chapter 5

A coroner may issue a direction to exhume a body lying within England and Wales according to the Coroners (Investigations) Regulations 2013, which came into force on 25 July 2013.

2.14 Legal procedures in death investigation: Other systems

2.14.1 Scotland

A death certificate may be issued by any doctor who knows the cause of death, even if not in attendance during the last illness. It has no notice to informant and can be delivered within seven days to the registrar.

2.14.1.1 View and grant A 'view and grant' procedure may be followed where it is felt that an external examination without the need for a dissection of the body will suffice. In such cases, the circumstances leading to death indicate clearly the most likely cause, even though a medical attendant may not have been present during the deceased's last illness.

2.14.1.2 Full autopsy The procedure for carrying out an autopsy in both the coroner and fiscal systems are similar where death is not thought to be due to suspicious circumstances. A single-doctor autopsy will generally take place. In suspicious cases, however, or where otherwise the fiscal feels it appropriate, e.g. deaths in custody, two doctors are requested to carry out the autopsy and are jointly responsible for their findings.

2.14.1.3 Fatal accident inquiry   A fatal accident inquiry (FAI) is held in Scotland and is conducted by Sheriff without a jury. It is mandatory in deaths involving industrial accidents and deaths in custody.

An FAI is discretionary and may be held in other categories of death provided that it is in the public interest to do so. The sheriff will make a determination (cf. inquest verdict).

2.14.2   Medico-legal death investigation in the United States

Medico-legal death investigations in the United States are performed under the provisions of state law, with either a coroner or medical examiner as the official primarily responsible for each investigation in a given jurisdiction, most often at county level.

The position now is that in the United States, where the responsibility for death investigation is with the individual states not the federal government and in many states is delegated to individual cities and counties, 22 states either have state medical examiners or have medical examiners in all their counties, 11 states have coroner systems, and in 18 states there is a mixture of the two. In Canada, there are medical examiner systems in four of the 12 provinces. Currently, approximately, half the US population is served by coroner systems and the other half by medical examiners.

With few exceptions, coroners are lay individuals who are elected to the office. They rely on whatever medical personnel are available to assist in investigations and perform autopsies. On the other hand, medical examiners are usually physicians and pathologists who are appointed and often have special training in medico-legal death investigations and forensic autopsy performance.

In the United States there had been considerable criticism of the coroner system that was introduced under English law during colonial rule and since 1877 there has been a trend to replace coroner systems with medical examiner systems (Hanzlick and Combs 1998). The best-known example of is the Office of the Chief Medical Examiner of New York City.

One of the main advantages of the medical examiner system is that a large proportion of all deaths are scrutinised by a trained medico-legal expert (cf. the establishment of medical examiners as laid down in the provisions of the Coroners and Justice Act 2009). Cases are scrutinised for any potential criminality and are subjected to a detailed autopsy. However, the system does not investigate non-criminal deaths to any depth and in such cases the investigation is less thorough than under the English coroner system.

2.14.3   The generic criminal investigation and judicial system

The generic criminal investigation and judicial system (also known as the continental (European) system), which is used in continental Europe and elsewhere, examines deaths of suspect or uncertain cause through the same systems that are used to investigate suspected crime. Deaths are investigated by the official with responsibility for investigating crime and bringing prosecutions, for example the *procureur* in France. Judicial involvement is from the examining magistracy, which has in most such countries an inquisitorial role and takes responsibility for directing the investigation.

There are provisions in all such countries for the authorities to order unconsented autopsies, although they are generally used only where there is suspicion of crime around the death. Such autopsies are carried out by forensic autopsy specialists, in some countries two doctors being required to participate in each case.

Generally, public judicial hearings into deaths in these countries are not held unless the investigations lead to criminal prosecutions, or there is a court challenge to a decision not to prosecute. They do not usually have special procedures around deaths in prison or detention of other kinds. There would not normally be any public examinations of self-inflicted deaths or traffic deaths, unless the vehicle driver is prosecuted.

These systems do not, characteristically, concern themselves with deaths that are considered to be natural but where the causative disease is not known, although at least in some countries there are powers to investigate and carry out autopsies in deaths from some defined communicable diseases.

In summary, systems of this kind concern themselves primarily with deaths that are suspicious in a criminal sense and not with a wider range of inquiry. They do not set out to cover deaths where the cause is natural but the specific disease is unknown.

References

Births and Deaths Registration Act 1874.
Births and Deaths Registration Act 1926, s.1.
Births and Deaths Registration Act 1953.
Cardiff Corporation Act 1894, 57 & 58 VICT. Ch. clxi, section 71.
Coroners Act 1887.
Coroners Act 1980.
Coroners Act 1988, c13.
Coroners and Justice Act 2009.
Coroners Rules 1977.
Coroners Rules 1980.
Coroners Rules 1984, SI 552.
Coroners Society England and Wales (2013). Implementation of the new provisions of the 2009 Act, 25 July 2013. https://www.coronersociety.org.uk/the-coroners society/history (accessed February 2016).
Cremation Act 1902, 2 Edw. 7 ch. 8.
Cremation Act 1952, 15 & 16 Geo. 6 & 1 Eliz. 2 c. 31.
Cremation, England and Wales 1930, Statutory Rules and Orders, No. 1016.
Criminal Law Act 1977.
Death Certification and Investigation in England, Wales and Northern Ireland (2003) The Report of a Fundamental Review 2003 Cm 5831.
European Convention of Human Rights 1950, Article 2. Rome.
European Qualifications (Health and Social Care Professions) Regulations 2007, Regulation 31.
Hanzlick, R. and Combs, D. (1998). Medical examiner and coroner systems: history and trends. *JAMA* 279 (11): 870–874. http://Coronersociety.org.uk/history (accessed 14 February 2016).
Human Rights Act 1988, c14.
Human Tissue Act 2004.
Human Tissue (Scotland) Act 2006.
Ministry of Justice 2015 Coroners Statistics 2014 England and Wales. Ministry of Justice Statistics Bulletin, 14 May 2015.
Report of the Committee of Death Certification and Coroners (1971) Cm 4810.
Report of the Departmental Committee on Coroners (1936) Cm 5070.

The Coroners (Investigations) Regulations 2013

The Cremation Regulations 2008, SI 2841.

The Registration of Births and Deaths Regulations 1987, Regulation 41. SI 2088.

The Shipman Inquiry, Third Report. Death certification and the investigation of deaths by coroners 14/07/2003. Cm 5854.

The Still-birth Definition Act 1992, c9.

3

The Duties of a Registered Medical Practitioner and the General Medical Council

Peter Vanezis

Queen Mary University of London, London, UK

3.1 Medical Acts

Medical professional responsibility in the United Kingdom is principally regulated by the General Medical Council (GMC), which receives its authority from the Medical Act 1983. It also falls within the judicial system in its broadest sense, which encompasses both English and Scots law.

The GMC was first established under the Medical Act 1858 and has been updated by Parliament on many occasions since then. The purpose of this first Act was to create the body now known as the GMC (previously the General Council of Medical Education and Registration of the United Kingdom) '… so that Persons requiring Medical Aid should be enabled to distinguish qualified from unqualified Practitioners'.

The Act created the position of Registrar of the GMC, still in existence today, whose duty is to keep up-to-date records of those registered to practise medicine and to make them publicly available.

In 1950 a further Medical Act introduced disciplinary boards and a right of appeal to the Council. It also introduced a compulsory year of internship for doctors after their university qualification, where doctors were only allowed to practise and prescribe drugs in National Health Service (NHS) hospitals and under the supervision of a hospital consultant. They were temporarily registered by the GMC for that year before moving to full registration if they successfully completed their training. Currently this internship has lengthened to two years, known as Foundation Years 1 and 2.

Essential Forensic Medicine, First Edition. Edited by Peter Vanezis.
© 2020 John Wiley & Sons Ltd. Published 2020 by John Wiley & Sons Ltd.

The Medical Act 1983, together with a number of more recent amendments, the last being in 2010, provides the current statutory basis for the GMC's functions which includes governance and responsibilities in relation to medical education and registration of doctors and also ensures that medical regulation changes reflect the changing needs of the society within which physicians work.

GMC regulation also takes into account common law, the Data Protection Act 1998, the Human Rights Act 1998, and the Health and Social Care Act 2001 (England and Wales only). Additionally, the Council is also bound by laws that implement a European directive on mutual recognition of professional qualifications from European Economic Area countries.

3.2   Role of the GMC

In essence therefore the role of the GMC includes:

- setting the standards of good medical practice that it expects of doctors throughout their working lives
- assuring the quality of undergraduate medical education in the UK and co-ordinating all stages of medical education
- administering systems for the registration and licencing of doctors to control their entry to and continuation in medical practice in the UK, including the introduction of revalidation, which started in 2012, and
- dealing firmly and fairly with doctors whose fitness to practise is questioned.

The GMC regularly publishes guidance on all the above matters which is regularly mailed to all doctors or made available on their website at www.gmc-uk.org.

A doctor is required to set an example to the rest of society as a model of a caring, compassionate individual with special skills acquired through training, which allow him/her to deliver a high standard of care to patients. However, this altruistic view where doctors are placed on a pedestal is unrealistic and most, unsurprisingly, do not meet such high expectations. It goes without saying that both the GMC and the judicial system will take into account in their deliberations and judgements, whether the issues in question are based on real expectations of a doctor's professional responsibility rather than a standard which can only be achieved by very few in the profession, if by anyone.

Where a doctor is thought to have breached his/her professional medical responsibility in relation to confidentiality issues, performance, incompetence and so on, redress might be sought by the complainant through the civil courts and will also come to the attention of the GMC either directly or indirectly. The latter will then also examine the issues involved and may well subject the doctor to its disciplinary proceedings at some stage.

If a doctor has failed in his/her professional responsibility through commission or omission to the extent that the authorities feel that he/she may have committed a criminal act, then it is possible that doctor may be prosecuted and tried in a criminal court. In such instances there is automatic notification to the GMC by the court or the police.

The most extreme punishment is erasure from the medical register, which therefore does not allow the doctor to practise, although they can appeal against this decision.

Before the GMC can stop or limit a doctor's right to practise medicine, it needs evidence of impaired fitness to practise. This might be, for example, because they:

- have not kept their medical knowledge and skills up to date and are not competent
- have taken advantage of their role as a doctor or have done something wrong
- are too ill, or have not adequately managed a health problem, to work safely.

A warning can also be issued to a doctor where the doctor's fitness to practise is not impaired but there has been a significant departure from the principles set out in the GMC's guidance for doctors, *Good Medical Practice* (General Medical Council 2013). A warning will be disclosed to a doctor's employer and to any other enquirer during a five-year period. A warning will not be appropriate where the concerns relate exclusively to a doctor's physical or mental health.

After a complaint is received about a doctor and preliminary enquiries have been carried out, the GMC decides whether to refer the doctor to a Fitness to Practise Panel hearing with the Medical Practitioners Tribunal Service (MPTS). This is the new adjudication service for UK doctors which was launched on 11 June 2012 as a new impartial adjudication function for doctors and a key part of the GMC's fitness to practise reforms.

Based in a dedicated centre in Manchester, the MPTS is part of the GMC but operationally separate from the regulator's complaint handling, investigation, and case presentation.

The MPTS is led by an independently appointed Chair, who is a senior judge and is responsible for appointing, training, appraising, and mentoring MPTS panellists and legal assessors.

This provides an important safeguard should allegations against the doctor be considered to present a risk to the public.

The GMC will consider both the seriousness of the allegations and the likelihood of being able to prove the case at a hearing. If the case examiners or the Investigation Committee are satisfied that there is a realistic prospect of establishing that the doctor's fitness to practise is impaired, the doctor will appear before an MPTS panel hearing.

Sometimes, if the GMC believes it is necessary, the doctor will be asked to appear before an Interim Orders Panel, which has the power to suspend or impose conditions on the doctor's registration while questions about the doctor's fitness to practise are resolved.

The decisions in the adjudication process are made by medical and lay panellists appointed to sit on Interim Orders and MPTS panels. The panellists are independent, but are required to take account of the Council's policy and guidance.

Interim Orders panels consider whether a doctor's registration should be restricted, either by suspension or by imposing conditions on their registration, while questions about the doctor's fitness to practise are resolved. This ensures that action can be taken to protect patients while enquiries are carried out into the doctor's fitness to practise. This panel meets in private, unless the doctor requests a public hearing.

The MPTS Fitness to Practise panels hear evidence and decide whether a doctor's fitness to practise is impaired. These hearings are the final stage of the GMC procedures. If the panel concludes that a doctor's fitness to practise is impaired, it may:

- take no action
- accept undertakings offered by the doctor provided the panel is satisfied that such undertakings protect patients and the wider public interest

– place conditions on the doctor's registration
– suspend the doctor's registration
– erase the doctor's name from the Medical Register so that they can no longer practise.

If a panel concludes that the doctor's fitness to practise is not impaired, it may issue a warning to the doctor.

MPTS Fitness to Practise panels meet in public, except when considering evidence relating to a doctor's health.

The GMC, in relation to its various hearings, employs both specialist and non-specialist doctors and other health professionals and lay panellists to adjudicate. All panellists undergo regular training by the GMC to assess their suitability for such work and to ensure that they are up to date with procedures.

The GMC and Royal Colleges have concurred that good practice should be measured against established guidelines and have stressed the importance of robust mechanisms to identify and maintain high standards in medical care. The GMC has emphasised that in order to promote the required standards of professional practice, there must be effective quality assurance and clear professional accountability. To ensure good practice, doctors must remain responsible for their own performance and conduct, and should share responsibility for the quality of care provided by their team. Good practice includes:

– ensuring that the care of the patient is the first concern
– treating every patient politely and considerately
– respecting patients' dignity and privacy
– listening to patients and respecting their views
– giving patients information in a way they can understand
– respecting the rights of patients to be fully involved in decisions about their care
– keep professional knowledge and skills up to date
– recognising the limits of one's professional competence
– being honest and trustworthy
– respecting and protecting confidential information
– making sure that one's personal beliefs do not prejudice the patients' care
– a doctor acting quickly to protect patients from risk if there is good reason to believe that he/ she or a colleague may not be fit to practise
– avoiding abusing one's position as a doctor
– working with colleagues in the ways that best serve patients' interests.

Good Medical Practice (General Medical Council 2013) was updated on 29 April 2014 to include a new duty about doctors' knowledge of the English language.

3.3   Consent

Consent should always be freely given and fully informed. The GMC's guidance to doctors emphasises the role of informed consent within a doctor–patient relationship based on trust. The person seeking consent must ensure that they provide both a clear explanation of the scope of consent being sought and an honest answer to all questions. The person from whom consent is sought must be provided with sufficient information to make an informed choice. Information must be offered in an accessible form, for example by avoiding the use of technical terms. Verbal communication skills are important for face-to-face interviews, particularly when answering questions, together with good interpersonal skills to ensure that the person from whom consent is sought feels comfortable about asking questions and does not feel pressured.

Consent should be written where possible. If written consent cannot be obtained, non-written consent must be formally documented and witnessed. In certain situations, for example where a patient visits a doctor for minor routine and non-invasive examinations, it may be implied that consent has been given for such examination to be carried out, such as rolling up a sleeve to have blood pressure taken. Nevertheless, it is always better to obtain oral consent before proceeding with any investigation.

A key principle underlying the notion of informed consent is respect for patient autonomy; it is for the patient, not the doctor, to determine what is in the patient's own best interests.

The information that is needed to obtain informed consent might include the following:

- Details of the diagnosis and prognosis, including what will happen if the condition is left untreated.
- Any uncertainties about the diagnosis, including what options there are for further investigation before treatment.
- Options for the treatment or management of the condition, including the option of not treating.
- The purpose of any proposed investigation or treatment – details of the procedures involved, including any additional treatment such as pain relief, how the patient should prepare, what they can expect during or after the procedure, including common or serious side effects.
- The likely benefits and probabilities of success for each option – what the likely risks are and what changes the patient may have to make to their lifestyle.
- Whether the treatment is experimental and how the patient's progress will be monitored.
- Who has overall responsibility for the treatment and who are the other senior members of the team.
- To what extent students or trainees will be involved.
- A reminder that patients can change their minds at any time.
- A reminder that patients can request a second opinion.
- Details of any charges that there may be for the treatment.

3.4 Decisions involving children and young people

A young person's ability to make decisions depends more on their ability to understand and weigh up options rather than on their age. When assessing a young person's capacity to make decisions, it should be borne in mind that:

- a young person under 16 may have capacity to make decisions, depending on their maturity and ability to understand what is involved
- at 16 years of age a young person can be presumed to have capacity to make most decisions about their treatment and care.

The case of Gillick (1986) tested whether children were competent to give consent on their own to treatment without their parents' knowledge. Mrs Gillick challenged the lawfulness of Department of Health guidance that doctors could provide contraceptive advice and treatment to girls under the age of 16 without parental consent or knowledge in some circumstances.

The House of Lords held that a doctor could give contraceptive advice and treatment to a young person under the age of 16 if:

- she had sufficient maturity and intelligence to understand the nature and implications of the proposed treatment
- she could not be persuaded to tell her parents or to allow her doctor to tell them
- she was very likely to begin or continue having sexual intercourse with or without contraceptive treatment
- her physical or mental health were likely to suffer unless she received the advice or treatment
- the advice or treatment was in the young person's best interests.

This case was specifically about contraceptive advice and treatment, but Axon (2006) makes it clear that the principles apply to decisions about treatment and care for sexually transmitted infections and abortion too. As a result of this decision, a young person under 16 with capacity to make any relevant decision is often referred to as being 'Gillick competent'.

3.5 Consent and capacity

It is a fundamental principle of English law that adults have the right to make decisions on their own behalf and are assumed to have the capacity to do so, unless it is proven otherwise. The responsibility for proving that an adult lacks capacity falls upon the person who challenges it.

The Mental Capacity Act 2005 provides a comprehensive framework for decision making on behalf of adults aged 16 and over who lack capacity to make decisions on their own behalf. This Act applies to England and Wales; Scotland has its own legislation, the Adults with Incapacity (Scotland) Act 2000. The approach in Northern Ireland is currently governed by common law. The Act applies to all decisions taken on behalf of people who permanently or temporarily lack capacity to make such decisions themselves, including decisions relating to medical treatment.

Decision-making capacity refers to the everyday ability that individuals possess to make decisions or to take actions that influence their life, from simple decisions about what to have for breakfast, to far-reaching decisions about serious medical treatment. In a legal context it refers to a person's ability to do something, including making a decision, which may have legal consequences for the person themselves or for other people.

For the purpose of the Mental Capacity Act, a person lacks capacity if at the time the decision needs to be made he or she is unable to make or communicate the decision because of an 'impairment of, or a disturbance in the functioning of, the mind or brain'. The Act contains a two-stage test of capacity: is there an impairment of, or disturbance in the functioning of, the person's mind or brain? If so, is the impairment or disturbance sufficient that the person is unable to make that particular decision?

The assessment of capacity is 'task-specific'. It focuses on the specific decision that needs to be made at the specific time the decision is required. It does not matter if the incapacity is temporary, or the person retains the capacity to make other decisions, or if the person's capacity fluctuates. The inability to make a decision could be the result of a variety of factors, including mental illness, learning disability, dementia, brain damage, or intoxication. The important point is that the impairment or disturbance renders the individual unable to make the decision in question. If the impairment is temporary and the decision can realistically be put off until such a time as he or she is likely to regain capacity, then it should be deferred. While it is clear that an unconscious patient will lack capacity, most other categories of patient will retain some decision-making capacity, however slight.

The Police Reform Act 2002 and The Criminal Justice (Northern Ireland) Order 2005 permit the taking of blood from incapacitated drivers for future consensual testing, therefore putting them in the same position with respect to testing for drug and alcohol levels as drivers with capacity.

3.6 Medical confidentiality

Confidential information is the information obtained by a doctor in their professional capacity to their patient. The following basic principles apply:

- Information about patients must be properly protected to prevent malicious, thoughtless, or inadvertent breaches of confidentiality.
- All people who come into contact with personal health information in their work should have training in confidentiality issues.
- Patients must be informed properly about the way information about them is used.
- Consent should usually be sought for the use or disclosure of personal health information. Occasionally, when it is not possible to obtain consent, information may be disclosed with strict safeguards.
- Data should be anonymised wherever possible.
- Disclosure should be kept to the minimum necessary to achieve the purpose.
- When patients request disclosure, their wishes should be respected.
- Doctors must always be prepared to justify their decisions about the use of personal health information.
- Disclosure may be required by law and includes:
  - public health legislation, e.g. notifiable diseases
  - National Drugs Treatment Monitoring System
  - coroner/fiscal
  - if required to do so in court.
- Disclosure where there may be an overriding public interest, e.g.:
  - where there is a serious risk to others
  - to protect a patient from harm
  - in relation to a serious crime.
- Anonymous information may be used for legitimate purposes without consent.
- The confidentiality of deceased persons must be respected.

3.7 Consent for disclosure

- Patients must be informed as to what is being disclosed.
- Patients must be given a choice and be competent to make a decision.
- Decisions must be conveyed to those seeking consent.
- Implied consent is generally acceptable for sharing information required for patient care.

– Express consent is needed for other uses of information.
– People with parental responsibility may give consent for the sharing of information about children who lack the capacity to decide.
– Proxy decision makers may give consent for disclosure of information about incapacitated adults.

When considering disclosing information to protect the public interest, doctors must:

– consider how the benefits of making the disclosure balance against the harms associated with breaching a patient's confidentiality
– assess the urgency of the need for disclosure
– consider whether the person could be persuaded to disclose voluntarily
– inform the person before making the disclosure and seek his/her consent, unless to do so would enhance the risk of harm
– reveal only the minimum information necessary to achieve the objective
– seek assurances that the information will be used only for the purpose for which it was disclosed
– be able to justify the decision.

References

Adults with Incapacity (Scotland) Act 2000.
Axon, R. (on the application of) v Secretary of State for Health [2006] EWHC 37.
Data Protection Act 1998.
General Medical Council. Good Medical Practice: Guidance for Doctors. (2006, 2009 and 2013) accessed at http://www.gmc-uk.org.
Gillick v West Norfolk and Wisbech AHA (1986) AC 112.
Health and Social Care Act 2001.
Human Rights Act 1998.
Medical Act 1858.
Medical Act 1950.
Medical Act 1983.
The Mental Capacity Act 2005.
The Police Reform Act 2002 and The Criminal Justice (Northern Ireland) Order 2005.

4
General Principles of Scene Examination

Peter Vanezis

Queen Mary University of London, London, UK

The scene is central to any forensic investigation. Its assessment, together with the collection of trace evidence and other relevant findings, will assist in determining the circumstances and type of death under consideration. Handling the scene or scenes in an appropriate way by forensic investigators, be they police, scientists or medical practitioners, will hopefully ensure that evidence is satisfactorily collected, contamination is prevented and all necessary information is comprehensively recorded.

4.1   Concept of the scene

The scene is often referred to as the 'crime scene' in the media and essentially this is a broad, popular, but possibly simplistic way of referring to the place of discovery of a dead body in suspicious circumstances. This may be appropriate in the majority of cases but it should be understood that where a body is found may not be where death occurred or where the incident or crime occurred which led to death. The forensic investigators frequently have to assess a number of possible 'crime scenes', taking into consideration the circumstances in which the body is discovered. The scene of discovery of a body may be related to the actual incident leading to death and the place of death in a number of ways, although it has to be borne in mind that there may be further scenarios and scenes in addition to the situations shown in Table 4.1 and the corresponding examples given below. Most commonly, the place where the person is killed is the same as where the body is found. In one study (Vanezis 1996) this was found to be the case in 471 of 634 deaths (74%).

Essential Forensic Medicine, First Edition. Edited by Peter Vanezis.
© 2020 John Wiley & Sons Ltd. Published 2020 by John Wiley & Sons Ltd.

Table 4.1 Different types of scenes commonly encountered, taking into account where the incident leading to death occurred, the place of death, and where the body was discovered.

	Scene 1	Scene 2	Scene 3
A	Incident leading to death + death + body	–	–
B	Incident leading to death + death	Body	–
C	Incident leading to death	Death + body	–
D	Incident leading to death	Death	Body

Example of A: Male prisoner battered about the head in his cell and found dead where he was assaulted. The blood spatter is able to confirm that he did not move significantly from the position where he was struck on the bunk bed.

Example of B: Female strangled by her husband inside their house. After death he transported her with a wheelbarrow to a neighbour's garage, where he positioned her body so that it would appear that she had been sexually assaulted by another person.

Example of C: Male stabbed in the car park of a public house during an altercation. He ran about 100 m and collapsed in the nearby road, where he was found.

Example of D: Male kidnapped and assaulted when he was forcibly dragged out of his vehicle. He was taken to an unknown location, where it transpired that the assault had caused a severe head injury from which he subsequently died in captivity. His captors then disposed of his body by dumping it in bushes by the side of a road and informed the police of its whereabouts.

4.2   Scene investigation and Locard's principle

Edmond Locard (1877–1966), who was head of the Institute of Criminalistics at the University of Lyon coined his 'theory of interchange' at the scene (Locard 1923, 1928): 'the person or persons at the scene when a crime is committed will almost always leave something and take something away'.

His principle to this day is the enduring fundamental guide which underlies the approach to any scene examination. His doctrine of exchange or transfer is based on the following observations:

1. The perpetrator will take away traces of the victim and the scene.

2. The victim will retain traces of the perpetrator and may leave traces of him/herself on the perpetrator.

3. The perpetrator will leave behind traces of him/herself at the scene (Wagner 1986).

4.2.1   Management of the scene

Satisfactory management of a scene involves a number of important actions that need to be carried out.

– If a person has been reported as missing, the circumstances may dictate searching for a body which may have been concealed in a particular location. This frequently involves substantial resources both in manpower and machinery, occasionally of a highly specialised nature. In such circumstances, particularly if burial is suspected, an archaeologist will be able to advise on methods of locating graves and assist in the recovery. A pathologist will also be able to advise on the possible condition of the remains that are being sought.

- Discovery of a body and preliminary assessment will be made to ascertain whether there are suspicious circumstances or overt evidence of a criminal act. The person making the discovery, who in many cases is a member of the general public, may cause contamination, move an obviously dead body or attempt resuscitation where inappropriate.

- The most urgent and prime consideration on finding someone who is apparently lifeless is to maintain life if there is any chance that the victim may still be alive. Thus, a doctor or paramedic may enter a scene to try and revive an injured person before any precautions are taken to prevent contamination of the body and its immediate environment.

- Ascertaining whether or not there is or might be criminal involvement in the victim's death is in some cases a straightforward matter and advice may be initially sought from the clinical forensic medical examiner who has been called to certify the fact of death. If the death is one that requires the assistance of a forensic pathologist, then usually he/she will be contacted and informed of the circumstances so as to give advice to the police. It should be appreciated that there are other deaths which require special examination of the scene, which may not involve a criminal offence but may nevertheless be in the public interest for an investigation along such lines, e.g. deaths in custody.

- Having ascertained that a forensic investigation is required, a senior officer will be appointed with the formation of a scene team, including relevant specialists. On arrival at the scene the senior investigating officer (SIO) and his/her team will carry out a preliminary assessment, draw up a plan of action, set up an incident room and assemble the scene team.

- The first action that will be taken will be to ensure that the scene is secured to protect it from intruders. It is extremely important that access to the scene is limited and takes into account the need to prevent contamination and/or the loss of vital evidence. This includes securing a wide perimeter around the scene. In an indoor scene as opposed to outdoors, the limits are well defined. Aerial cover such as a tent over the body, or even a marquee if one is dealing with multiple deaths, may be used to prevent unauthorised photography of the scene and the deceased from long-distance, high vantage points or from light aircraft. Once the scene is secured then the senior investigating officer with the advice of the scene team will decide the best way to approach a scene to minimise disturbance.

- Only personnel authorised to be at a scene by the investigating officer should attend, with access being restricted to a small but well-trained group of professionals. Each scene team member will carry out their own particular role and must be aware of the each other's tasks and especially the need for preservation and collection of different types of evidence by the various specialist examiners. It is imperative that protective clothing be worn to protect the examiner from materials at the scene and also to protect the scene from the examiner.

- It is necessary to photograph the scene from an early stage to provide a record of the position of items within a room for example, so that that any subsequent movements of furniture can be recognised. Sometimes furniture or other items are moved by a paramedic attempting resuscitation or by the person who found the body.

4.2.2 Health and safety

It is essential to ensure the safety of the team working at the scene and wherever possible certain circumstances and locations require care and assessment as to their safety and possible risk to the scene team.

–   An obvious example is a building which has been on fire and has been rendered structurally unsafe, or buildings subjected to other forms of disruption such as in an explosion.

–   There may have been the release of noxious substances into the environment such as in certain industrial incidents involving chemicals or radiation.

–   Another type of scene which poses a real risk of causing death to the investigators is an atmosphere where the air is irrespirable, e.g. a mine shaft. Special breathing equipment will be required in such circumstances.

–   Occasionally, booby traps may have been laid at a scene to cause injury to the investigators and to prevent them from carrying out their tasks, particularly in situations where there is civil disturbance.

–   The terrain where a body is discovered may be relatively inaccessible and hazardous, for example when recovering bodies from mountainous terrain in an air crash where the investigators will need to be adequately acclimatised to lower oxygen saturation in the atmosphere at high altitudes.

–   Careful consideration should be given to the risk of infection from microbial agents such as HIV or hepatitis B or C, which may be present in body fluids, or from blood-contaminated discarded hypodermic syringes and needles in death scenes involving intravenous drug abuse. The risk is minimal provided protective clothing is worn and the examiner is careful when moving the body where there may be an excess of blood or other fluids associated with it. It should also be noted that the risk of infection from the exhumation of human remains is minimal unless internment was recent and death has resulted from an epidemic disease such as cholera (Morgan and Tidball-Binz 2006).

–   Attack by predators may also be a risk where there are venomous snakes or wild animals in the vicinity.

4.2.3   Climatic conditions

The weather conditions prevailing at the scene may dictate the approach that needs to be adopted for investigation at the location.

–   Adverse conditions may require the body to be moved to the mortuary as soon as possible. If this cannot be done, appropriate steps such as erecting a tent should be taken to protect the body from the elements.

–   In a particularly hot environment, decomposition would be rapidly accelerated and the body should be removed at the earliest opportunity for autopsy.

4.3   Scene location and associated problems

4.3.1   Types of scenes encountered

Scenes are so varied that one can only categorise them in very broad terms. The examination of each type of scene frequently requires a different type of approach, with the attendance of appropriate forensic expertise. The senior investigator when assessing a scene will decide on the approach and the various types of experts that might be required. This will depend on the location, type of incident, number of deceased, health and safety aspects, urgency of examination and climatic conditions.

The location may be in a building or enclosed within a structure, such as a residence or workplace. It is essential to understand the connection if any between the location and the deceased, i.e. is the location the deceased's residence. An outdoor scene may be in either an urban or countryside environment and in a number of situations involves some degree of concealment, particularly in homicide cases where there has been an attempt to dispose of the body. Occasionally a body is disposed of by burial and there may well be the need to locate the deceased. A body found in water will present further problems. A number of issues need to be resolved, such as where the deceased entered the water in relation to where the body was found and whether the deceased was dead or alive on entry (see Chapter 10).

4.3.2 Indoor location

Most scenes involve an indoor location, usually at the deceased's residence, and it is important in all such cases to seek a full medical history of the deceased from the local community hospital, health centre, general practitioner, and/or community nurse to assess whether one is dealing with an unnatural death or one due to natural causes. In particular, it should be appreciated that an indoor scene is seen most commonly in homicide cases involving family or acquaintances (Figure 4.1).

Police officers dealing with cases that appear prima facie to be somewhat unusual should be encouraged to obtain a second opinion at an early stage; evidence of unclothing, injury or signs of a disturbance should require an early visit from officers trained in homicide investigation.

It is extremely difficult, if not impossible, to attempt to retrieve the situation when a scene has already been variously altered and disturbed from its original state.

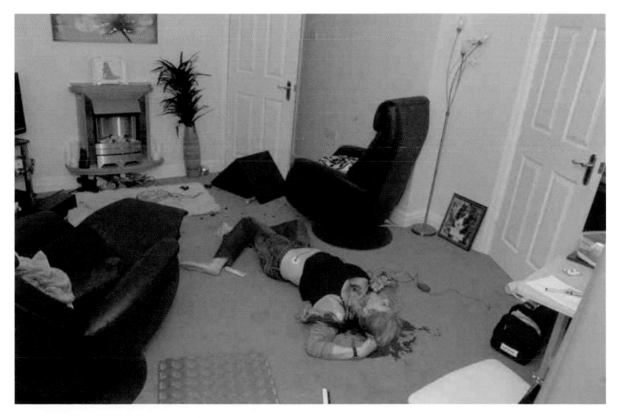

Figure 4.1 The deceased was found stabbed in the lounge by her husband. Signs of a disturbance are seen.

When a body inside a house is found to be partially or totally concealed, or is in an unusual location within the house, such as in an attic, outbuilding, garage or cellar, or perhaps concealed within a wardrobe or underneath floor boards or up a chimney, then the possibility of foul play must be considered at a very early stage and every effort made to collect carefully and methodically as much evidence as possible to exclude this. The discovery of the bodies of infants, children and/or younger adults, particularly in similar circumstances, should always raise strong suspicion. The same is perhaps more obvious when there had been attempts at disposal of the body as by partial burning, the use of chemicals or acids or by dismemberment. In all such circumstances a full scene of crime investigation is imperative.

Tissue damage of a very extensive nature can be produced by pets who are locked inside the house with no other access to food (Rossi et al. 1994). Animals will start off by licking away at secretions emerging from the body orifices but soon after will eat away at the soft tissues.

Access to the body by rodents and by ants may cause further injuries after death, which may be quite confusing to interpret.

A particular situation of an indoor location in which the presence of a pathologist at the scene may prove invaluable involves death occurring in a *bathroom*, especially when the deceased is found in the bath. In such circumstances there are a number of possibilities which one must be aware of:

1.   Is the bath relevant to the death or is it coincidental?

2.   Did the deceased get into the bath voluntarily and die thereafter or did they fall in or were perhaps forced in?

Devos et al. (1985), in a retrospective study of deaths in baths spanning 50 years, found that 52% were due to carbon monoxide poisoning, 20% were suicides, 8.5% were due to natural causes, 8.5% were accidental drownings (mainly infants that were left unattended), and 6% were homicides. Examination of the deceased in situ, the rest of the bathroom, and indeed the other areas in the residence may provide valuable pointers to the forensic team as to the true nature of the death. Initially it is important to note whether there is water in the bath and its depth, and the degree to which the body is covered. The position of the head in relation to the water level may be relevant, particularly if one is considering drowning as a possibility. It should be appreciated, however, that unless the body is discovered very early, the water level will fall and indeed may be very low or non-existent. This will be accelerated if water is leaking through the plug. It is helpful in such cases to establish where the original water level may have been by looking carefully for a possible line of deposit around the bath. This is particularly easy to see if the water is dirty. It is also important to measure the temperature of the water. The position of the plug itself should be noted. Did someone let the water out after death? It may also be relevant to retain a sample of water for analysis. It is also important to note the position of the taps and other objects attached to the bath and their relevance to any injuries on the body.

Examination of the bathroom should take into account how the water supply and room are heated, and whether there is a gas-fuelled heater and a possible source of carbon monoxide. Examination of the type of ventilation and its adequacy is important. The floor of the bathroom may be wet, particularly if there has been a struggle which has resulted in spillage of water onto the floor. This may not be immediately obvious, particularly if the floor is carpeted and some time has passed. One would need to lift any top floor covering and note the dampness underneath.

4.3.3 Outdoor location

Bodies will often be discovered out of doors, on many occasions accidentally by members of the public, who will then call the police. A decision should be made by the officers who are first to arrive at the location on the procedure which should be adopted to protect the scene (Figure 4.2).

(a)

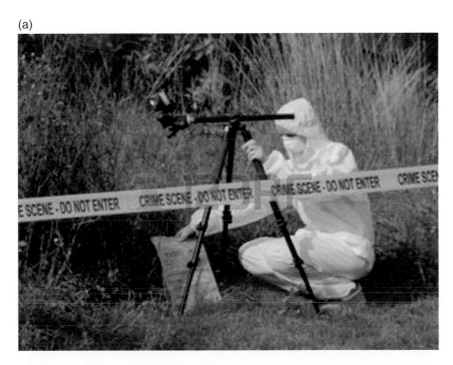

(b)

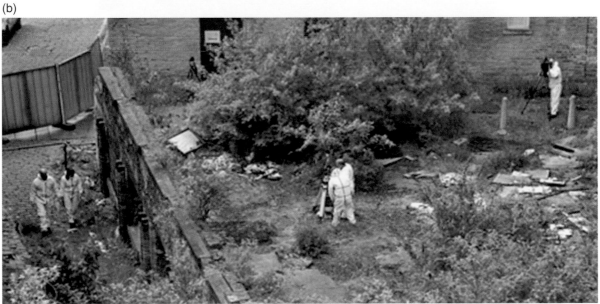

Figure 4.2   (a) Scene cordoned off. (b) Back yard of apartments being examined by suited investigators.

In those instances when the discovery of the body is the result of an anonymous tip-off to the police, more caution is required from the outset.

The person may have died there or could have been transported to or deposited at such a site from another location some distance away.

4.3.4   Outdoor location with Case study

Elderly male deceased was found covered by a tent and the scene cordoned off at the river bank. Figure 4.3 shows various views of the body with feet facing the river. His face contains soil and vegetation. After the face was cleaned in the mortuary scratches were seen from his face being forced into the ground covered with vegetation. The deceased had been suffocated.

In the case of a deceased found by the seashore, the question arises as to whether the person died at the site of discovery or had been washed up by the tide from out at sea.

Persons intent on committing suicide often try to conceal their deed and secrete themselves in woods or undergrowth, often many miles away from their neighbourhood, to avoid detection or disturbance of their plans. In such very secluded circumstances they may take overdoses, hang themselves, or less commonly fatally injure themselves by firearms or cutting implements,

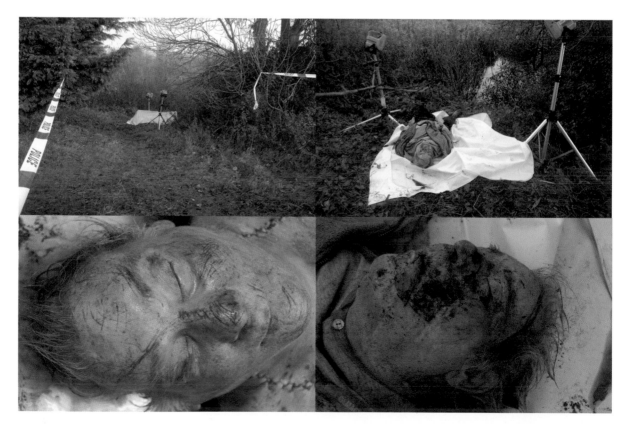

Figure 4.3   Elderly male near river bank showing the area cordoned off, his feet facing the river, and close-up of his face showing scratches.

well out of the way of the public gaze. Months may elapse before such human remains are discovered.

The mode of death may be quite obvious in such cases from the examination of the scene, in the shape of empty bottles of tablets or syringes close by the body or ligatures from which the body is still suspended. If sufficient time has elapsed, ligatures made of organic material may deteriorate by moisture or less sturdy ones may snap, with the body being found on the ground with only the remnants of the ligature around the neck and on the suspension point above the body and these changes would be superimposed on the putrefactive changes, thus causing further potential difficulties in interpretation (Hill 1977; Haglund et al. 1988; Bruce and Rao 1991; Hyams and Rao 1991; Haglund and Reay 1993). Bodies may be dismembered and partially unclothed in such circumstances, with different parts of the body being found at separate locations.

An early search of the pockets may reveal a suicide note or some other form of identification through which the identity of the missing person can be traced and any predisposing psychiatric background identified at an early stage. Persons may die from exposure; this is either induced by cold and/or moist weather on its own or aided by exhaustion or the liberal use of alcohol, and less frequently of other substances. It is important to remember the well-documented association of such deaths from hypothermia with 'paradoxical undressing' (Gormsen 1972; Wedin et al. 1979; Sivaloganathan 1986). The body may be partially undressed or totally naked in such instances and this often raises the possibility of a sexual crime and foul play on initial examination. However, certain cases which at first sight appear to have been death from exposure in hikers or bikers, may turn out to be homicides, often with a robbery or sexual motivation.

4.3.5 Recovery of buried remains from clandestine graves

In the instance of bodies transported to a site to effect their disposal and to prevent their discovery, it is often the case that there will be an attempt to dispose of or conceal the body further by covering it with vegetation, burning it or by burying it in a shallow grave (the investigation of mass graves is dealt with in Chapter 11). Chemical agents such as acid or quicklime may be added in an attempt to accelerate decomposition. In such instances it should be borne in mind that if a weapon has brought about the death, it may be left with the body or discarded very close to it. It is therefore important that any search of the scene should not be limited to the site where the body is found but should also be expanded further afield as circumstances dictate. Blood-stained clothing belonging to the assailant may also be disposed of close by and must be collected and submitted for DNA profiling.

At the scene of a body which has been concealed, either partially or fully buried, it is essential to proceed to recover the remains in a systematic way to ensure its complete removal, together with other necessary material retained from the area immediately surrounding the deceased and frequently within a wider area.

4.3.6 Attendance at a scene where a decomposed body is found

The discovery of a body after the lapse of a period of days or weeks from the time of death frequently raises the possibility that foul play may be involved. The pathologist who attends may thus be able to indicate that the cause of death was natural, accidental or suicidal at the earliest possible phase of the investigation, with little further cause for major concern or the deployment of specialist investigative teams, preventing unnecessary resources being used in a spurious murder investigation. It would be foolhardy to deny that the examination of a scene where a decomposed body is found is particularly difficult and unpleasant, and it must be reiterated from the outset that such investigations are perhaps the most difficult. It is essential to understand the changes of decomposition and the order in which they occur, in particular the production of post-mortem artefacts and how their appearance may simulate ante-mortem injuries.

Protective clothing must be made available to all those who are directly involved in such an investigation. In addition to the unsuitability of the terrain and the general unpleasantness of the cadaver, various micro-organisms thrive in great abundance throughout decomposed bodies. However, unless in the very unlikely event one is dealing with bodies which have a contagious disease such as anthrax or small pox, where the length of survival time after death is significant, the risk to the scene investigators is negligible (Health and Safety Executive 2005).

4.4 Type of incidents

The general principles underlying any scene investigation will guide the forensic investigators to a carry out a comprehensive and professional assessment, although it goes without saying that each type of scene in relation to the type of incident as well as location will be required to be tailored to meet the needs of each particular situation. Location has been discussed above and deaths involving multiple bodies are discussed elsewhere. Different types of scenes according to the type of incident are discussed in detail in other chapters.

4.4.1 Number of deceased persons

Most scenes involve the discovery of one body and it should be appreciated that an investigation where one body had been initially discovered may lead to the finding of further human remains, as in the case of the notorious serial killers Fred and Rosemary West. They were responsible for the deaths of at least 11 women between 1967 and 1987. The majority of the murders occurred between May 1973 and September 1979 at their home in 25 Cromwell Street, Gloucester and the human remains were discovered in 1994 when their garden was excavated. John Reginald Halliday Christie, an earlier necrophiliac serial killer, was responsible for several murders, including his wife. During the Second World War, Christie committed the first of his gruesome murders, which took place at 10 Rillington Place in West London. There were at least seven victims in total, all of which were women and included his wife. Christie moved out of Rillington Place on 20 March 1953 and the bodies were discovered a few days later by the new tenant, hidden in a wallpapered-covered coal cellar in the kitchen. Tests later revealed carbon monoxide in their bodies (Camps 1953).

It may also be suspected from the outset that the scene or a number of related loci contain a number of sets of human remains. It is incumbent on the forensic investigators when the scene examination is carried out to ensure that all such possibilities are considered. Situations where a number of bodies are encountered may include fire death with multiple casualties, transportation incidents, and multiple clandestine graves, including serial killings in a number of related sites and burials in mass graves of genocide victims.

4.5   The forensic pathologist and other medical personnel at the scene

4.5.1   Introduction

There appears to be a wide regional variation in the frequency of attendance at a scene by a pathologist, depending on local practice and to some extent on the volume of casework. In some areas the pathologist will be expected to go to every scene involving a suspicious death or obvious homicide. On the other hand, in other regions attendance is not obligatory, but rather is at the discretion of the investigating officer, in consultation with the pathologist. It is under the latter circumstances that there is always the possible risk of evidence crucial to the investigation being lost or misinterpreted if the pathologist does not attend. Visiting every scene may not be practicable, but one should not underestimate the wealth of invaluable information and experience that may be gained by regular attendance. Indeed, even if the body has been removed to the mortuary, every effort should be made to allow the pathologist full access to the scene. When a pathologist is attempting to reconstruct the chain of events leading to death, an awareness of the scene of the fatal incident, the objects within such a scene, type of location and so on, may help to explain, for example, minor injuries which are found, as well as the more obvious major fatal wounds.

In a substantial number of cases a scene visit followed promptly by a post-mortem examination to ascertain whether or not foul play is involved, enables the investigating officer to make an appropriate early decision regarding deployment of manpower and thus keep the cost of the investigation to a minimum.

Certification of the fact of death is usually carried out by the clinical forensic medical examiner or occasionally by the pathologist. The latter, however, usually arrives some time after the police have made their initial assessment of the scene and the body.

The purpose of examination of the body at the scene before transportation to the mortuary for autopsy is essentially fourfold:

1.   Preliminary assessment where possible as to the type of death, i.e. whether it is a homicide, accident, suicide or due to natural causes.

2.   Aid the investigation of a crime (if one has been committed) by collecting information which leads to the arrest of a suspect and provides evidence against that person.

3.   Collect such information about the body that will corroborate statements of witnesses and the suspect (where a crime is involved).

4.   Maintain the integrity of the chain of custody of evidence.

4.5.2   The pathologist

The pathologist should take into account the following when visiting the scene:

1.   The environment.

2.   The condition and position of the body at the locus, also taking into account attempts at resuscitation.

3. Consideration of the circumstances surrounding death in relation to the body and the scene.

4. Interpretation of post-mortem findings in light of the scene examination.

4.5.3 The pathologist's approach

A systematic approach to the task in hand, such as the following, should be adopted.

1. Preparation: The pathologist should ensure that he/she has a dictaphone, note paper, writing implements, and a rectal thermometer. Body charts, pen torch, and a small ruler are also useful and can be easily carried on one's person.

2. Record the time requested to attend the scene and the name and status of the person making the request. Custom will vary within different medico-legal systems as to the person contacting the pathologist; in England and Wales it may either be a coroner's officer or senior police officer, whereas in Scotland the pathologist is contacted by the procurator fiscal.

3. On arrival at the scene the pathologist should in all circumstances report to the officer at the entrance to the scene in order that the time of arrival and their identity can be recorded.

4. The pathologist should then don protective clothing and wait to be guided to the body via the agreed access route. At this stage the chief scene investigator or one of his colleagues should be available to describe the circumstances of the discovery of the body.

5. The pathologist should then ascertain from the senior investigating officer what is required of him/her. Under no circumstances should the pathologist go straight to the body and start examining it without leave to do so. There are many reasons for this, contamination of the scene and irredeemable loss of trace evidence being the two principal ones. Adequate lighting, e.g. from a portable generator, will ensure that such errors are not made.

6. The body should then be described as found in situ, together with its immediate environment, including its posture, clothing, and relationship to the other objects in its immediate vicinity.

7. Examine the body for the purposes of preliminary assessment of marks and/or injuries to the body.

8. Assess the time of death, if appropriate.

9. Advise the scene investigators on protection of trace evidence on the body during transportation to mortuary.

10. Compile a description of other areas near the body, e.g. other rooms in the house.

11. Supervise removal of the body from the scene.

12. In addition to the above, care must be taken when attending the scene to avoid:
    a. giving 'off the cuff' and premature views to investigating officers
    b. being influenced by senior investigating officers into assuming death has occurred in a certain manner, particularly when all the relevant facts surrounding the case are not yet to hand and examination of the body is incomplete
    c. having any contact with members of the mass media. This is the responsibility of the chief scene investigator through the appropriate press liaison officer.

4.5.4   Examination of the body and its environment

1. Examination of the body, its position, condition (state of preservation), distribution of injuries, and distribution of blood stains should be carried out in conjunction with a description of the scene and not in isolation.

2. It is necessary to appreciate that where the body is discovered may not be where death occurred. It is essential therefore to establish what the scene of discovery of the body represents. Is it where death occurred or was the deceased transported from elsewhere? By careful examination of the body at its location there may be obvious signs that the body has been transported in some way. There may be binding of hands and feet to facilitate this, or there may be drag marks, clothing on the body inappropriate for the scene of discovery or evidence of storage in one particular environment for some time before transportation to another type. It may be necessary, where appropriate, for the pathologist to visit other related scenes.

3. The investigating officer may be able to give the pathologist a comprehensive account of the circumstances leading to death and the pathologist should always satisfy him/herself of whether or not his/her examination supports the account given.

4. One of the first things that a pathologist may be asked to ascertain at the scene is whether or not he/she feels that foul play had occurred. He/she may feel able to say with confidence that the death was due to natural causes and thus curtail a potentially expensive homicide investigation. In practice, however, in the majority of suspicious deaths this is not resolved until the autopsy is carried out. In such cases where the situation is not clear either way, one should expedite the post-mortem examination and ensure that the scene meanwhile remains fully secured and undisturbed.

5. It is usually difficult to examine the body externally in a comprehensive manner at the scene and indeed there is no point in attempting to do so. The body, which may be clothed, is usually not undressed until its arrival at the mortuary and then only by the pathologist or under his/her direction. If it is felt, however, that movement of the clothed body may cause contamination of the clothing, then the removal of the clothing is justified, provided the pathologist is fully aware of the type and distribution of such clothing on the body and is able to examine it fully. This procedure should be documented fully and carried out carefully to avoid loss of trace evidence.

6. The position of the body, the distribution of rigor mortis, and the position of hypostasis, where possible, should also be noted. Minimal disturbance should be the aim of the pathologist at this stage. The main part of the external examination is much better left until the post-mortem

examination is carried out in the mortuary. It should be appreciated that the position of the body when examined by the pathologist may be different from its initial position on discovery for a number of reasons. These include attempts at resuscitation, as outlined below, by medical personnel or others. The body may be moved to a different position to enable access to a scene, particularly if the deceased is wedged against a door, for example, or moved to a position to enable a safer approach and access or for the collection of essential samples or removal of clothing to maximise trace evidence collection and prevent contamination.

7. Examination of the immediate environment (where the body is lying) is essential and will assist the pathologist in gaining a better understanding of the scenario leading to death. There may be pooling of blood which can be matched later with injuries, vomited material, and other body substances such as saliva, urine, and faeces which by their position and quantity may be of assistance to the pathologist in his/her investigation. The type and extent of damage to furniture or structures within a room may assist in reconstructing the various positions and movement of persons at a scene during a fatal attack, particularly when related to the distribution of injuries on the body.

8. A general examination of the scene by the pathologist may be valuable, particularly if blood stains and other indications of injury are found away from the body, for example in other locations in a house. It may be necessary to give explanations for some injuries found which may, for example, fit with falling down a flight of stairs even though the deceased may have been found in the lounge.

4.5.5   Ascertaining the fact of death

When a body is discovered, the initial action is to ascertain whether or not the person found at the scene is in fact dead. Anyone can presume death, but only a medically qualified practitioner should certify the fact of death according to standard practice, even though this may be plainly obvious.

Usually, it is the clinical forensic medical examiner (formerly police surgeon) who is called to the scene to carry out such an examination, and indeed may also be in a position to give some guidance as to the nature of the death (whether suspicious or otherwise). Strictly speaking, however, once death has been ascertained, the involvement of the forensic medical examiner ends and the pathologist should then be called if the death is thought to be suspicious. Occasionally, where it is more expedient, the pathologist may be asked to certify death (for further details on diagnosis of death see Chapter 16).

4.5.6   Assessing the post-mortem interval (time of death)

In a substantial number of cases, the question of the post-mortem interval, i.e. the period elapsed between death and discovery of the body, comes into question and the investigating officer may need some guidance.

The following factors are taken into account:

-   cooling of the body and associated climatic conditions of environment
-   rigor mortis
-   hypostasis

– putrefactive changes
– infestation by insects.

Post-mortem interval estimation is dealt with in detail in Chapter 16.

4.5.7   Artefacts due to resuscitation attempts

First aid, and occasionally major surgery, may have been carried out at the scene and one must always bear this in mind. In attempting to save life, the doctor or paramedic is not going to concern themselves with the need to preserve trace evidence or worry whether a thoracotomy incision is going to modify or incorporate a particular wound. The medical attendant's thoughts will be directed solely to saving the victim's life. Consequently, when life is deemed to be extinct and the medical team have left the scene, it is inevitable that they will have altered the body and the scene to a certain extent. The pathologist should therefore be made aware that resuscitation attempts have been carried out so that any resulting artefacts (such as the examples given below) may be given due consideration during the course of the investigation. The resuscitation team should be questioned as to what they found initially and what they did.

1. Drainage wounds, particularly on the chest, may resemble stab wounds. If examined at the scene in relation to any blood pattern, erroneous conclusions may be drawn. On the other hand, a stab wound may on occasions have a drain inserted into it and initially may not be thought of as significant.

2. A surgeon frequently incorporates a stab wound into a thoracotomy or laparotomy incision and the injury may therefore not be immediately apparent at the scene.

3. Wounds resulting from placing drips, either punctures or 'cut down' wounds, are common and need to be differentiated from needle punctures in the arms due to recent intravenous drug abuse.

4. The position of the body is frequently substantially shifted from its original position and it may also have been turned over.

5. Foreign bodies may have been left in a body cavity or in the air passages.

6. Surfaces may be smeared with transferred blood or other fluids from the body by medical personnel.

7. Extraneous material may be left behind by the medical team such as syringes, packaging etc.

4.5.8   Retrospective scene visit

It should also be appreciated that the body may have been removed to hospital before, or soon after, death and hence cannot be viewed in situ at the scene. Nevertheless, much valuable information is frequently gained by a retrospective visit to the scene. Some would even argue that on occasions a visit after rather than before the post-mortem examination may be more beneficial to the pathologist, bearing in mind that he/she will have thoroughly assessed injuries and other significant marks at autopsy and as a result be better placed to accurately reconstruct events leading to death and/or advise as to the type of instrumentation causing trauma. In addition, there are occasions when, because of prevailing climatic conditions or poor lighting, it is necessary to return to the scene at a later stage, in some cases after the autopsy has been completed.

4.5.9 Documentation of the scene

An accurate record of the scene is vital for the investigation and subsequent use as evidence in court. The body may be moved and objects shifted around at the scene; it is therefore essential that a full visual and written record is made from the moment the body is discovered. Such documentation comprises:

Notes (written or dictated, including the use of a dictaphone). It should be borne in mind that all notes and other material produced may be required to be presented as evidence in court. All material is in any event disclosable.

Still photography (the most essential element of scene documentation). The role of the scene of crime stills photographer is to provide a high-quality permanent record of the scene which will be essential for reference during the course of the investigation and will ultimately be used as evidence in court.

Video-recording. This allows good overall coverage and a permanent record of the scene, which is particularly useful for the pathologist and others who for whatever reason cannot attend the scene with the body present, or indeed wish to refresh their memory. It should nevertheless be appreciated that for best definition and detail, the stills photographer is as yet unsurpassed in being able to produce images of the highest possible quality. It is always good practice to warn all those in the vicinity of the video recorder that the microphone used on these occasions will pick up any conversation over a very wide area.

Plans and sketches. Body charts, templates with the outline of rooms, vehicles etc. are always useful as an aid memoire for producing reports. Occasional use has also been made of scale models of crime scenes in murder trials in order to facilitate the presentation of a particularly complex case (Eckert 1981; O'Brien 1989) and more recently a number of systems have been developed which enable virtual scene of crime tours for court presentation (Ursula et al. 2012).

References

Bruce, A.H. and Rao, V.J. (1991). Evaluation of dismembered human remains. *Am. J. Forensic Med. Pathol.* 12: 291–299.

Camps, F.E. (1953). *Medical and Scientific Investigations in the Christie Case*. London: Medical Publications, Ltd.

Devos, C., Timperman, J., and Piette, M. (1985). Deaths in the bath. *Med. Sci. Law* 25: 189–200.

Eckert, W.G. (1981). Miniature crime scenes. *Am. J. Forensic Med. Pathol.* 2: 365–368.

Gormsen, H. (1972). Why have victims of death from a cold environment undressed? *Med. Sci. Law* 12: 201–202.

Haglund, W.D. and Reay, D.T. (1993). Problems of recovering partial human remains at different times and locations: concerns for death investigators. *J. Forensic Sci.* 38: 69–80.

Haglund, W.D., Reay, D.T., and Swindler, D.R. (1988). Tooth mark artefacts and survival of bones in animal-scavenged human skeletons. *J. Forensic Sci.* 33: 985–997.

Health and Safety Executive (2005). Controlling the risks of infection at work from human remains. A guide for those involved in funeral services (including embalmers) and those involved in exhumation. Health and Safety Executive, Crown Copyright. Published June 2005, accessed at www.hse.gov.uk/pubns/web01.pdf.

Hill, A.P. (1977). Disarticulation and scattering of mammalian skeletons. *Palaeopathology* 5: 261–274.

Hyams, B.A. and Rao, V.J. (1991). Evaluation and identification of human remains am. *J. Forensic Med. Path.* 12: 291–299.

Locard, E. (1923). *Manual of Police Technique*. Paris:Payot.

Locard, E. (1928). Dust and its analysis: an aid to criminal investigation. *Police J.* 1: 177–192.

Morgan, O. and Tidball-Binz, M. (eds.) (2006). *Management of Dead Bodies after Disasters: A Field Manual for First Responders*. Washington, DC: PAHO.

O'Brien, M.W. (1989). Scale model use in crime trials. *J. Forensic Ident.* 39: 359–366.

Rossi, M.L., Shahrom, A.W., Chapman, R.C., and Vanezis, P. (1994). Postmortem injuries by indoor pets. *Am. J. Forensic Med. Pathol.* 15: 105–109.

Sivaloganathan, S. (1986). Paradoxical undressing in hypothermia. *Med. Sci. Law* 26: 225–229.

Ursula, B., Silvio, N., Beat, R. et al. (2012). Accident or homicide – Virtual crime scene reconstruction using 3D methods. *Forensic Sci Int.* [Epub ahead of print].

Vanezis, P. (1996). General principles of scene examination. In: *Suspicious Death Scene Investigation* (ed. P. Vanezis and A. Busuttil), 8–10. London: Arnold.

Wagner, G.N. (1986). Crime scene investigation in child abuse cases. *J. Forensic Med. Pathol.* 7: 94–99.

Wedin, B., Vanggaard, L., and Hirvonnen, J. (1979). Paradoxical undressing in fatal hypothermia. *J. Forensic Sci.* 24: 543–553.

Further reading

Fisher, B.A.J. (2005). *Techniques of Crime Scene Investigation*, 7e. Boca Raton, FL: CRC Press.

5
The Medico-legal Autopsy

Peter Vanezis
Queen Mary University of London, London, UK

5.1 Introduction

An autopsy (Figure 5.1) may be carried out for either clinical or medico-legal reasons. The purpose of a clinical autopsy is to determine the manner and cause of death, evaluate the disease process, and assist in advancing medical research and informing healthcare delivery. A medico-legal autopsy will be carried out in cases under the authority of the coroner or procurator fiscal to assess whether there are issues arising of forensic interest. Medico-legal autopsies in adults will be the subject of detailed discussion in this chapter, with some reference made to clinical (hospital) autopsies. Deaths in children are dealt with in Chapter 13.

The term *autopsy* originates from the Greek 'to look at oneself'. One can also use the term *post-mortem examination, necropsy* (Greek for 'look at a corpse') or *necrotomy* (Greek for 'dissect a corpse'). The author of this text will use both *autopsy* and *post-mortem examination* throughout the text.

5.2 Historical background

Galen (131–200 CE), a Greek physician in the Roman empire, who was arguably the greatest physician in the ancient world, performed dissection of animals and humans. He was determined to demonstrate that Hippocrates' theory that disease was due to four circulating humours (phlegm,

Essential Forensic Medicine, First Edition. Edited by Peter Vanezis.
© 2020 John Wiley & Sons Ltd. Published 2020 by John Wiley & Sons Ltd.

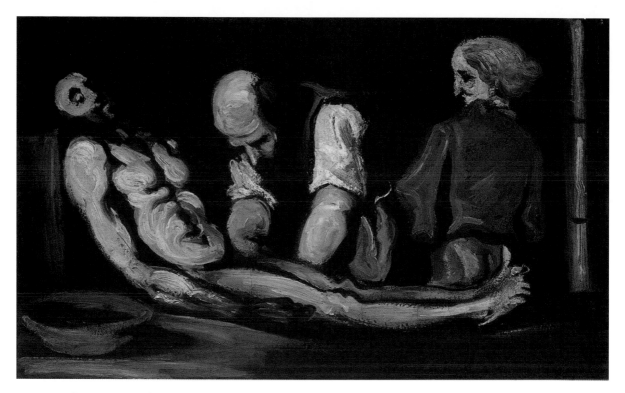

Figure 5.1   Paul Cézanne: *Preparation for the Funeral (The Autopsy)* 1867–1869 (private collection).

blood, yellow bile, and black bile) was correct. Because of his influence, the four-humour doctrine held back medical science for about 1400 years.

Before 1700, dissection of the human body was looked upon in a negative way, although it was carried out by the ancient Egyptians, Greeks, Romans, and medieval Europeans for religious reasons or to learn anatomy. There were, however, notable exceptions. In the late 1200s the law faculty dominated the University of Bologna and would order autopsies to be performed to help solve legal problems (Figure 5.2). In the late fifteenth century in Padua and Bologna, Italy, the sites of the world's first medical schools, Pope Sixtus the IV issued an edict permitting dissection of the human body by medical students. By the sixteenth century, the autopsy was generally accepted by the Catholic Church, marking the way for an accepted systematic approach for the study of human pathology.

Giovanni Bathista Morgagni (1682–1771) is considered generally to be the father of the modern autopsy. He correlated pathological findings with clinical symptoms, marking the first time that autopsies made major contributions to the understanding of disease in medical science. He laid the foundation for great strides to be made in autopsy practice for medical education during the nineteenth century. In that century the foremost advocates of the autopsy were Karl Rokitansky of Vienna (1804–1878) and Rudolph Virchow (1821–1902) of Berlin. From the legacies they have left, their names, together with Morgagni's, are well known in the development of modern autopsy practice today (Figure 5.3).

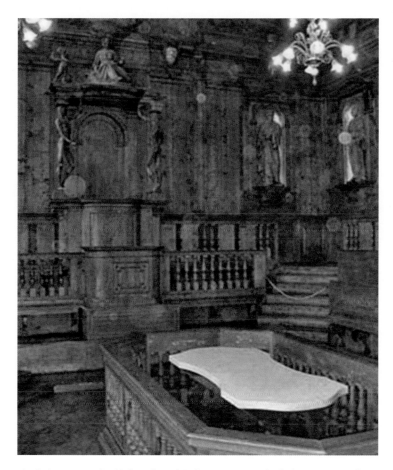

Figure 5.2 The anatomical theatre at the University of Bologna. It was built in 1637. Students sat to observe surgical operations and autopsies.

5.3 Types of autopsy

There are different categories of autopsies, which fall into two general groups in the UK and indeed many other jurisdictions:

- Clinical, non-coronial cases are carried out in hospital in order to assist in understanding and clarifying the extent of a known disease, such as a carcinoma which has metastasised, and the effect of medical intervention. Autopsies in such cases play an important role in clinical audit. Such cases can only be made with the consent of the next of kin.

- Medico-legal autopsies, which include all cases which come under the authority of HM coroner, are discussed in detail below.

- Verbal autopsy is a method of gathering health information about a deceased individual to determine his or her cause of death. Health information and a description of events prior to death are acquired from conversations or interviews with a person or persons familiar with the

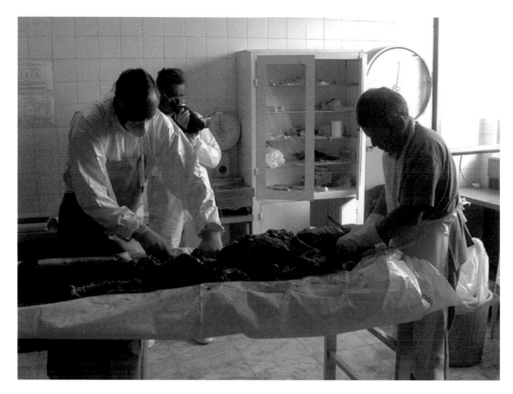

Figure 5.3 Autopsy being performed in a modern hospital setting.

deceased and analysed by health professionals or computer algorithms to assign a probable cause of death. Verbal autopsy is used in settings where most deaths are undocumented. Estimates suggest that the majority of the 60 million annual global deaths occur without medical attention or official medical certification of the cause of death. This method attempts to establish causes of death for previously undocumented subjects, allowing scientists to analyse disease patterns and direct public health policy decisions (WHO 2016). Noteworthy uses of the verbal autopsy method include the Million Death Study in India (Jha et al. 2006), China's national program to document causes of death in rural areas (Yang 2006), and the Global Burden of Disease Study 2010 (Lozano et al. 2012).

5.4 Types of autopsy in the Coroner system

The coroner has a duty under section 1 of the Coroners and Justice Act 2009 to investigate a death if he/she has reason to suspect that:

a.   the deceased died a violent or unnatural death
b.   the cause of the death is unknown *(although may be found to be due to natural causes)* or
c.   the deceased died while in custody or state detention.

This is similar to the wording of section 8(1) of the Coroners Act 1988, except the requirement to investigate where the death is 'sudden' has been removed.

The 2009 Act also refers to deaths in 'state detention' as meaning a person who is 'compulsorily detained by a public authority within the meaning of section 6 of the Human Rights Act 1998'. This, in effect, extends the definition of state detention to institutions such as immigration detention centres and secure mental health hospitals. It would also appear to extend to deprivation of liberty orders (Schedule A1, Mental Capacity Act 2005). All deaths in custody or state detention must be investigated and go to inquest but not necessarily with a jury.

The 2009 Act has given more flexibility in the way in which an autopsy can be made in order to give an opinion as to the cause of death. The type of autopsy will depend on the circumstances surrounding the death. Clearly most information regarding not just the cause of death, but other disease processes in the body can only be achieved by a thorough external and internal dissection of the cadaver accompanied by various ancillary investigations. Before the autopsy, such investigation might include imaging (depending on the circumstances), and during the dissection sampling of tissues for further examination is regarded as good practice, although it is not always carried out if the cause of death is plainly obvious on gross examination.

Furthermore, it is common practice in many coroners' jurisdictions to allow for only a partial (restricted) examination where, if an obvious cause of death is suspected and found in one area of the body such as a ruptured abdominal aortic aneurysm, the Coroner may request that examination should be restricted to the abdominal cavity.

It is also becoming more acceptable with the rapid progress of post-mortem computerised tomography (CT) scanning and magnetic resonance imaging (MRI) to confidently diagnose the cause of death without the need for an internal examination. The demand for a minimally invasive alternative to traditional autopsy has come mainly from the Jewish and Muslim communities, who have religious objections to post-mortem dissection. In response to requests from faith communities, post-mortem imaging services have developed in several centres around the UK in both hospitals and a few public mortuaries. An early validation study of the use of post-mortem MRI in adults identified important weaknesses, notably an inability to visualise coronary artery disease, which is the single most common cause of death found at coroner's autopsy (Roberts et al. 2003). There has been only one study to determine objectively the relative accuracy of CT and MRI when compared with the traditional autopsy (Roberts et al. 2012). This concluded that CT was more accurate than MRI in identifying the cause of death in adults, and that radiologists were better able to identify those cases in which the imaging diagnosis was correct using CT. The most frequent diagnostic errors made on both CT and MRI were in the diagnosis of coronary heart disease and pulmonary embolism. In light of these findings, Roberts and Traill (2014) developed a method of minimally invasive targeted CT coronary angiography that has high sensitivity for detection of significant coronary artery stenosis and when combined with CT is comparable in accuracy with a full autopsy in identifying the cause of sudden adult death.

An external examination without the use of imaging may be another option if the pathologist is prepared to examine the circumstances surrounding the death and give a cause of death on the balance of probabilities. This indeed is an everyday feature of the so called 'view and grant' examination in Scotland.

5.5   Autopsy procedure

A general description of the procedure for medico-legal autopsies is given here. All medico-legal autopsies can only be carried out at the direction of the appropriate authority: the coroner in England, Wales and Northern Ireland or the procurator fiscal in Scotland.

5.5.1   Review of the circumstances surrounding death and other information

An essential preliminary to examination of the body is to be appraised of the circumstances surrounding the demise of the deceased. In cases where the police are involved there will be a briefing by one of the officers of the situation as known at the time. The pathologist must always keep an open mind on the accuracy of an initial brief, bearing in mind that the account and veracity of the circumstances may change as more information comes to hand. There are also frequently other sources of information which necessarily the pathologist should be aware of and these include the following:

– Available statements from witnesses who were present at the time of the incident leading to death. Statements may come from bystanders and other lay persons or from police or paramedics, doctors or indeed anyone who has any pertinent information to offer. It may also be the case that interviews and witness statements are available from persons thought to be involved in some way in the circumstances leading to death. For example, if the deceased became involved in a fight with a number of persons, statements would be taken from all those involved, amongst which may be the person or persons responsible for causing the death. It should be appreciated that information in such statements may vary considerably in accounts given of events. The pathologist must therefore be aware of, but not be influenced by, them when making his/her examination, remaining objective in his/her findings at all times.

– It is essential that the pathologist be provided with information regarding any medical care that the deceased has received. This will include providing him/her with healthcare records dealing with the current medical intervention and past medical history. The examination of such records may be time-consuming, particularly in complex cases involving concerns regarding the quality of healthcare given to the deceased. In relation to medical intervention, consultation with medical colleagues and other relevant personnel prior to the autopsy may be necessary to fully discuss treatment rationale and particularly to explain complex surgical procedures. In some post-operative deaths it is useful for one of the surgeons present during surgery to be present at the autopsy to give some explanation of the findings and the procedure involved.

5.5.2   Identification procedure

The pathologist, prior to beginning his autopsy, will need to have the body identified to him/her. In Scotland, in suspicious deaths or where deemed necessary, two doctors will carry out the autopsy and usually have the body identified to them by two next of kin. The essential goal of the identification procedure is that the correct identification be made to the pathologist, whether directly by an acquaintance of the deceased or indirectly via the anatomical pathology technician or police.

5.5.3 Documentation of the post-mortem examination

Making a record of the autopsy procedure and findings is an essential process which requires careful consideration and teamwork, particularly in more complex forensic cases. It will involve photography or other imaging such as video recording, the use of radiography, and dictation of the findings and of the procedures (e.g. for sampling and retaining tissue for further examination).

– *Photography*
  Photographs are taken at the direction of the pathologist at all stages of the examination.
  It is essential to take full-length views of the body, first within the body bag in which it arrived in the mortuary and showing the label on the bag containing details of the deceased. Once the bag is opened, views are taken of the body dressed and undressed, front and back.
  This is followed by views of all relevant external findings (including negative findings). All injuries and other marks should be photographed both with and without a scale, and the location documented. It is advisable when taking external photographs of the deceased for this to be carried out so that the images follow the order of the external examination so as to enable easy identification of all images. Even with the most experienced eye, it may be difficult to ascertain on occasions the location of the body that has been photographed, such as whether it is the left or right side and even whether one is viewing, for example, the upper or lower limbs. In order to avoid such errors, it is important to instruct the photographer to take a location shot at a further distance prior to the intended view. The location shot should be such that the region of the body from which the intended view of a particular finding is taken is immediately obvious. Albums of images, either as hard copies or electronically, should always be provided to the pathologist with an index detailing the views taken. However, it is essential that the pathologist always confirms this information with the notes he/she has made at the autopsy.
  Internal photographs of the body are also taken. Such views are not usually shown in court, but are nevertheless essential as part of the record of all findings and for review by other pathology colleagues where necessary. As with external photographs, location views may be necessary.
– *Video recording*
  An edited video recording, highlighting the relevant parts of the examination without sound, may be a useful adjunct, particularly where there may be a need for a review of the procedure of the autopsy and to verify findings which might be difficult at a further post-mortem examination due to post mortem changes, or indeed to avoid the need for a further examination.
– *Imaging*
  CT, MRI or radiography should be available to be used if necessary as dictated by the circumstances of the case (see above).
– *Pathologist's documentation of the autopsy findings*
  A documentation of the autopsy procedure and findings is made either by the use of a voice dictation recorder or in written note form. The original notes should be retained for inspection in court if required. When a recorder is used, a literal transcript should be made from the recording and retained. With digital recorders, the file can be downloaded onto a computer and stored securely. In this way, the original documented findings of the pathologist are available prior to a final witness statement being produced.

5.5.4   External examination of the body

The examination of the body begins with observing, assessing, and documenting what can be seen before any dissections are made. The external examination will thus involve description and assessment of the following:

– *Clothing*

- *Type of clothing*
  It is important, particularly in suspicious deaths, that the type and quantity of clothing (if worn) should be examined and evaluated. For example, when assessing the force used to produce stab wounds, the thickness and material constituents of clothing are very important considerations.

- *Damage and other marks*
  Tears, cuts, and other findings on clothing, such as flakes of paint, blood stains, body fluids and other material, should be assessed in conjunction with the injuries and other marks to the body. It is not the province of the pathologist to carry out detailed examination of the clothing, but he/she should examine the clothing in order to assist in obtaining a clearer picture of the circumstances leading to death.

- *Arrangement of clothing*
  The body may have been dragged, in which case clothing may be rucked up and there may be drag marks reflecting the type of surface on which it has been dragged and any material and contaminants with which the body may have come into contact. There may be sexual interference, with movement or repositioning or occasionally re-dressing the body after death.

– *Property*
  It is essential to consider the contents of the deceased's pockets for a number of reasons, including identification, clue to motive for death, e.g. suicide note, weapon, and other objects which may assist the investigation. In addition, the lack of property and pockets turned inside out may indicate a deliberate attempt to prevent identity and/or theft. Marks on the body itself may indicate whether rings and other jewellery have been forcibly removed, before or after death.

– *General examination*
  Once the body has been undressed, it is essential for the pathologist to measure the height and weight and assess the nourishment, noting the body mass index (BMI). The hair distribution, colouration, and general state of the body are described and should also include an assessment of rigor mortis, body temperature where relevant, distribution of hypostasis, state of cleanliness, and distribution of any blood and other body fluids or marks on the body. The deceased should not be washed before all the above have been assessed and any relevant samples collected which may be lost during washing.

– *Regional description*
  Injuries and other marks on the body should wherever possible be examined and documented systematically, region by region. It is wise where there are injuries with the same mode of causation that they are grouped together for the purposes of documentation, e.g. stab wounds.

– *Labelling and numbering of injuries*
Annotation of injuries with numbers or letters is useful where there is a number of similar wounds. This will aid description of the injuries and facilitate referral to photographs. Large numbers of wounds may be annotated as groups rather than have a large number of labels obscure the injuries when photographs are taken. All injuries should also be accompanied by a scale when photographed.

– *Classification and assessment of injuries*
Injuries should be examined and described in terms of their location and morphological appearance and assessed as to mode of causation; occasionally there may be a pattern which will assist in identifying the type of object or surface causing the injury. Injuries should also be assessed as to their age and severity and whether they are ante-mortem or post-mortem. They should also be distinguished from marks associated with medical intervention.

– *Time of death*
It is occasionally relevant to attempt to make a reasonable estimate of the time of death, despite the limitations of all the available methods. This subject is discussed in detail in Chapter 16.

5.5.5 Internal examination of the body

The internal examination is aimed at:

* determining the extent and severity of injury in cases involving trauma; if there are a number of injuries, assessing the role of each in causing death

* reconstructing the mode of infliction of any injuries

* assessing whether there is any natural disease present and whether it is relevant to the death

* determining the cause of death

* determining whether in deaths involving suspicious circumstances if a particular suggested mode of causation can be excluded or confirmed.

Internal examination requires that incisions are made which will facilitate the exposure of the underlying structures (Figure 5.4) and at the same time enable the technician to adequately reconstruct the body for viewing by relatives if required.

a. A single vertical incision is made from below the chin (usually prominence of the thyroid cartilage).
b. Y incision giving good exposure of the neck region is started medial to each shoulder and meets at the upper part of the manubrium sternum.
c. Subclavicular incision (T-shaped) starts from the tips of both shoulders in a horizontal line across the region of the collar bones to meet at the sternum in the middle.
d. The head incision is behind the crown and the ears and extends to both the sides of the neck.

In a, b, and c the cut extends down to the suprapubic region (making a deviation to either side of the umbilicus).

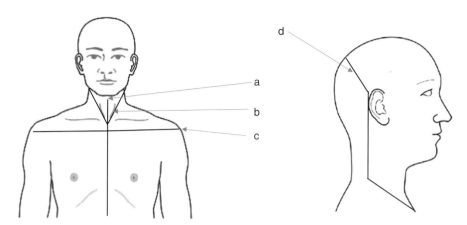

Figure 5.4   Common types of post-mortem incisions for dissection of the deceased.

A full autopsy will involve exposure and examination of the internal structures of the head and neck, thorax, abdomen, pelvic cavities as well as the musculo-skeletal structures. In addition, depending on the circumstances of the case, further specialist dissection and examination may be required. The list detailed here is not exhaustive.

– *Eyes*

  In most autopsies the eyes are examined during the external examination although there may be situations where it is required to carry out evisceration of the eyeball for further examination by an ophthalmic pathologist. Most such examinations are carried out in cases of physical child abuse, or occasionally other cases in relation to trauma to the eye which may be of high significance in the investigation, for example in penetrating injuries.

– *Neck*

  Cervical spine and associated structures

  Detailed examination of the cervical spine where trauma to this region is suspected requires careful exposure of the underlying musculature, the cervical spine, and the cord. In such cases imaging may be of assistance in demonstrating any injury such as a fractured or dislocated vertebra. In cases of vertebral artery trauma, exposure and excision of the posterior neck structures followed by imaging will be required to assess such injury.

  Anterior structures

  Layered detailed dissection of the front of the neck within a bloodless field is particularly important in cases of suspected compression of the neck, with attention directed to the hyoid bone and laryngeal cartilages and their associated musculature.

– *Pelvic organs*

  It is necessary in many cases of sexual violence to make a systematic examination of the ano-genital areas. This may well involve dissecting en block the genital structures within the pelvic cavity, including the rectum and anus, to enable a detailed examination of this region.

– *Subcutaneous tissue dissection*

  It is very common, particularly in trauma cases, to carry out subcutaneous dissection of different parts of the body (back, upper and lower limbs, and face) to look for bruising, which may not be visible on the skin surface, or to assess the depth and extent of bruising which may have been detected on external examination.

– *Heart*

Specialist examination of the heart by a cardiac pathologist may need to be carried out. In addition to detailed morphological examination both macroscopically and microscopically, genetic testing may need to be carried out as shown in Figure 5.5. This is common practice in cases of sudden arrhythmogenic(arrhythmic) heart disease in young adults, particularly when there are no other findings at autopsy, i.e. in sudden arrhythmic death syndrome (SADS). This genetic testing approach is also referred to as a 'molecular autopsy' (Semsarian et al. 2015). The impact on other family members who may be at risk will also need to be considered since it would be incumbent on the physician to clinically evaluate and manage them.

The heart may also need to be assessed in detail in relation to sudden adult death where the deceased had been involved in an altercation, for example, with or without physical violence shortly before death.

– *Brain and spinal cord*

A pathologist will retain the brain and spinal cord as necessary in homicides involving head injury and other special cases such those related to restraint, or other cases where there may be an issue regarding the role of any condition of the brain in contributing to death.

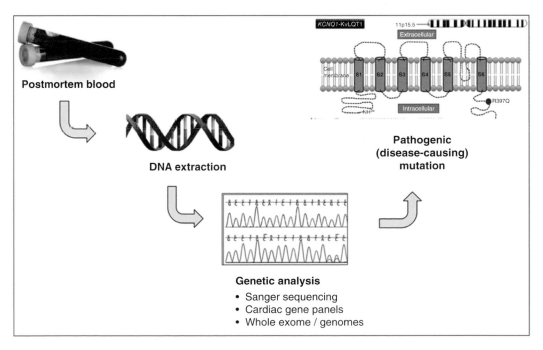

Figure 5.5 Steps in the molecular autopsy process. Deoxyribonucleic acid is extracted from blood collected at post-mortem. Subsequent DNA analysis of selected genes by Sanger sequencing or newer parallel next-generation sequencing platforms. (Source: Published with permission of Semsarian et al. *European Heart Journal*, 2015.)

5.5.6   Other Investigations

– *Imaging prior to dissection*

  Imaging prior to dissection of the body may be a useful adjunct in all post-mortem examinations and essential in others. The types of cases where imaging is essential include:
  - paediatric deaths, particular those involving young infants where there is a necessity to assess whether physical abuse has taken place
  - fire deaths to identify whether there is ante-mortem injury and differentiate from post-mortem artefacts
  - deaths from explosions to identify foreign bodies and assess trauma
  - deaths from firearms to identify missiles, wound trajectory, and trauma
  - dismembered remains and otherwise mutilated remains to assist with identification and assessment of trauma
  - other bodies on an individual basis to assess trauma when there is advanced decomposition and skeletal remains.

– *Laboratory investigations following the post-mortem*

  It is good practice in all cases, even in natural deaths where the pathologist is entirely confident of the cause of death, to take samples of body tissues for histological examination to assess whether there is natural disease present and occasionally in order to age injuries. The need for other types of investigation will depend on the circumstances of the death. The types of samples taken shown in Table 5.1 are not exhaustive and should be regarded as a general guide only.

Table 5.1   Type of samples taken at autopsy and further investigations.

Type of sample	Type of investigation
Blood	For conventional grouping and DNA profile
	Essential for comparison with other samples of blood found e.g. blood stains at scene
	Toxicology: Alcohol and drugs analysis, other noxious substances
	Microbiology
	Biochemistry
	Genetic testing in SADS
Urine	Toxicology, biochemistry
Other fluids or tissues, e.g. vitreous humour, stomach contents, bowel contents, muscle, brain, kidney, lung, bone marrow, hair, nails	Toxicology, biochemistry, DNA, diatoms
Swabs	
Oral	Semen, vaginal material
Genital (anal, rectal, penile, vaginal, perineal)	Semen, lubricant, saliva
	Vaginal material, faeces, saliva, lubricant
	Fluid drained from anus or vagina
Fingernail clippings or scrapings	Transfer of material from suspect
Head hair	Compared with other transferred hair, DNA, drugs
Pubic hair	Transfer of semen or comparison with hair at scene

5.6   Examination of the exhumed body

5.6.1   Exhumation of legally interred remains

It should be appreciated that the legal procedure for exhumation varies, in some cases significantly, between different countries and jurisdictions. The Coroners (Investigations) Regulations 2013 came into force on 25th July 2013. Part 5 refers to powers in relation to bodies. With respect to exhumation, Regulation 22 (1) states that a coroner may issue a direction to exhume a body lying within England and Wales. Where such a direction is made the coroner must use Form 4.

In order to fully investigate a case which has been legally disposed of by burial, it is necessary to exhume the body. A typical situation may concern the burial of a deceased with the usual formalities of disposal adhered to (death having been thought to have been due to some non-suspicious cause) which at a later date, in the light of further information, may indicate that there could be some element of foul play involved.

In addition to conducting an examination for the purposes of a criminal investigation, exhumations may also be carried out for a number of other reasons:

- possible civil proceedings

- identification

- redevelopment of graveyard (most common)

- for ancient or historical reasons.

5.6.2   Investigation of single or multiple clandestine graves

– *Procedure at the burial site*
  - The procedure for the recovery of a fully buried body is essentially similar in many ways, whether from a clandestine grave or as part of the process of an exhumation of a person who has been legally interred (Vanezis et al. 1978). As with other outdoor scenes it is essential to work in an environment free of interference from unwanted onlookers. For this reason, and also to avoid the procedure interfering with the daily routine of the cemetery, exhumations are normally carried out in the early morning at first light, with the site being screened off.
  - Initially, if the burial site is unknown and requires detection, this may require the expertise of a number of disciplines (France et al. 1992). There are a number of different ways in which cadavers may be located. Information, if available, from witnesses and suspecting where the grave or graves may be from other information, is the important first step. Aerial photography might be used to see any changes in the terrain, as well as the use of geophysics to observe changes to vegetation, thermal imagery, and cadaver dogs to name but a few.
  - If the investigation is of forensic interest the pathologist will work as part of a multi-disciplinary team of experts, usually including an archaeologist and/or anthropologist, and most probably a palynologist, botanist, and entomologist to ensure that the remains are recovered as completely as possible and with minimal or no damage to them, or any clothing or other items on or around them.

- Initially the grave site is dug to a sufficient depth to expose the coffin. The coffin plate should then be identified, preferably by the original undertaker who interred the body. The coffin is then lifted and should be removed to the mortuary after removal of excessive mud; care must be taken in removal of a coffin which is disintegrating.

- With a body that is not within a coffin, once it has been exposed the soil is cleaned off it then plastic sheeting and sometimes hard board is placed beneath it to aid removal. Contamination of the body, which may interfere with the autopsy, should be taken into account. Removal of the body in a complete state may be difficult, especially if virtually skeletonised. Bones must therefore be collected and placed in separate bags and labelled for ease of recognition.

- The earth surrounding the body may reveal considerable information and should therefore be dug up systematically and in layers. Initially, the soil must be removed from all sides of the burial site and placed in bags which are then labelled with the area of retrieval. The need to take soil samples not only from the area around the body, or coffin, but from other locations in the cemetery, for instance, was emphasised by Camps (1962). This is particularly important in excluding any noxious substances, especially arsenic. He described a case where the presence of arsenic in soil samples completely invalidated estimates of the poison within the remains in the coffin.

- Vegetation may prove to be extremely useful for estimating the length of internment. Roots that have grown through parts of the body may prove particularly invaluable. The advice of a botanist in such cases should be sought at an early stage and indeed a botanist should attend the site wherever possible (Vanezis et al. 1978).

- The coverings of the body, which must be carefully collected, will often provide invaluable evidence as to identification of the body. They may also sometimes give invaluable pointers as to the manner of trauma leading to death, particularly if the remains are skeletonised and are incomplete as a result of action by predators.

- As with recoveries from clandestine graves, in legally interred graves certain precautions must be observed and procedures adhered to. The most important aspect of the procedure at the graveside is to exhume the correct body. Stringent requirements for identification must therefore be adhered to. Positive identification of the grave wherein lies the deceased in question is the responsibility of the cemetery authorities. The graveyard superintendent or some other cemetery official must therefore be present at the graveside to do this and the official should indicate the actual plot that is to be opened.

- *Procedure in the mortuary*
  - Once the body has been removed to a nearby mortuary, it is essential when there is a forensic investigation involved that imaging should be carried out before it is disturbed more than is necessary. CT scanning of the whole body and of remains which are in a fragile state and partially skeletonised will greatly assist the pathologist.

  - Identification of a legally interred individual must be made known to the pathologist by the mortuary technician, the police or the funeral director who has brought the body to the mortuary. Further confirmatory evidence of identity in the mortuary will take place by a number of means (see below) once the body has been removed from its coffin or unwrapped from its shroud.

  - Detailed examination of the remains will depend on the degree of decomposition of the deceased, which can vary considerably from a well-preserved state to total skeletonisation. The aim of this part of the examination is to determine whether there are any obvious significant findings such as injuries and to differentiate them from post-mortem artefacts.

- *Further and more detailed investigation in the laboratory*

The next stage is the laboratory stage of the examination where the remains are subjected to a number of investigations with the assistance of a number of different experts. These investigations frequently include imaging (see above), both to assess injuries and to assist identification), dental examination, full anthropological assessment (age, ancestry sex, stature), DNA analysis, toxicology (where possible), histology, dating the remains, and in relation to deceased which cannot be identified through comparison with ante-mortem data, possibly facial reconstruction.

5.7 Safety in the mortuary and dealing with high-risk cases

A mortuary is a potentially hazardous workplace. It is thus vital that stringent procedures exist and are adhered in order to ensure the safety of staff and visitors. Potential risks may occur from handling high-risk infected bodies, or those contaminated with chemicals or radioactive material. The building and its facilities should be appropriate and provide a safe working environment, and working practices which are safe must be followed. A detailed description of the various facilities that are essential in a mortuary for carrying out work in a safe environment is beyond the scope of the text and the reader is referred to the publication on safety in mortuaries by the Health and Safety Executive (2003).

A high-risk case, as noted above, is defined as a case where there is serious infectious disease that can be caught by those present at the autopsy.

Serious infections that cause concern include:

- human immunodeficiency virus (HIV)

- slow viruses such as Creutzfelt–Jacob disease (CJD)

- Lassa fever

- Ebola

- hepatitis A, B or C

- tuberculosis

- anthrax and tetanus

- typhoid and paratyphoid

- meningococcal infections.

In terms of the likelihood of developing an infection from making an autopsy, tuberculosis is the most common cause of both illness and fatality. Hepatitis remains a serious hazard and immunisation against HBV for those who work in the mortuary is essential. HIV is high risk, but recorded cases of infections occurring in the mortuary are very rare.

It is necessary to take precautions when a case is recognised as high risk from the history, e.g. history of drug addiction, including the following:

- Wherever practical blood should be tested prior to the autopsy for HIV and hepatitis status.

- Wherever possible, Category 3 infections should be examined in separate rooms with a restriction on the number of persons present so that an anatomical pathology technician and a circulator are present with the pathologist. Category 4 infections must only be carried out if absolutely necessary in specially equipped rooms, otherwise a post-mortem examination must not be carried out in such cases (e.g. CJD, haemorrhagic viral fevers, e.g. Ebola, Lassa fever).

- Protective clothing must be worn, including double gloves with heavy over gloves and total body suits.

- Instruments should be kept to a minimum and blades should be sharp but sturdy.

- Electric saws should only be used if aerosol spray can be confined by vacuum attachment and/or by working under plastic.

- Jagged ends of bones should be avoided.

- Cleaning agents and disinfectants such a bleach, formalin, cidex, and sodium hydroxide should be readily available for cleaning up and for soaking organs.

- Care must be taken with sewing up after autopsy. This is the most common type of penetrating injury seen in the mortuary.

References

Camps FE (1962). Soil – some medico-legal aspects. In Soil. British Academy of Forensic Sciences, Teaching Symposium, No. 1. Sweet & Maxwell, London, pp. 47–51.

Coroners Act 1988. http://www.legislation.gov.uk/ukpga/1988/13/contents.

Coroners and Justice Act 2009. http://www.legislation.gov.uk/id/ukpga/2009/25.

France, D.L., Griffin, T.J., Swanburg, J.G. et al. (1992). A multidisciplinary approach to the detection of clandestine graves. *J. Forensic Sci.* 37: 1445–1458.

Health and Safety Executive (2003). Safe working and the prevention of infection in the mortuary and post-mortem room, 2nd ed. Health and Safety Executive. www.hse.gov.uk.

Human Rights Act 1998. http://www.legislation.gov.uk/ukpga/1998/42/section/6.

Jha, P., Gajalakshmi, V., Gupta, P.C. et al. (2006). Prospective study of one million deaths in India: rationale, design, and validation results. *PLoS Med.* 3 (2): e18.

Lozano, R., Murray, C.J., Naghavi, M. et al. (2012). Global and regional mortality from 235 causes of death for 20 age groups in 1990 and 2010: a systematic analysis for the Global Burden of Disease Study 2010. *Lancet* 380: 2095–2128.

Mental Capacity Act 2005. Schedule 1. http://www.legislation.gov.uk/ukpga/2005/9/schedule/1.

Roberts, I.S.D. and Traill, Z.C. (2014). Minimally invasive autopsy employing post-mortem CT and targeted coronary angiography: evaluation of its application to a routine coronial service. *Histopathology* 64: 211–217.

Roberts, I.S., Benamore, R.E., Benbow, E.W. et al. (2012). Post-mortem imaging as an alternative to autopsy in the diagnosis of adult deaths: a validation study. *Lancet* 379: 136–142.

Roberts, I.S.D., Benbow, E.W., Bisset, R. et al. (2003). Accuracy of magnetic resonance imaging in determining cause of sudden death in adults: comparison with conventional autopsy. *Histopathology* 42: 424–430.

Semsarian, C., Ingles, J., and Wilde, A.A.M. (2015). Sudden cardiac death in the young: the molecular autopsy and a practical approach to surviving relatives. *Eur. Heart J.* 36: 1290–1296.

Vanezis, P., Sims, B.G., and Grant, J.H. (1978). Medical and scientific investigations of an exhumation in unhallowed ground. *Med. Sci. Law* 18: 209–221.

World Health Organisation (2016). Verbal autopsy standards: ascertaining and attributing causes of death. The 2016 WHO Verbal Autopsy Instrument. http://www.who.int/healthinfo/statistics/verbalautopsystandards/en (accessed March 2018).

Yang, G. (2006). Validation of verbal autopsy procedures for adult deaths in China. *Int. J. Epidemiol.* 35: 741–748.

Further reading

Burton, J. and Rutty, G. (2010). *The Hospital Autopsy: A Manual of Fundamental Autopsy Practice*, 3e. CRC Press.

Rutty, G.E. (2001). *Essentials of Autopsy Practice*, vol. 1. Springer.

6

Interpretation of Injuries: General Principles, Classification, and Age Estimation

Peter Vanezis
Queen Mary University of London, London, UK

6.1   Introduction

A wound or injury is best defined as 'damage to any part of the body by the impact of a physical object/ surface against it.' The interpretation of the various types of injuries produced from the impact of different surfaces, weapons, and other objects and in differing circumstances according to the type of incident and forces applied can be a complex task, but one that is central to any examination of a trauma victim. The aim of the text is to give a better understanding of different types of injury and their interpretation, although the range of types and combination of injuries that can be caused is extensive, and there will inevitably be some injuries which might be difficult to associate confidently with a particular type of weapon or surface, even by the most experienced practitioner. Consultation with colleagues and reference to established databases is useful and appropriate in such circumstances. In addition to assessing how a wound may have been caused and by what type of implement, on occasions it is necessary to give an opinion on the age of an injury and this is also discussed in this chapter.

6.2   General aspects

6.2.1   Mechanism of injury

A wound occurs when the applied force exceeds the ability of the tissue to adapt or resist.

The tissues of the body have different biomechanical properties which affect how they respond to trauma. Furthermore, the location of the same type of tissue at different parts of the body may also

Essential Forensic Medicine, First Edition. Edited by Peter Vanezis.
© 2020 John Wiley & Sons Ltd. Published 2020 by John Wiley & Sons Ltd.

affect the response to trauma. For example, skin, which is elastic, is more easily damaged over bone than where there is no bony surface directly beneath. Underlying soft tissues are less resistant to impact and this can be seen particularly in some abdominal injuries where impact to the skin surface has not left any surface bruising but the underlying organ or organs may be significantly injured.

Injury to bone requires significant force to cause a fracture or joint dislocation in the absence of primary or secondary bone disease.

Although the brain is protected to a great extent by the skull, it is vulnerable to direct impact and more so to forces resulting in rotational movement, which may in turn cause various degrees of nerve fibre shearing (axonal injury either localised or diffuse).

We can summarise the following important factors which affect whether an injury will occur, and its appearance and severity:

- mass of the weapon

- surface characteristics, e.g. carpet, concrete

- velocity at the point of impact

- area over which force acts

- type of tissue.

6.2.2   Strength of force at impact

In terms of the amount of force applied at impact, its intensity varies directly with the mass of the impacting implement/surface and the square of the velocity at impact and can be expressed as follows:

$$\text{force} = \frac{1}{2}\text{mass} \times \text{velocity}^2.$$

6.2.3   Types of injuries

The classification of different types of injuries should be according to their appearance and method of causation. Flexibility in approach is necessary, bearing in mind that frequently combinations of different types of injuries may be seen, for example a graze, laceration or incision may be accompanied by bruising.

The following is a brief list of the different types of injuries based on their external appearance. These external injuries and their related internal manifestation are discussed in detail in the relevant chapters elsewhere.

- Blunt force trauma
  - Abrasions
  - Bruises
  - Lacerations

- Sharp force trauma
  - Cuts (incised/slash, stabs)

- Other penetrating injury (mainly firearm)

- Thermal
  - Burns
  - Scalds

- Cold injury

- Chemical

- Radiation

- Atmospheric pressure

6.2.4 Development and ageing of injuries

In the investigation of a case in many instances there is a requirement to provide an opinion as to when an injury occurred in relation to the time at which the injury is examined in a living individual or from when death occurred in a deceased person. There are many factors which affect the development and resolution of injuries.

Wound healing occurs through the following broad successive phases with overlap between them and subject to large intra- and inter-individual variations:

Inflammatory phase (1–3 days after injury): vascular, haemostatic, and cellular response. During the inflammatory phase, platelet aggregation at the injury site is followed by the infiltration of leukocytes such as neutrophils, macrophages, and T-lymphocytes into the wound site.

Proliferative phase (up to 10–14 days after injury): epithelial and connective tissue regeneration. In the proliferative phase, re epithelialisation and newly formed granulation tissue begin to cover the wound area to complete tissue repair. Angiogenesis is indispensable for sustaining granulation tissue.

Reorganisation or remodelling phase (several months after injury). Advanced cell biological studies have demonstrated that many cytokines, growth factors, proteases, and so on are closely involved in the wound-healing process to complete normal tissue repair after damage (Martin 1997; Singer and Clark 1999).

From the 1960s to 1980s, Raekallio (1980) (Table 6.1) and others (Oehmichen 2004; Grellner and Madea 2007; Cecchi 2010) investigated the application of histology and the activity of several enzymes at a wound site by enzyme histochemistry, including the levels of serotonin and histamine at the wound edges, which are indicative of vital phenomena. Thereafter, with the advance of immune-histochemistry, the application of immune-histochemical techniques opened up a new field of wound age investigation by forensic pathologists.

More recently, many bioactive substances have been found to be essentially involved in skin wound healing to assist in timing of injury and vitality (whether caused before or after death). These include collagens, cytokines, and growth factors (a good review of the subject is provided by Kondo 2007). These substances are potentially useful as markers for timing wounds and, where

Table 6.1 Suggested schema for histological estimation of time interval from infliction of injury to death in open skin wounds and abrasions (after Raekallio 1980).

Time	Observations
<4 hours	No distinct signs of inflammation
	Histological distinction between ante-mortem and post-mortem skin wounds not possible
4–12 hours	4 hours: some polymorph leucocytes first appear perivascularly
8–12 hours	Polymorphs, macrophages, activated fibroblasts form distinct peripheral wound zone
	Polymorphs more than macrophages, 5:1; imminent necrosis in central zone
12–48 hours	12–24 hours: relative number of macrophages increases (polymorph:macrophage) falling to 0.4:1
After 16 hours	Older fibrin stains bright red with Martius scarlet blue, whereas before 16 hours 'newer' fibrin stains yellow
24 hours	Number of polymorphs and amount of fibrin increase to maximum (remain at this level for 2–3 days
	Cut edge of epidermis shows cytoplasmic processes
24–48 hours	Epidermis migrates from the incised edge towards centre of wound
32 hours onwards	Necrosis apparent in central wound zone
48 hours	Macrophages reach maximum concentration in peripheral zone
2–4 days	Fibroblasts migrate from the nearby connective tissue to wound periphery
3 days	Epithelialisation of small wounds and abrasions complete; thereafter regenerated epidermis becomes highly stratified and thicker than normal surrounding epidermis
3–4 days	Capillary buds appear
4 days	First new collagen fibres seen
4–5 days	Profuse ingrowth of new capillaries; capillaries continue to proliferate until the eighth day
6 days	Lymphocytes reach maximum concentration in wound periphery
8–12 days	Decrease in number of inflammatory cells, fibroblasts, and capillaries; increase in the number and size of collagen fibres
>12 days	Definite stage of regression of cellular activity in both epidermis and dermis
	Vascularity of dermis diminishes
	Collagen fibres restored
	Epithelium shows stainable basement membrane
14 days	Fibroplasia reaches its peak, thereafter there is gradual shrinkage and maturation of connective tissue in the wound

required, their vitality. Studies are still in the experimental stage that have tried to apply gene expressions in wound age determination. It appears that in future determination of wound vitality or wound age will be established at the molecular as well as the protein level.

6.2.5   Factors affecting the development of bruises

There are many variables which influence the development and absorption of bruises as well as their appearance and extent of spread, thus adding to the difficulty in their interpretation.

6.2.5.1   Site of injury   Bruising will occur more easily where there is loose tissue, e.g. over the eyebrow, than where the skin is more strongly supported. In addition, bruising occurs more easily where there is an excess of subcutaneous fat.

6.2.5.2   Type of agent inflicting injury and force used   The type of surface and force which impacts on the body will influence the intensity, size, and shape, including pattern, of the resulting bruise. In a healthy individual this will assist with assessment. Accompanying lacerations or abrasions will be useful pointers in assessing the force of an impact.

6.2.5.3 Age of the subject In infants and the elderly, bruising tends to occur more easily. In the very young the skin is looser, more delicate, and there is an increased amount of subcutaneous fat. In old people, although there is loss of subcutaneous fat, blood vessels are also more poorly supported and bruises take longer to absorb.

6.2.5.4 Sex Females tend to bruise more easily because of increased subcutaneous fat.

6.2.5.5 Skin pigmentation Skin colouration modifies the appearance of a bruise to the naked eye. It is much easier to observe the extent and colour of bruising in lighter-skinned individuals.

6.2.5.6 Conditions in which bruising occurs more easily or spontaneously It is essential to carefully consider the existence of any condition which may either give rise to spontaneous tissue haemorrhage/bruising or render the individual more likely to bruise easily and out of proportion to the force of impact (Figure 6.1). Such conditions fall into a number of categories and apart from various bleeding disorders, one must also consider hypertension, cardiovascular degenerative changes, and a host of collagen and other supporting tissue disorders that may result in an increase in the amount of blood extravasating from vessels.

6.3 Timing of bruises

For the clinical forensic medical examiner, the assessment of bruises in living subjects is limited of necessity to their external gross appearance, including photographs and history given by the victim where available. The pathologist, on the other hand, has more available options for an objective assessment which involves microscopic examination as well as closer gross assessment by dissection. In addition both the pathologist and clinical practitioner will need, in any case, to assess and corroborate or refute accounts given by eyewitnesses where available.

An assessment of a bruise to ascertain when it occurred may be made in a number of different ways:

- direct gross examination of the victim (external and by dissection)
- conventional and special photography
- conventional histological examination

Acquired
Liver disease, vitamin K deficiency, severe renal failure, hypothyroidism, DIC from any cause, diseases of bone marrow, myeloma, myeloproloiferative disorders, myelodysplasia.
Use of antithrombotic medications: Heparin, warfarin, aspirin, non-steroidal anti-inflammatory drugs
Thrombocytopenia: In bone marrow failure, autoimmune, hypersplenism, HIV infection, massive transfusion, haemolytic uraemic syndrome, thrombotic thrombocytopenic purpura

Congenital
Von Willebrand's disease, haemophilia

Figure 6.1 Some conditions associated with increased bleeding.

- various histochemical techniques
- biochemical methods
- objective colour assessment.

6.3.1   Dating bruises at the post-mortem examination

A great deal of information can be obtained from gross examination of the body in the mortuary, for example differentiation of a fresh from an older bruise is usually not difficult. It is important, however, to bear in mind that the location of a bruise needs to also be taken into account when assessing its age. For example, a deep bruise in thigh muscle may not appear for a day or two after its infliction and have a fresh appearance, whereas a bruise over a bony prominence and where tissue is lax, for example the eyebrow, will appear very quickly and with accompanying swelling.

Larger bruises remain visible longer than smaller ones. The development and rate of disappearance of a bruise will also depend on the state of health and age of the person. Bruises take much longer to disappear in the elderly.

6.3.2   Gross naked eye and photographic assessment

Studies of bruising carried out in living subjects which are based on their appearance in photographs illustrate the difficulties involved in timing such injuries. Langlois and Gresham (1991) in their study of 369 photographs found that the most significant change was the development of a yellow colour, which was also found to develop significantly faster in those under 65 years. They concluded that a bruise with a yellow colour was more than 18 hours old and that the appearance of the other colours was of less significance. In a further similar study (Stephenson and Bialas 1996), in which photographs were assessed of children who suffered accidental bruising, the authors did not observe a yellow colouration in those bruises that were under 1 day old. A number of authors of textbooks of forensic medicine over the years have made various observations and published guidelines on when colour changes in bruises occur (Table 6.2).

It is clear that the red/blue/purple colour in bruises may persist for days and even longer. The green colour is difficult to interpret as it may well reflect a combination of blue and yellow, but it is nevertheless seen as an intermediate stage between the initial appearance and the later yellow

Table 6.2   Summary of colour change in bruises with time (adapted from various authors' observations, excluding studies from photographs).

Source	0–24 hours	1–3 days	4–7 days	1–2 weeks	Over 2 weeks
Camps (1976)	Red, dusky/ purple, black		Green	Yellow	Resolution
Glaister (1962)	Violet	Blue	Green	Yellow	Resolution
Polson and Gee (1985a,b)	Red, dark or red/ black		Greenish tinge (day 7)	Yellowing	Resolution
Smith and Fiddes (1955)	Red, purple/black	Yellow (begins)	Yellow	Yellow/Resolution	
Spitz and Fisher (1974)	Light blue/red	Dark purple	Dark purple, greenish/ yellow	Brown	Resolution
Adelson (1974)	Red/blue, purple	Blue/brown	Yellow/green	Resolution	Resolution

appearance. One of the interesting findings is the time at which the yellow colour first appears and can be seen naked eye. Most authors writing in textbooks and referring, in the main, to anecdotal evidence of their own personal experience state that the yellow colour does not appear for at least several days, usually 1 week, afterwards. A comprehensive study of bruises (Moritz 1942) demonstrated that deep bruises may take 12–24 hours to appear and that a brown colour would indicate that the bruise was over 24 hours old. This contrasts with other authors' views, e.g. Spitz and Fisher (1974), who did not find a brown colour until the end of the first week.

It is important in dark-skinned individuals to pay particular attention to the subdermal appearance and spread of a bruise.

6.3.3 Microscopical changes in bruises

Most of the basic observations used for the timing of haemorrhages have been known for over 150 years. Virchow in 1847 first described pathological pigments in old haemorrhagic areas inside and outside cells as diffuse, granular, and crystalline structures which he called haematoidin, which was later identified as bilirubin (Fischer and Reindel 1923). In 1869 erythrophagocytosis was detected in haemorrhages (Langhans 1869) and in 1888 the iron-containing pigment in old haemorrhages was named haemosiderin and differentiated from haematoidin (Neumannn 1888).

6.3.3.1 Histological changes The changes seen in the reaction to haemorrhage mirror and overlap with the description of injury to other tissues as described above.

- *Non-exudative phase:* Initially, as a result of fluid exudation, there is oedema within the vicinity of the haemorrhage. Histologically, widening of fibrous septa is seen.

- *Leucocyte reaction:* This early, non-cellular exudative phase merges into the leucocyte reaction. It should be appreciated that it is not only the white blood cells which extravasate with the haemorrhage that are detected but also the granulocytes that migrate from neighbouring blood vessels. Recent observations give times for leucocyte reaction in both haemorrhages and wounds varying between 1 and 24 hours. With regard specifically to subcutaneous haemorrhages it was found that the first influx of polymorphonuclear leucocytes was detected after about 4 hours (Berg and Ebel 1969).

- *Macrophage reaction:* The first leucocytes to migrate, become increasingly necrotic after about 15–30 hours, and are superseded by phagocytic mononuclear cells (macrophages).

- Erythrocytes are seen in macrophages after 15–17 hours from infliction of the injury in the skin or brain whereas the corresponding findings in the human lung are seen as early as 30 minutes. Haemosiderin laden macrophages have been seen in the skin and subcutaneous tissue as early as 24–48 hours after the infliction of trauma and more commonly from 4 to 8 days (Figure 6.2).

- In brain, haemosiderin has been observed in macrophages as early as 3–4 days, but more commonly between 5 and 15 days. In human subdural haematomas, haemosiderin has been described as occurring after 5 days. In the human lung haemosiderin on the other hand, is found much earlier – the earliest being at 17 hours.

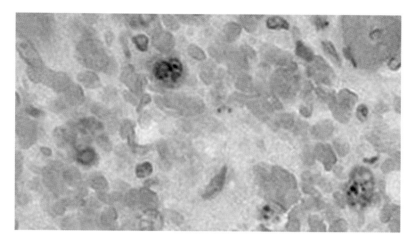

Figure 6.2 Haemosiderin-laden macrophages in a 4-day-old subdermal bruise (Perl's stain).

6.3.3.2 Histochemical changes Enzyme-histochemical investigation of subcutaneous bruises from routine autopsy material (Berg and Ebel 1969) showed an increase in ATPase activity in the vascular walls after 2.5 hours. Aminopeptidase and esterase activity increased at 4.5 hours and 7 hours, respectively. Polymorphs appeared within 4 hours and mononuclear cells within 9 hours. Using several histochemical methods (Alcan blue-PAS and dialysed iron-PAS, both controlled by enzyme digestion) acid glycosaminoglycans, after having shown an initial decrease, were demonstrated in several days-old bruises, together with an increase in the cellular elements of the connective tissue (Nevelös and Gee 1970).

6.3.3.3 Biochemical methods Biochemical methods are of little practical use in routine forensic practice.

Although the measurement of the increase in bilirubin content in some day-old haematomas is possible and seems to correlate with the age of the haematoma (Mostafa et al. 1957; Laiho 1982), there are serious methodological difficulties with this approach.

Extraction of haem and extractable iron from homogenate is straightforward. The ratio of extractable iron per haem content reflects the change between the amount of haem or haemoglobin actually present in the tissue and the degraded extractable iron, but is more influenced by the amount of blood originally present than the ratio based on the total iron. When the haemorrhage in the tissue is very small and the values of extractable iron, total iron, and haem are nearly the same as in the control tissue, the evaluation of the age of a haematoma by ratio comparison would give unreliable results.

6.4 Colour measurement of bruising

Dating a bruise from its colouration is problematical for a number of reasons. One of these is that in general forensic practice the colour of a bruise on a cadaver or a living person is assessed by naked eye examination, which by its nature is subjective and conditions for assessment are virtually impossible to standardise.

Despite the limitations of relating colour change to date of trauma infliction, it is useful to apply a standardised method for measuring the colour and intensity (lightness) of a bruise.

There are two standard techniques which are used to measure colour and have been applied to bruising: colourimetry and spectrophotometry.

6.4.1 Colorimetry

Measurement of skin colour by colorimetry was initially used to assess hypostasis in relation to time of death estimation (Vanezis 1991; Vanezis and Trujillo 1996) and was subsequently applied to colour changes in bruising (Trujillo et al. 1996; Vanezis et al., personal communication). A colorimeter is designed to allow an accurate non-subjective assessment to be made of a colour, giving a numerical value based on the internationally recognised colour system CIE (Commission Internationale de l'Eclairage) L*a*b* (Figure 6.3). Any object can thus be described in terms of its spatial position on a three-dimensional axis. The vertical axis L* describes the lightness (luminance) of the image, the horizontal a* value describes position of the red–green axis, and the b* value describes the position on the yellow–blue axis. The technique is easy to perform, fast, gives reproducible results, and is non-invasive (Figure 6.4). A series of formulae are required to convert the raw data into the L*a*b* format which is the conventional form for communicating the results.

Unpublished data (Vanezis et al., personal communication) was in broad agreement with naked eye observations in relation to colour changes. It was noted in this unpublished study of 93 live subjects examined in a casualty department that there was great variability in colour change but it nevertheless followed the general pattern of change seen in other studies. Furthermore, in common with the observations from photographs (Langlois and Gresham 1991; Stephenson and Bialas 1996), yellow colour was not seen until towards the end of the first day.

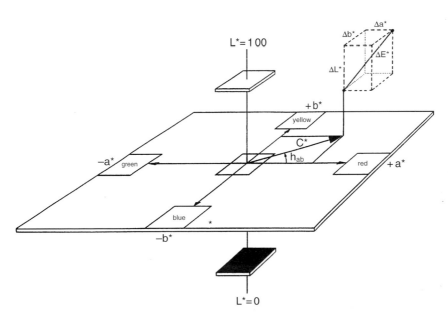

Figure 6.3 CIE LAB colour system.

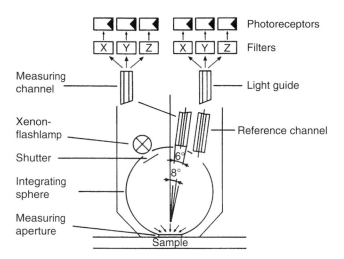

Figure 6.4   Colorimeter optical system. The equipment is placed onto the test surface, which is lit up by a standard illuminant produced by a xenon flash lamp that approximates to the same conditions as daylight. The diffuse reflection from the surface is normally measured at an angle of 8° in the measuring head and then split up into three equal parts by a light guide. Light is then directed to three measuring filters for the three standard tristimulus values X, Y and Z.

6.4.2   Spectrophotometry

Spectrophotometry is used in many branches of science and its principal use is to identify any substance by its colour properties. Different substances absorb, reflect or emit light in different ways and a spectrophotometer is an optical instrument for measuring the change in light intensity relative to its wavelength after it has interacted with the sample. To summarise the process, a spectrophotometer emits light from a lamp onto a test sample. The sample absorbs some of the light, with the rest passing through. In the spectrophotometer a diffraction grating disperses the light from the sample by wavelength and the spectrum formed is observed with a detector. Reflectance spectrophotometry (light measured on the same side of the sample as the source of light and used on opaque samples such as solids) is now commonly used in dermatology. It was first used to analyse skin colour in 1929 (Brunsting and Sheard 1929) and has since been developed to quantify colour changes in skin under various circumstances (e.g. the application of corticosteroids). The technique was applied to colour changes in subcutaneous bruises over time (Klein et al. 1996). The authors performed measurements between wavelengths 450 and 700 nm (visible wavelength 360/380–750/780 nm) and found the best results between 540 and 580 nm. Although they were not able to produce unambiguous ageing of bruising, they concluded that the technique could be used as an objective non-invasive technique for bruise analysis. In a study using both excised post-mortem samples and live subjects it was found that spectrophotometry was of limited use because of the large number of variables involved (Carson 1998).

6.5   Differentiation from artefacts and other post-mortem appearances

The pathologist must take care when examining a bruise to establish whether the discolouration is bruising or caused by some other means. Even in the non-decomposed cadaver there are a number of normal manifestations and alterations after death that resemble bruises.

6.5.1 'Post-mortem bruising'

It is essential to understand the mechanism of production of any post-mortem injury and how it may be distinguished from its ante-mortem counterpart. The extravasation of blood into the tissues after death, for whatever reason, is no exception and in certain circumstances may give rise to misinterpretation.

This problem is more than of academic interest and, as most forensic pathologists will confirm, the distinction between true ante-mortem bruising and pseudo-bruising can sometimes be difficult, if not impossible, both in the autopsy suite and sometimes even after routine histological and immuno-histochemical examination.

At this point it is appropriate to consider whether blunt trauma delivered after death and causing tissue disruption can result in extravasation of blood which has an appearance that is indistinguishable from bruising produced before death. This problem was addressed by Polson and Gee (1985a,b), who observed that the production of post mortem 'bruises' (sometimes known as pseudo-bruises) required the application of considerable violence, with the resulting bruise almost always being small or wholly disproportionate to the force delivered. Interestingly, however, they found that a blow with a wooden mallet delivered after death to the occiput (moderate force was used so as not to fracture the skull) may well cause blood extravasation involving the full thickness of the scalp up to 1 in. (2.54 cm) in diameter. Bearing in mind that the scalp is rich in blood vessels and that by storing cadavers in the supine position, it is perhaps not such an unusual phenomenon, but one that nevertheless, requires careful interpretation.

6.5.2 Hypostasis and congestion

Post-mortem lividity or hypostasis which results from pooling of blood after death as a result of gravity gives a reddish purple appearance to the areas where the blood is pooled. Usually there is no difficulty differentiating hypostasis from bruising except where the hypostasis has a patchy appearance or bruising is on the back (cadavers stored in a mortuary in a supine position are usually found with a substantial proportion of lividity on the back). The situation may be compounded by congestive changes to the body, particularly where congestion is seen in association with deaths involving some kind of trauma.

Cases involving a mechanical asphyxial mode of death, e.g. manual strangulation or postural (positional) asphyxia, may show areas of congestion and genuine bruises whose sizes are larger than would be expected because of the increased volume of blood in surrounding vessels which will escape and contribute to the bruised area. In addition, congested areas may show post-mortem ecchymoses, which resemble petechial haemorrhages. These are particularly seen within areas of hypostasis (Figure 6.5).

Although it is recommended that a careful dissection of the involved area be carried out to assess whether, as in the case of a bruise, the blood has been noted to escape from blood vessels into the surrounding tissue, this on occasions, particularly with marked congestion, can still be problematical. It is sometimes useful to move the cadaver into another position to allow drainage of pooled blood to a secondary position. True bruising will remain in the same position.

6.5.3 Post-mortem injuries

All pathologists are familiar with the typical appearance of post-mortem injuries, which have a tendency to a yellowish brown 'bloodless' appearance and lack vital reaction (Figure 6.6). To the naked eye, bruising accompanying injuries such as lacerations has the appearance of extravasated

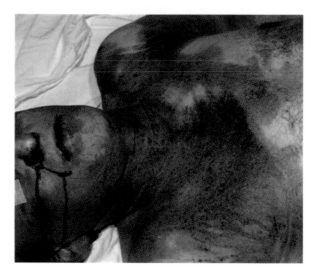

Figure 6.5 Male who died from postural asphyxia as a result of alcohol intoxication. The deceased is very congested and ecchymoses are extensive within the florid hypostatic areas.

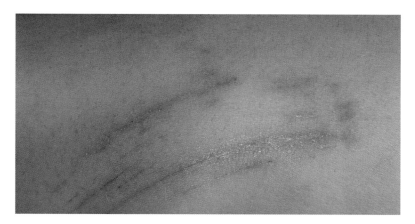

Figure 6.6 Yellow-brown appearance of drag marks on the back produced when the victim was moved after death.

blood (red/purple/blue when fresh) and other changes such as tissue oedema and swelling reflecting reaction to injury and which is dependent on the interval between the infliction of trauma and death. However, in many instances where there is congestion of the cadaver, blood escapes from vessels damaged after death sufficiently to give an appearance of bruising that is indistinguishable from a fresh injury occurring shortly before death.

The post-mortem dissection procedure will also produce artefactual bruising, which may be indistinguishable from ante-mortem bruising. This is particularly problematic when marked congestion is present or where the area in question is very vascular. An example where difficulties may arise is in the assessment of neck bruising associated with neck compression.

The pathologist carrying out a second autopsy must be wary of this and not over-interpret findings. Furthermore post-mortem dissection will also facilitate the migration of genuine bruising. Against this background, ante-mortem bruises will be modified after death, as discussed in the next section.

A particular situation which may lead to misinterpretation concerns the examination of the neck structures in asphyxia deaths involving compression, e.g. manual strangulation. In such cases it is important to bear in mind that the neck structures are, in all probability, congested. The assessment of bruising and its distribution is of paramount importance to the pathologist in their examination. As stated above, bleeding from vessels which are cut or pulled away from other structures occurs as part of the post-mortem dissection and evisceration, and results in collections of blood in soft tissues and organs which may be thought erroneously to be ante-mortem bruises. With regard to neck structures, even with careful dissection of the anterior neck structures to separate them from the cervical vertebral column, significant extravasation of blood may be produced. Artefactual production of bleeding in such circumstances is known as the Prinsloo–Gordon effect after the two authors who described this artefactual production of bruising in detail (Prinsloo and Gordon 1951). They recommend that a bloodless field be produced in the neck region prior to examination and removal of the anterior structures. This is achieved by opening the skull as well as the chest and abdomen to allow free flow of blood from these areas, prior to dissection of the neck.

The differentiation between haemorrhage which has occurred before or after death as stated above may be impossible where injuries are inflicted just before, during the agonal phase of dying or within a short time after death. It used to be considered that the finding of clotted blood was considered to be a vital reaction in bruising, but it has been shown that coagulation in blood may occur as late as 6 hours after death (Mueller 1964). To further complicate matters, another study (Laiho 1967) concluded that the standard histological staining methods for fibrin do not give conclusive evidence that a haemorrhage contains fibrin and that the absence of fibrin does not mean that the haemorrhage occurred after death. Even with immuno-histochemical studies the same author was not able to distinguish with certainty post-mortem from ante-mortem fibrin. It was also observed that well-preserved fibrin networks found at autopsy performed 2–3 days after death pointed to an ante-mortem or agonal haemorrhage (Pullar 1973). The reason for this was that a large proportion of a post-mortem subcutaneous haemorrhage undergoes fibrinolysis within 1 day of its production.

6.5.4 Resuscitation injuries and handling after death

Another area of practical difficulty for the pathologist is the differentiation of bruises from marks caused by resuscitation. Because resuscitation in most instances occurs around the time of death, with some degree of maintenance of a circulation, or at least intermittent forced movement of blood within vessels, there is every possibility of producing extravasation of blood to the tissues which is indistinguishable from true bruising. Care should therefore be taken in the interpretation of injuries in areas of the body where resuscitation is said to have taken place. These areas include the face, neck, and chest, and occasionally the abdomen, particularly in children. Frequently the question arises in cases involving pressure to the face and neck, especially in manual strangulation, where fingertip-type bruising as well as other marks such as abrasions due to fingernails are commonly found. The problem is compounded in areas where there is intense congestion.

6.6 Decomposition

With the increasing post-mortem interval, bruises become more diffuse and are frequently accentuated in intensity due to the degradation products of haemoglobin (Figure 6.7). Indeed, it is well-known to pathologists that if they return a day or two after their post-mortem examination, bruises

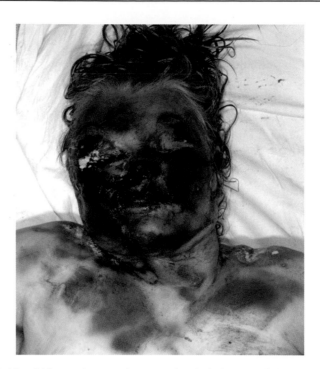

Figure 6.7   The bruising of this middle-aged woman has spread to include most of the face. Note the post-mortem desiccation of the upper chest and neck admixed with bruising which had spread.

may appear de novo or may be seen more easily. Fingertip bruises indicative of grip marks are a particularly good example of this phenomenon.

With the onset of putrefaction, the body becomes discoloured and bruises become further modified in their appearance so as to render their accurate assessment difficult. Glycorphin A, a constituent of red cell membranes, has been demonstrated as a useful marker (Kibayashi et al. 1993) to differentiate between true bruising and putrefactive discolouration. Although haemoglobin pigments readily filter through blood vessels, erythrocyte membranes do so less easily because of their molecular size. Therefore bruises will contain a greater amount of erythrocyte membrane material as compared to areas of discolouration resulting from putrefactive change. Glycorphyn A, however, will not allow differentiation between ante-mortem and post-mortem injury because extravasated blood from vessels includes the erythrocytes, regardless of the damage produced before or after death.

References

Adelson, L. (1974). *The Pathology of Homicide*, 382. Springfield, IL: Charles C Thomas.

Berg, S. and Ebel, R. (1969). Altersbestimmung Subcutaner Blutungen. *Münch Med Wochenschr* 111: 1185–1190.

Brunsting, L.A. and Sheard, C. (1929). The colour of skin as analysed by spectrophotometric methods. *J. Clin. Invest.* 1: 559.

Camps, F.E. (1976). *Gradwohl's Legal Medicine*, 2e, 265. John Wright.

Carson D O (1998). The reflectance spectrophotometric analysis of the age of bruising and livor. MSc thesis. University of Dundee.

Cecchi, R. (2010). Estimating wound age: looking into the future. *Int. J. Legal Med.* 124 (6): 523–536.

Fischer, H. and Reindel, F. (1923). Über Haematoidin. *Hoppe-Seyler Z Physiol. Chem.* 127: 299–316.

Grellner, W. and Madea, B. (2007). Demands on scientific studies: vitality of wounds and wound age estimation. *Forensic Sci. Int.* 165 (2–3): 150–154.

Glaister J. (1962). The medico-legal aspects of wounds. In: *Medical Jurisprudence and Toxicology*, 11th Ed. E & S Livingstone, Edinburgh 220-234

Kibayashi, K., Hamada, K., Honjyo, K., and Tsunenari, S. (1993). Differentiation between bruises and putrefactive discolorations of the skin by immunological analysis of glycophorin a. *Forensic Sci. Int.* 61: 111–117.

Klein, A., Rommeiss, Fischbacher, C. et al. (1996). Estimating the age of hematomas in living subjects based on spectrometric measurements. In: *The Wound Healing Process: Forensic Aspects* (ed. M. Oehmichen and K.H. Schmidt-Römhild), 283–291. Lubeck: Schmidt–Römhild.

Kondo, T. (2007). Timing of wounds. *Legal Med.* 9: 109–114.

Laiho, K. (1967). Immunohistochemical studies on fibrin in vital and postmortem subcutaneous haemorrhages. *Ann. Acad. Sci. Fenn.* 128: 1–85.

Laiho K (1982). Biochemical and morphological changes in experimental subcutaneous hematomas. In Proceedings of the 8th Meeting of the Scandinavian Forensic Society, Vedbaek, Denmark, pp. 141–146.

Langhans, F. (1869). Beobachtungen über die Resorption der Extravasate und Pigmentbildung in denselben. *Virchows Arch. Pathol. Anat.* 49: 66.

Langlois, N.E.I. and Gresham, G.A. (1991). The ageing of bruises: a review and study of the colour changes with time. *Forensic Sci. Int.* 50: 227–238.

Martin, P. (1997). Wound healing – aiming for perfect skin regeneration. *Science* 276: 75–81.

Moritz, A.R. (1942). *The Pathology of Trauma*, 21–34. London: Henry Kimpton.

Mostafa, K., Hamdy, F.E., Deatherage, F.E., and Shinowara, G.Y. (1957). Bruised tissue I. Biochemical changes resulting from blunt injury. *Proc. Soc. Exp. Biol. Med.* 95: 255–258.

Mueller, B. (1964). Zur Frage der Unterscheidung von vitalen bzw. agonalen und postmortalen Blutungen. *Acta Med. Leg. Soc. (Liege)* 17: 43–46.

Neumannn, E. (1888). Beiträge zur Kenntnis der Pathologischen Pigmente. *Virchows Arch.* 111: 25.

Nevelös, A.B. and Gee, D.J. (1970). Vital reaction in the epithelial connective tissue ground substance. *Med. Sci. Law* 10: 175–177.

Oehmichen, M. (2004). Vitality and time course of wounds. *Forensic Sci. Int.* 144 (2–3): 221–231.

Polson, C.J. and Gee, D.J. (1985a). Injuries: general features. In: *The Essentials of Forensic Medicine*, 4e, 102–104. Oxford: Pergamon.

Polson, C.J. and Gee, D.J. (1985b). Injuries: general features. In: *The Essentials of Forensic Medicine*, 4e, 104–105. Oxford: Pergamon.

Prinsloo, A. and Gordon, I. (1951). Post-mortem dissection artefacts of the neck; their differentiation from ante-mortem bruises. *S. Afr. Med. J.* 25: 358–361.

Pullar, P. (1973). The histopathology of wounds. In: *Modern Trends in Forensic Medicine*, 3e (ed. A.K. Mant). London.: Butterworths. 64.

Raekallio, J. (1980). Histological estimation of the age of injuries. In: *Microscopic Diagnosis in Forensic Pathology* (ed. J.A. Perper and C.H. Wecht), 3–16. Springfield, IL: Charles C Thomas.

Singer, A.J. and Clark, R.A. (1999). Cutaneous wound healing. *N. Engl. J. Med.* 341: 738–746.

Smith, S. and Fiddes, F.S. (1955). *Forensic Medicine*, 110–111. London: Churchill.

Spitz, W.U. and Fisher, R.S. (1974). *Medicolegal Investigation of Death*, 124. Springfield, IL: Charles C Thomas.

Stephenson, T. and Bialas, Y. (1996). Estimation of the age of bruising. *Arch. Dis. Child.* 74: 53–55.

Trujillo, O., Vanezis, P., and Cermignani, M. (1996). Photometric assessment of skin colour and lightness using a tristimulus colorimeter: reliability of inter and intra-investigator observations in healthy adult volunteers. *Forensic Sci. Int.* 81: 1–10.

Vanezis, P. (1991). Assessing hypostasis by colorimetry. *Forensic Sci. Int.* 52: 1–3.

Vanezis, P. and Trujillo, O. (1996). Evaluation of hypostasis using a colorimeter measuring system and its application to assessment of the post-mortem interval (time of death). *Forensic Sci. Int.* 78: 19–28.

Virchow, R. (1847). Die Pathologischen Pigmente. *Virchows Arch. Pathol. Anat.* 1: 379–486.

Further reading

Vanezis, P. (2001). Bruising: concepts of ageing and intrerpretation. In: *Essentials of Autopsy Practice*, vol. 1 (ed. G.N. Rutty), 221–240. Springer.

Vanezis, P. (2001). Interpreting bruises at necropsy. *J. Clin. Pathol.* 54: 348–355.

7
Blunt Impact Trauma

Peter Vanezis
Queen Mary University of London, London, UK

Blunt impact trauma is caused by a surface which does not have a sharp edge as its predominant feature and impacts on a body with blunt force. Such a force is compressive in nature and any injury that is produced depends on the length time of compression, its force, and the area compressed. Injuries produced which are visible on the surface include bruises, abrasions (with tangential impact) or lacerations, depending on the severity of the impacting force, the part of the body upon which the impact has occurred, the condition of the part of the body struck, and the nature of the impacting surface. Such injuries may be found alone or in combination. Furthermore, the type of impacting surface sometimes leaves a patterned injury which might assist in identifying the object or surface in question.

Blunt trauma, depending on its severity, may cause serious internal tissue damage to organs and supporting musculo-skeletal elements, which includes fractures, contusions, lacerations, and perforations. In a recent study, Yartsev and Langlois (2008) found that the correlation between external and internal injuries was poor, and the most severe external injuries were the most reliable predictors of lethal internal injuries. External injuries of the head were more predictive of internal damage than external injuries elsewhere. The authors determined that minor external injuries (such as bruises, small abrasions or small lacerations) did not predict lethal internal injuries. It should also be appreciated that there may not be any surface injuries overlying severe internal injuries, particularly where there are no bony prominences underlying the skin surface, such as in the abdominal region.

There are also many situations where both blunt impact and sharp force trauma may occur at the same time, for example in road traffic collisions and bomb explosions. In other situations, blunt impact trauma is predominantly or exclusively the type of injury seen, as in severe beating using hands and/or shod feet (kicking/stamping).

Essential Forensic Medicine, First Edition. Edited by Peter Vanezis.
© 2020 John Wiley & Sons Ltd. Published 2020 by John Wiley & Sons Ltd.

7.1   External surface injuries

7.1.1   Abrasions

An abrasion is a superficial scuffing injury of the skin caused by tangential motion (Figure 7.1).

There are different types of abrasions and these may indicate the type of surface and or the mechanism by which the abrasion was produced. Tangential contact which causes a superficial breach of the skin characteristically gives rise to piling up of the lifted skin at the other end of the wound away from where the contact was first made. Such injuries are commonly seen in a pedestrian who brushes against a vehicle in a road traffic collision or in falls where there is tangential movement across a surface. Examples of abrasions caused by contact with the ground are shown in Figures 7.2 and 7.3.

Other types of abrasions combined with bruising may have a pattern/imprint component, e.g. from a fall or from an object such as a shoe caused by vertical impact and causing crushing of the epidermis with an imprint of the impacting object (Figure 7.4). A comprehensive study by Strauch et al. (2001) demonstrated the usefulness of the close examination of surface characteristics caused by stamping, including abrasions, bruises, and contact traces such as blood and dirt.

Other types of abrasions occurring in certain situations include those caused by fingernails by direct compression against the skin or by dragging the fingers across the skin surface (Figure 7.5). Such marks are frequently seen in compression of the neck or other situations where the hands have been applied to the body combined with movement against the skin in a tangential manner.

Abrasions may also be classified as drag marks if there is a directional parallel distribution of the linear components of these marks, in conjunction with their position on the body. Drag or friction abrasions may be either ante-mortem or post-mortem and can be seen commonly from a road surface in road traffic collisions and elsewhere where a person is dragged or has scraped along a surface (Figure 7.6a–c). They are frequently seen in combination with marks to clothing, contaminants on the body from surfaces, and blood smearing both on the body and on the surface where the body has been dragged.

7.1.2   Bruises

A bruise is a collection of blood seen in the surrounding tissues which has leaked from blood vessels damaged by mechanical impact (Vanezis 2001). It occurs within the dermis (the epidermis is bloodless) (Figure 7.7). Bruising demonstrates evidence of ante-mortem blunt force injury. Real

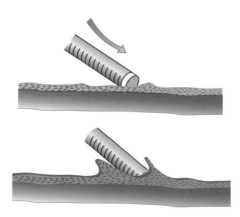

Figure 7.1 Blunt object stretching the skin, causing an abrasion. The arrow shows the tangential direction of travel.

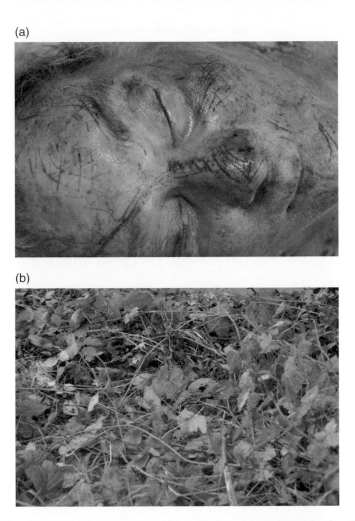

Figure 7.2 Sixty-year-old male with multiple criss-cross facial abrasions (a) caused by his face being pushed into ground covered with thick vegetation (b).

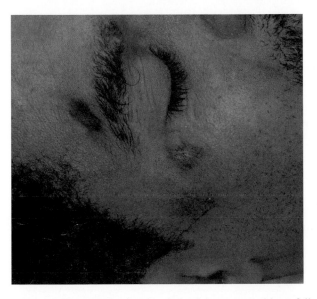

Figure 7.3 Abrasions on the right forehead and cheek bone caused by a fall to the ground.

(a)

(b)

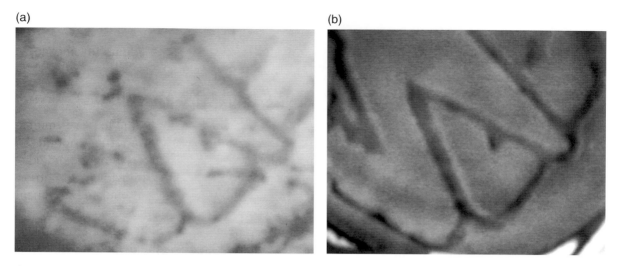

Figure 7.4   Imprint abrasions and bruising on the head (a) which has been stamped upon with the heel of a trainer (b).

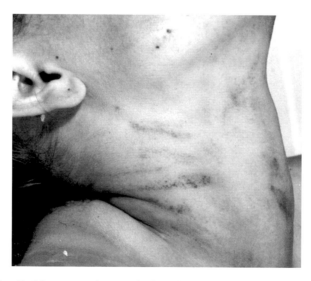

Figure 7.5   Young woman who died from manual strangulation. The right side of her neck shows linear fingernail abrasions extending to the hairline and right ear. They were caused by movement of the neck against the grip of the assailant.

bruising should not be confused with so-called 'pseudo bruising', which results from oozing of blood from vessels after death or during life as a non-traumatic manifestation of bleeding (Advenier et al. 2014). Furthermore, it should also not be confused with hypostasis (lividity, livor mortis).

Bruising is caused by blunt impact and commonly by the following:

– blows by hands or feet: fists, slaps, kicks, stamps
– blows by various weapons, e.g. bars, hammer, etc.
– falls against surfaces
– gripping/pinching
– bites.

(a)

(b)

(c)

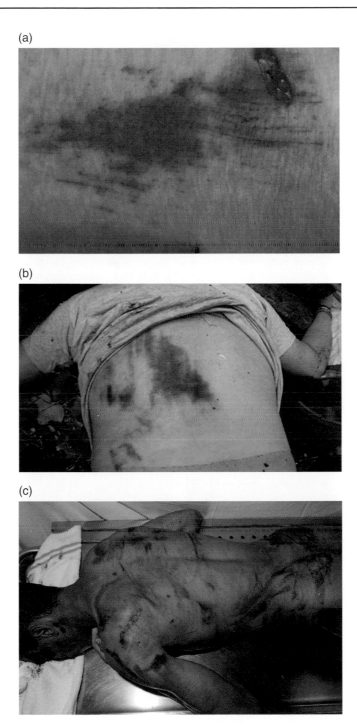

Figure 7.6   (a) Post-mortem grazes marks from dragging the body after death. The marks have a yellow-brown appearance. (b) Grazing and bruising caused by scraping along the wall of a building whilst falling from a height. Note clothing has been rucked up. (c) Bruising and grazing whilst trapped under a car and dragged for a short distance.

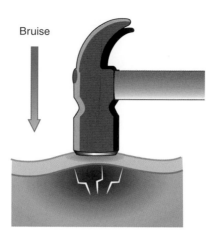

Figure 7.7   Bruising caused by blunt force impact on to skin. The arrow shows the direction of impact (cf. the tangential direction of abrasions causing tearing of the skin in Figure 7.1). Note that bruising occurs within the subepidermal layers because the epidermis contains no blood vessels.

(a)   (b)

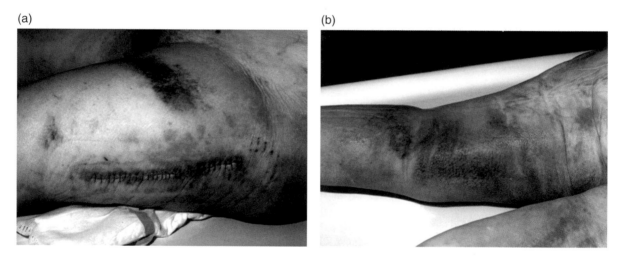

Figure 7.8   (a) Operation site to repair a fracture of the left neck of the femur in an elderly woman. (b) The bruising from the operation site has spread through tissue planes to below the popliteal fossa.

Bruising may be associated with significant internal organ contusions or bone fractures.

Unlike a laceration, the position of a bruise does not necessarily indicate the site of impact as bruising can spread through tissue planes. This is noticeable where the site of bruising is within loose or thin skin and is particularly seen in the elderly (Figure 7.8a and b).

Some bruising, particularly when deep and in areas away from bone surfaces such as the thighs and buttocks, may appear some days later.

The nature of the agent causing a particular bruise is central to assessing the circumstances of injury and thus assisting in the reconstruction of events. On occasions, depending on the site of injury and nature of the impacting agent, it may be possible to match a patterned bruise with an object such as the sole of a shoe (see Section 7.1.1).

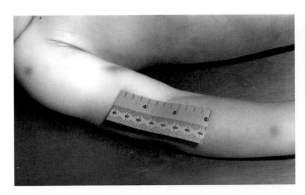
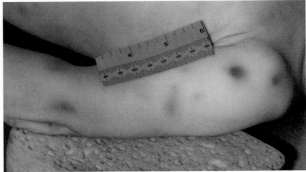

Figure 7.9 'Fingertip' bruising on both upper arms of a young child that had been gripped forcefully.

(a)   (b)

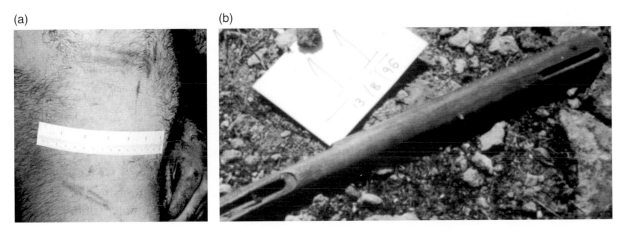

Figure 7.10 (a) Two 'tramline' bruises caused by (b) the cylindrical wooden object found at the scene.

Other bruises, although not producing a 'mirror image' of the offending agent, will nevertheless produce characteristics typical of the type of impacting agent. For example, round or discoid small bruises may well be due to fingertips (Figure 7.9) and tramline bruising may be caused by objects that have a longitudinal cylindrical surface, e.g. a rod or baseball bat (Figure 7.10).

7.1.3 Lacerations

A laceration is a wound produced by tearing or splitting of the skin due to crushing or shearing forces produced as a result of impact with a blunt surface (Figures 7.11 and 7.12).

The following features are typical of lacerations:

– irregular ragged edges (sometimes clean edges if over bone)
– abraded and bruised edges
– tissue bridging in wound
– heal less easily than cut wounds
– seen commonly over bony prominences

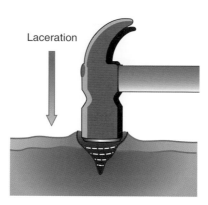

Figure 7.11   Bruising seen within the dermis since the epidermis is bloodless.

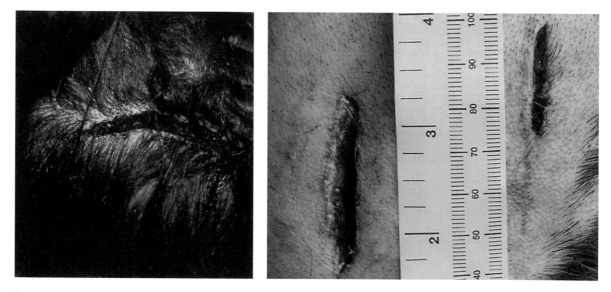

Figure 7.12   Lacerations to the crown of the head. Over the scalp, they may have 'clean cut' edges as they are crushed closely against bone. In the examples shown they have both 'clean cut' and ragged edges.

As with bruising, the shape of the laceration may assist with identifying the type of impacting surface/weapon and may also indicate the direction of a blow. Unlike bruising, the site of the laceration indicates the site of impact. A laceration also indicates that there was more force used than would be used to cause only a bruise in the same region and by a similar surface/object. A laceration may also contain fragments of evidential value such as splinters of wood, glass, paint, etc.

It is important here to emphasise that the use of the word 'laceration' (instead of stab or incised wound) is often used erroneously in describing wounds that have been caused by sharp force trauma, particularly by medical staff not trained in forensic medicine. When perusing through medical records it is important to bear this in mind so that the cause of such wounds is correctly interpreted. As Milroy and Rutty (1997) state 'courts rely to a greater or lesser extent on the medical profession to determine the cause of wounds. The difference in sentencing for conviction for an assault with a punch, which produces a laceration, and a slash with a knife, which results in an incised wound, could be the difference between non-custodial and custodial punishment'.

7.2 Types of incidents in which blunt impact trauma is the predominant feature

7.2.1 Road traffic collisions and other transportation-related incidents

7.2.1.1 Incidence Injuries and deaths from vehicular collisions and other types of transportation incidents are amongst the most common causes of morbidity and mortality globally, and are seen frequently by healthcare staff. The worldwide estimate of road traffic deaths in 2010 was approximately 1.24 million people. Road traffic injuries are the leading cause of death amongst young people aged 15–29 years. Ninety-one percent of the world's fatalities on the roads occur in low-income and middle-income countries, even though these countries have approximately half of the world's vehicles. Half of those dying on the world's roads are 'vulnerable road users': pedestrians, cyclists, and motorcyclists. Only 28 countries, representing 416 million people (7% of the world's population), have adequate laws that address all five risk factors: speed, drink-driving, helmets, seat-belts, and child restraints (WHO Fact Sheet 2013).

7.2.1.2 Types of injuries and their assessment in road users The forensic practitioner will be required to assess injuries from vehicular collisions and to relate them to the findings of the crash investigation team to enable a full understanding of their causation. These considerations include whether the person was a vehicle occupant (driver or passenger) or pedestrian. This may be obvious and in keeping with the type of injuries seen or may require careful consideration where persons have been ejected from a car. Other important factors which may predispose to a collision include the roadworthiness of a vehicle. Human factors predisposing to collision include intoxication of through alcohol and/or drugs, other distracting activities such as the use of cellular phones, altercation with other vehicle occupants, and natural disease (e.g. epilepsy, cardiac disorders).

7.2.1.3 Injuries to vehicle occupants The types of injuries seen may differ significantly among occupants depending on where they were seated and who was driving at the time. The design of the car, safety features, and size will also be another relevant factor. Without doubt the speed just before impact is important. Furthermore, the direction from where the impact occurred with another vehicle is an essential consideration, i.e. whether it was frontal, side or rear. Furthermore, frequently there are impacts with other structures such as a nearby building or tree, as well as occasionally roll over or precipitation when coming off the road into a ditch, steeper terrain or falling onto much lower ground, e.g. from a flyover highway.

Frontal impact results in the occupant usually travelling in pathways relative to the dashboard either down and under or up and over. With down and under movement, the knees strike the dashboard and upper legs absorb the impact, whereas with an up and over direction, the body strikes the steering wheel and the momentum of the thorax is absorbed by the ribs and chest organs.

Side impact injury patterns differ depending on whether the vehicle remains in place or moves away from the impact.

Rear impact to a vehicle causes it to rapidly accelerate and move forward under the occupant. Such collisions cause relatively less damage than frontal collisions, taking into account that the speed just prior to impact is the difference between the two vehicles' speed whereas with frontal collisions it is the sum of both vehicles' speed.

Roll over movement of the vehicle results in the occupant(s) tumbling inside the vehicle, suffering multiple impacts at many different angles, and may cause multiple-system injuries. The type and distribution of trauma is thus difficult to predict and may produce any pattern seen in other types of collisions.

7.2.1.4 Types of injuries sustained by different body regions   *Head and neck*: When the head strikes a stationary object, the skull stops abruptly, but the brain continues moving and is compressed against the skull, which may cause fractures, intracranial haemorrhage, and cerebral injuries. Facial soft tissue trauma with associated underlying fractures may also be seen. The cervical spine is frequently subjected to excessive movement beyond its physiological limit as a result of axial compression, hyperextension or hyperflexion or a combination of these and one may see dislocations, fractures, and underlying spinal cord damage to varying degrees.

Thorax: The aorta is often torn by severe deceleration forces and in particular in the descending portion just below the arch near the ligamentum arteriosum attachment, resulting in rapid exsanguination. The lungs and heart are often involved in compression/crush injury to the thorax. Accompanying multiple rib and sternal fractures are commonly seen.

Abdomen: Compression injuries causing solid organ rupture are seen, including vascular laceration and haemorrhage, as well as hollow organ perforation into the peritoneal cavity. Common injuries include lacerations to the spleen, liver, kidney, and occasionally rupture of a full bladder. It should be appreciated from the foregoing that there is frequently more than one impact in many road traffic collisions which would account for the multiplicity and unpredictability of some of the injuries seen.

Although vehicles are fitted with harnesses, and more recently with air bags, it should be carefully assessed whether a harness had been worn by the vehicle occupants and whether air bags had been deployed on impact. Harnesses can reduce injuries significantly but can also produce significant trauma to the trunk. If an occupant has been ejected from a vehicle, further injuries may be seen depending on where further impacts have occurred.

7.2.1.5 Injuries from motorcycle collisions   It has been estimated that motorcycle riders have a 34-fold higher risk of death in a crash than people driving other types of motor vehicles (Lin and Kraus 2009). With a head-on impact, the rider may be thrown over the handlebars and the resulting injuries may include head and neck, chest and abdomen, femur, lower leg fractures, and perineal injuries. Whilst lower-extremity injuries most commonly occur in all motorcycle crashes, head and neck injuries are most frequent in fatal crashes (Figure 7.13). Helmets and helmet-use laws have been shown to be effective in reducing head injuries and deaths from motorcycle crashes. With an angular or side impact, the rider may be caught between the bike and another object. Injuries in this scenario may include crush injuries to the affected side resulting in open fractures of the long bones of the leg on the affected side as well as fracture dislocation of the ankle region. Where the motorcycle has turned over onto the ground with the rider in the seat, one frequently observes severe abrasions where there has been skidding along the ground and possibly fractures on the affected side.

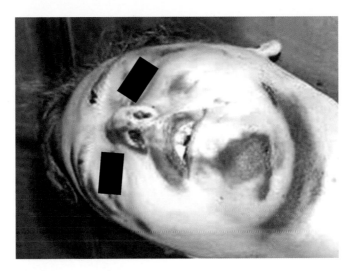

Figure 7.13 Motorcyclist who was thrown head first onto a tree trunk and died instantly from a hyperextension injury to the cervical spine. Note the abrasions on the face from the impact as well as the curved friction abrasion of his upper neck, caused by the strapping on his helmet.

The use of protective equipment will help to reduce the risk of injury. Helmets in particular will absorb energy and significantly reduce head and facial injuries (the risk of injury is increased over three times when a helmet is not used). Other equipment worn includes boots, leather clothing, and eye protection.

7.2.1.6 Injuries to pedestrians Injuries sustained by pedestrians will depend on a number of factors, including the size and velocity of the vehicle, and the age, height, build, and infirmity of the pedestrian, including whether they are under the influence of drink and/or drugs.

Injuries seen frequently result from primary, secondary, and sometimes further impacts according to where the initial impact occurred and whether the pedestrian was thrown further onto the car or onto other objects in the vicinity (e.g. ground, tree, building or into the path of further vehicles).

Common types of injuries include leg injuries frequently from primary impact with a vehicle, e.g. bumper injuries. Head injuries may also be primary but are more usually secondary impacts from being thrown onto the bonnet or roof of the car or hitting the ground. Sometimes soft tissue flaying is seen from being dragged along the road. There may be also be runover injuries with internal crushing of organs either from the original impact or from other vehicles (Figure 7.6c).

7.2.1.7 Injuries to pedal cyclists The injuries that are commonly seen in pedal cyclists result from the cycle being struck by a vehicle and the rider being thrown off. Head injuries are the most common fatal injuries, but occasionally one may see run over or crushing injuries to the head, chest or abdomen caused by a cyclist being trapped between their cycle and a car or larger vehicle and a building. This may happen when the cyclist tries to travel on the inside of a truck or car turning into a side road on the cyclist's side. A retrospective analysis in Denmark based on deaths in cyclists and moped riders that were struck by a right-turning HGV between1996 and 2005 (Munkholm et al.

2007) found that in 20 cases (80%) death had occurred instantly. Also in 20 cases (80%), injuries were found in at least three body regions. These results demonstrate that in such incidents the cyclist is more often run over rather than merely hit by the HGV.

7.2.1.8   Injuries from train collisions   Occasionally, one may see injuries caused by impact with a train. Many of these are self-inflicted, notwithstanding other types of fatalities involving trains, described in Chapter 17. Multiple injuries are commonly seen and include mutilating injuries with partial or complete severance of limbs or the head in the most severe cases. Runover injures are common. In other cases, the deceased may strike the train without being run over and in such instances injuries may resemble severe primary and secondary impact injuries as seen in road traffic pedestrian deaths.

7.2.2   Other incidents that involve blunt impact injuries

7.2.2.1   Serious assaults involving beating with objects, kicking, and punching   The victim of an assault may show extensive blunt impact injury. The injuries may be patterned to indicate the type of object used. In a stamping or kicking injury there may well be part of the pattern of the sole or other part of footwear such as the toe cap area. Such patterned injuries can be matched with the offending footwear and similarly with other objects matching may also be useful. For example, a curved laceration may indicate the head of a hammer and tramline bruising the use of a circular rod (Figure 7.10).

Target sites, particularly with kicking and stamping assaults, include the head and neck area, with mandibular and maxillary fractures being a common feature in such cases. Extensive bleeding from facial injuries is common and death frequently results from blood inhalation as well as blood loss against the background of an unconscious or semi-conscious victim with a compromised cough reflex (Strauch et al. 2001). Such cases may be further compounded by airway obstruction following crush injuries to the laryngeal-hyoid complex. Skull fractures and brain contusions from direct impact injuries from kicks may also be seen, together with intracranial haemorrhage (principally subdural and/or subarachnoid). Whether or not there are any obvious gross injuries seen to the brain or skull, axonal injury is frequently seen, either localised or diffuse, as well as cerebral oedema with secondary brain stem haemorrhages. Occasionally, a kick to the neck may result in trauma to the upper part of the vertebral artery with resulting basal subarachnoid haemorrhage (discussed in more detail below).

The thorax is also a commonly injured area, particular from stamping, resulting a flail chest following sternal and multiple rib fractures and accompanied by severe internal thoracic organ damage, including lung lacerations from displaced fractures and occasionally avulsions from attachment at the hilar regions. The heart may also be subjected to injury in this way and there is also occasional tearing of the aorta when the severest force is employed.

Abdominal, loin, and groin areas are also targeted, although injuries to these regions are less frequently seen. The common organs which are affected include the liver and spleen, where severe contusions/lacerations may be seen. The hollow organs, such as the bowel, may perforate, causing soiling of the peritoneal cavity. Kidneys may be lacerated, with resulting haematuria seen in the bladder or avulsed from the vascular attachments. The duodenum and pancreas may be crushed against the lumbar spine in someone who is lying supine or from a forceful kick to the middle of the abdomen when standing. Scrotal and testicular injuries may also be noted from kicks to the groin when the victim is standing.

7.2.2.2 Falls from a height The concept of 'falling from a height' is commonly understood to mean a fall at least greater than the distance of the victim's own height. Even such a distance is regarded by many as too short and they consider high falls as occurring from at least the average height of a single-storey apartment building (approximately 3 metres). In any event it is important to differentiate between a simple fall that involves falling onto the surface on which one is standing and a fall from a higher level. With higher level falls it is imperative that the distance of the fall should be assessed, as this will obviously need to be related to the type and extent of injuries seen (Türk and Tsokos 2004).

Falls from a height are commonly seen in countries such as Singapore and Hong Kong where most people live in high-rise apartments. A recent study in Singapore examined 1818 cases of death by unnatural causes and found that the majority (652 cases) resulted from falls from a height (Wang and Ching 2013). Most of these cases either fell from windows in apartments or from common corridors, which typically have parapets of 1.2 m high. The large majority of the cases were suicidal attempts as this is the most common method of suicide in Singapore. A very small minority were victims of homicides and accidents; the latter occurring in very young children.

The type of surface onto which the person has fallen should be noted and also the point of primary impact ascertained. Quite often due to the sudden deceleration of the body onto a hard surface in particular the victim may rebound off the surface to a secondary or even tertiary position. Furthermore, the victim may strike intermediate surfaces on the building during the fall, with resulting injuries, and this may affect the position of the primary impact with the ground.

The injuries that are seen in such falls reflect both the height and direction of the fall (Figure 7.14).

There are a number of important considerations when someone is found in an unwitnessed, assumed fall near, for example, the bottom of a high-rise building. The questions that need to be considered are whether the victim did indeed fall from a height or were they killed by some other means at ground level and found in that position, e.g. a road traffic collision? If they fell, were they alive when they fell or were they dead before they were thrown out? If alive, were they conscious, did they deliberately jump or were they in some way killed by another person(s) before being thrown in some way out of the building? A careful examination of the scene, both on the ground and from the place from where the fall is said to have taken place, the background of the individual, the type and distribution of injuries, and other post-mortem findings are all essential elements is assessing such a death.

In a person who is alive and conscious when they fall, multiple injuries are commonplace and also reflect the fact that a large proportion of individuals in such circumstances tend to fall with the lower part of the body impacting initially on the ground.

Common injuries seen include fractures to the skull (base, vault, and foramen magnum), spine, pelvis, and upper and lower limbs. Lacerations as well as grazes from dragging against the ground or building, and other abrasions and bruises are seen externally, with some appearing severe in relation to underlying fractures, and contusions and lacerations to organs such as the aorta, lungs, liver and pelvis in particular.

It is not uncommon to find injuries which reflect that the person tried either deliberately or instinctively to break their fall on impact. Such injuries are seen particularly at the upper and lower limb bones and shoulder joint and/or pelvic girdle. They include fractures and dislocations to the upper limbs at the wrist carpal bones, elbow joints and shoulder joints, and corresponding joints of the lower limbs and pelvic girdle.

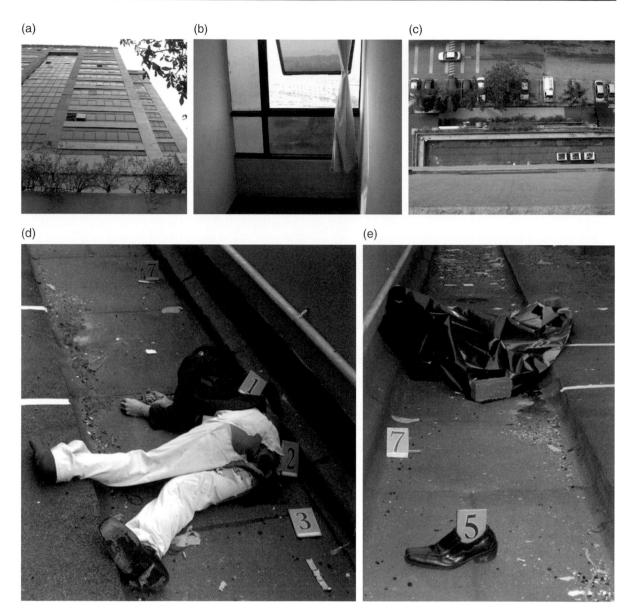

Figure 7.14   Young adult male who precipitated from a window of a high-rise building and landed on a lower roof top surface opposite a car park (a–c). He landed on his buttock area and the force of the impact tore his clothing and dislodged one shoe and his wrist watch (d and e). He sustained injuries to arms, legs, ribs, and pelvis, demonstrating that the force on impact was approximately vertical (f–i).

7.2.3   Head injuries from blunt impact trauma or non-impact forces on the head

In addition to all the injuries described above, head and associated neck injuries may be caused by simple falls or various types of blows or by a combination of both. Injuries may be caused by direct or indirect impact as well as by acceleration/deceleration forces as in shaken baby syndrome. As

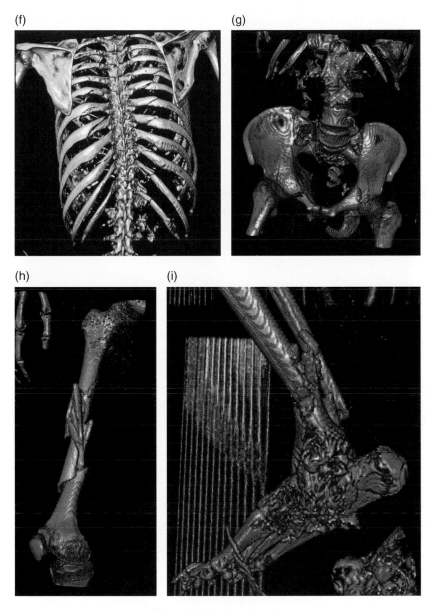

Figure 7.14   (Continued)

stated elsewhere, one type of injury is not mutually exclusive of one or more other mechanisms and it is essential that a full account is taken of the circumstances leading to death to understand how the trauma was caused.

It is also important to differentiate between natural conditions and those due to injury. Furthermore, as the intracranial contents are in a confined space with very little room for expansion, sequelae of injury may include cerebral oedema with potentially fatal effects resulting from hypoxia and space-occupying effects, including herniation of the hind brain and secondary (Duchet) brain stem haemorrhages.

7.2.3.1 Injuries to the head from blunt trauma   A skull fracture may be accompanied by varying degree of underlying intracranial injury or may be confined to the skull. It is an indication of significant force applied to the head.

7.2.3.2 Types of fractures to the skull   There are a number of types of fracture sustained by the cranium and it is beyond the scope of this book to describe them in more than brief detail. The type of fracture that will be sustained will depend on the type of weapon/surface on which the skull impacts, the position on the skull, and the magnitude of force and the area over the skull on which the force acts. If the fracture communicates with the outside environment through the overlying external injury, it is an open or compound fracture and it is closed if it does not.

There are essentially four types of fractures to the cranial part of the skull: linear or depressed fractures to the vault of the skull, fractures which involve and cross suture lines (known as diastatic and seen particularly in children and young adults when sutures have not yet closed), and fractures to the base of the skull, which include the so-called 'hinge' fracture running side to side across the base that is commonly seen in road traffic collisions.

7.2.3.3 Intracranial injuries   Intracranial injuries include brain trauma and/or intracranial haemorrhage and may or may not be accompanied by a skull fracture. Brain trauma can be broadly divided into focal or diffuse injury, or indeed can be a combination of the two. Intracranial haemorrhage may be extradural (epidural), subdural, subarachnoid or intracerebral or a combination.

7.2.3.4 Focal head injuries   Traumatic injury results from direct mechanical forces and is usually associated with focal brain tissue damage visible to the naked eye. It has symptoms that are related to the damaged area of the brain (Figure 7.15).

Blunt impact trauma to the head showing the position of coup (direct underlying injury) and the effect on the opposite side of the brain causing contrecoup injury.

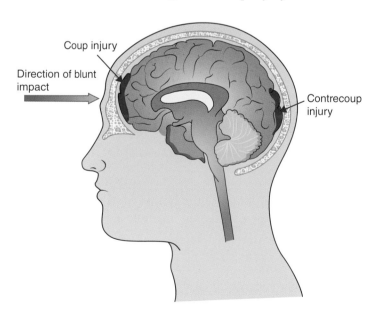

Figure 7.15 Blunt trauma impact to the head.

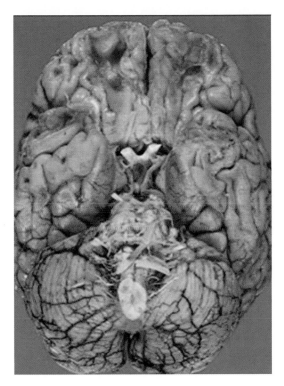

Figure 7.16 Old contusions on the underside of both frontal and temporal lobes in a chronic alcoholic caused by falling and hitting the back of his head on a hard surface.

Injuries include cerebral contusions that commonly result from contact of the brain with the inside of the skull (Figure 7.16). A cerebral laceration occurs as visible breach of the surface of the brain and this is accompanied by tearing of the pia-arachnoid membrane. Infarcts may occur secondary to trauma.

Contusions are seen in approximately 95% of head injuries and are usually found on the crest of gyri on the deep part of the brain. They maybe from direct impact (coup) and/or from indirect impact (contrecoup) (Figures 7.15 and 7.16). 'Gliding' contusions, i.e. haemorrhagic lesions in the parasagittal white matter, are a type of diffuse brain damage occurring at the moment of injury. Gliding contusions are significantly associated with road traffic collisions, with the absence of a skull fracture or a 'lucid interval', and with the presence of diffuse axonal injury (DAI) and deep hemispheric traumatic hematomas.

7.2.3.5 Diffuse injuries Diffuse injuries, also called multifocal injuries, include brain injury due to hypoxia and damage to blood vessels. Unlike focal injuries, which are usually easy to detect using imaging, diffuse injuries may be difficult to detect and define; often, much of the damage is microscopic. Diffuse injuries can result from acceleration/deceleration injuries. Rotational forces are a common cause of diffuse injuries and are common in diffuse injuries such as concussion and DAI. The term 'diffuse' has been called a misnomer, since injury is often actually multifocal, with multiple locations of injury. DAI is widespread damage to the white matter of the brain that usually results from acceleration/deceleration types of injury (see below). Vascular injury usually causes death shortly after an injury. Although it is a diffuse type of brain injury itself, diffuse vascular injury is generally more likely to be caused by focal than diffuse injury. Swelling, commonly seen after traumatic brain injury, can lead to dangerous increases in intracranial pressure. Though swelling itself is a diffuse type of injury, it can result from either focal or diffuse injury.

7.2.3.6 Diffuse axonal injury With DAI, a patient is unconscious from the time of the injury, and autopsy examination of the brain reveals a widespread axonal injury in the cerebral hemispheres, cerebellum, and brainstem. It is the most common consequence of diffuse traumatic brain injury (Adams et al. 1985; Andriessen et al. 2010; Johnson et al. 2013) and is caused by angular rotational acceleration in addition to contact forces. There is mechanical injury to the axon (mostly cytoskeleton) in the white matter tracts. It is most commonly seen in the corpus callosum, grey-white junction, rostral brainstem, internal capsule, and cerebellar peduncles. The severity of DAI is determined by the magnitude, duration, and onset rate of angular acceleration. Increased immunoreactivity (see below) of the neurofilament is seen 1 hour after injury and β-amyloid precursor protein is seen in damaged axons as soon as 3 hours after injury. Ubiquitin (a marker for neurons damaged severely enough to undergo degradation, seen in almost all neurodegenerative diseases) is seen within 6 hours of injury. Microglia are then activated after several days to clean up injured neuron debris.

Microscopic axonal injury is evidenced by disrupted axons which retract to form spheroid or axonal retraction balls, and develops over a period of days after initial injury. Haematoxylin and eosin (H&E) with silver impregnation is used to demonstrate retraction balls. They are most commonly found in the internal capsule, corpus callosum, and superior cerebellar peduncle. Apoptosis following closed head injury is noted at 3–4 days following trauma.

Axonal injury is graded as follows:

Grade 1: only microscopic evidence of axonal injury

Grade 2: corpus callosum focal injury as well as microscopic DAI

Grade 3: focal lesions of the corpus callosum and midbrain in addition to microscopic DAI.

7.2.3.7 DAI in children Mortality and morbidity is similar in adults and children under the age of 4, whilst children between 5 and 15 have a more favourable outcome. Diffuse cerebral swelling is two to five times more common in children than adults (probably due to vascular engorgement, cytotoxic oedema, and disruption of the blood brain barrier) but more commonly associated with poor outcome in adults.

7.2.3.8 Intracranial haemorrhage Intracranial haemorrhage is seen in about 60% of head injuries. The type of haemorrhages seen according to the compartment within the cranial cavity, include extradural (epidural), subdural, subarachnoid, and intracerebral haemorrhage.

Extradural haematoma/haemorrhage (Figure 7.17) is found in about 2% of head injuries and is usually associated with a fractured skull in adults. In children such haematomas are frequently found without a fracture. They are seen in the squamous temporal bone region and most frequently are associated with damage to the middle meningeal artery, although other veins and arteries may be involved. Characteristically, there is a lucid interval whilst the haematoma increases in size and causes significant intracranial pressure with secondary effects on the brain stem which if not alleviated by surgical intervention is fatal.

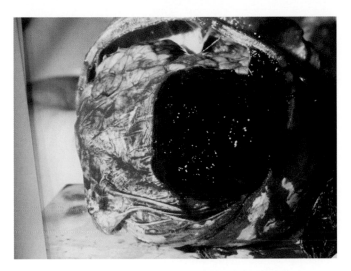

Figure 7.17   Extradural (epidural) haematoma.

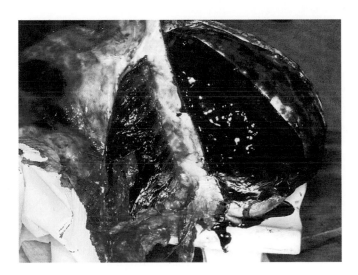

Figure 7.18   Fresh subdural haematoma.

Subdural haematoma haemorrhage (Figure 7.18.) is seen in approximately 13% of head injury cases and is caused as a result of rupture of dural bridging veins. It may be caused by whiplash injury and in the midline position may be associated with shaken baby syndrome. Subdural bleeding usually develops rapidly and covers the entire surface of the affected part of the brain. A haematoma of more than 40 ml will cause an increase in intracranial pressure. Ageing of a haematoma is not satisfactory as there is usually re-bleeding into an existing blood clot. A subdural haematoma should always be regarded as traumatic until proved otherwise. Around 72% of subdural haematomas result from a fall or an assault and 24% are seen in road traffic collisions.

The pathogenesis of *chronic subdural haematoma* is not clear (Figure 7.19). Such haematomas are encapsulated and slow growing. They are seen commonly in the elderly, where the space between the inner table of the skull and brain surface may be increased sufficiently to allow room to expand

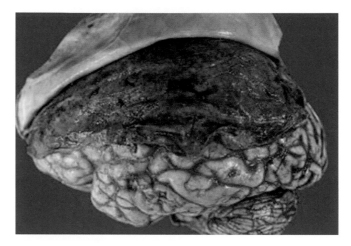

Figure 7.19 Chronic subdural haematoma showing formation of a membrane. The subdural membrane has been reflected to reveal a large subdural haematoma covering the left cerebral hemisphere. Bleeding is also seen within the temporalis muscle.

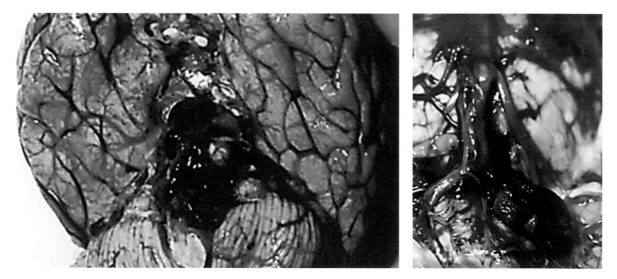

Figure 7.20 Basal subarachnoid haemorrhage caused by a ruptured left vertebral artery aneurysm.

slowly. Such cases frequently present at post-mortem and are not associated with any obvious clinical history during life.

Subarachnoid haemorrhage may result either from trauma or a natural condition. Trauma of different types may cause subarachnoid haemorrhage and it is frequently accompanied by other intracranial haemorrhage types, as well as cerebral contusions. Basal subarachnoid haemorrhage needs to be interpreted with particular caution because if caused by trauma, it is usually the upper part of the vertebral artery which is damaged (both intracranial and extracranial portions, nearly always C1 or C2 level). Occasionally one of the branches from the vertebral artery may be responsible, particularly the posterior inferior cerebellar artery. However, one must take care to examine the vessels at the base of the brain for any aneurysms or other vascular malformations (Figure 7.20). Some aneurysms may be very small and easily missed on gross examination.

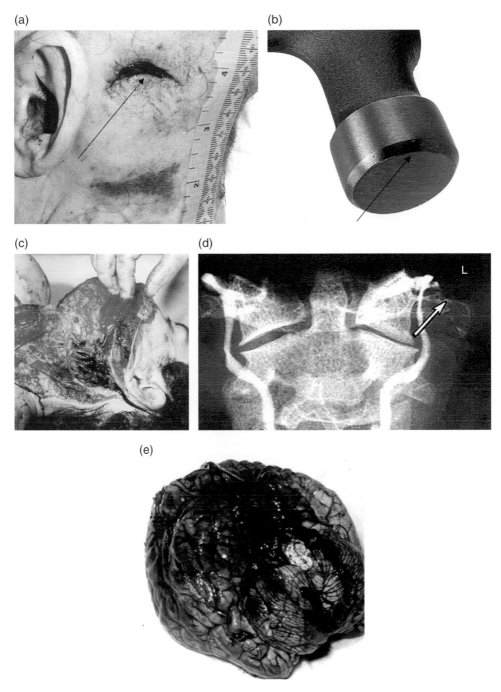

Figure 7.21   Blow to the left side of the neck resulting in a semicircular laceration and below it an abrasion (a) caused by a by a claw hammer with a flat circular face (b). Internal bruising is seen in the soft tissues of the left side of the upper neck (c). The blow caused stretching and tearing of the left upper vertebral artery within the fractured left transverse process of C1 (d), resulting in basal subarachnoid haemorrhage (e). Collapse was rapid and death followed within minutes. (Source: Courtesy Vanezis 1989.)

Vertebral artery trauma is caused by sudden stretching of the vessel from a blow delivered to the neck or the side of the face (Figure 7.21). There is usually a history of alcohol intoxication in the victim immediately prior to sustaining the injury (Vanezis 1989). A clotting disorder causing subarachnoid haemorrhage will frequently show evidence of bleeding elsewhere, e.g. disseminated intravascular coagulation.

Intracerebral bleeding may be seen in around 15% of head injuries and occurs as a result of direct rupture of intracerebral vessels at the time of trauma. Common sites of bleeding include the basal ganglia, thalamus, and deep white matter. Such bleeding is also associated with gliding contusions and axonal injury. Haemorrhage, if large and expanding, may rupture through the brain surface into the subarachnoid and subdural space.

Intracerebral haemorrhage from natural conditions must be differentiated from bleeding caused by trauma.

References

Adams, J.H., Doyle, D., Graham, D.I. et al. (1985). Microscopic diffuse axonal injury in cases of head injury. *Med. Sci. Law* 25: 265–259.

Advenier, A.S., Marchaut, J., and de la Grandmaison, G.L. (2014). Neck pseudo-bruising secondary to acute aortic dissection. *Med. Sci. Law* 54: 54–57.

Andriessen, T.M., Jacobs, B., and Vos, P.E. (2010). Clinical characteristics and pathophysiological mechanisms of focal and diffuse traumatic brain injury. *J. Cell. Mol. Med.* 14: 2381–2392.

Johnson, V.E., Stewart, W., and Smith, D.H. (2013). Axonal pathology in traumatic brain injury. *Exp. Neurol.* 246: 35–43.

Lin, M.R. and Kraus, J.F. (2009). A review of risk factors and patterns of motorcycle injuries. *Accid. Anal. Prev.* 41: 710–722.

Milroy, C.M. and Rutty, G.N. (1997). If a wound is 'neatly incised' it is not a laceration (letter). *BMJ* 315: 1312.

Munkholm, J., Thomsen, A.H., and Lynnerup, N. (2007). Fatal bicycle accidents involving right turning heavy goods vehicles – forensic pathological findings. *Ugeskr. Laeger* 169: 232–235.

Strauch, H., Wirth, I., Taymoorian, U., and Geserick, G. (2001). Kicking to death – forensic and criminological aspects. *Forensic Sci. Int.* 123: 165–171.

Türk, E.E. and Tsokos, M. (2004). Paythologic features of falls from height. *Am. J. Forensic Med. Pathol.* 25: 194–199.

Vanezis, P. (1989). *Pathology of Neck Injury*, Chapter 11, 103–111. London: Butterworths.

Vanezis, P. (2001). Interpreting bruises at necropsy. *J. Clin. Pathol.* 54: 348–355.

Wang, M. and Ching, C.K. (2013). Pattern of coroner's autopsies at health sciences authority, Singapore: a retrospective study (2009–2010). *Med. Sci. Law* 53: 149–153.

WHO Fact sheet No. 358: March 2013.

Yartsev, A. and Langlois, N.E. (2008). A comparison of external and internal injuries within an autopsy series. *Med. Sci. Law* 48: 51–56.

8
Sharp Force Trauma

Peter Vanezis
Queen Mary University of London, London, UK

8.1   Introduction

The term 'sharp force trauma' includes all kinds of injury caused by a weapon or an implement with a sharp edge or point and include knives, scissors or indeed any type of implement with a sharp edge or point, including objects made of materials which may break to produce sharp edges such as glass from, for example, a bottle, vessel, windscreen or from other rigid, brittle, and breakable material such as porcelain (e.g. plates cups, ornaments, and similar objects). Certain tools, such as axes or machetes, combine a sharp edge with heavy weight and produce injuries with sharp and blunt impact elements.

A sharp edge can produce, broadly, two basic types of wounds: stab and incised/slash. There are of course gradations between the two and frequently both types of wounds are seen on the same person, particularly when the victim has been attacked with a sharp weapon such as a knife.

Incidence of sharp force trauma (figures for England and Wales are from the ONS CSEW Statistical Bulletin released in April 2018) (ONS 2018):

- The police recorded 39 598 offences involving a knife or sharp instrument in the year ending December 2017, a 22% increase compared with the previous year (32 468) and the highest number in the 7-year series (from year ending March 2011). The past 3 years have seen a rise in the number of recorded offences involving a knife or sharp instrument, following a general downward trend up to March 2011.

Essential Forensic Medicine, First Edition. Edited by Peter Vanezis.
© 2020 John Wiley & Sons Ltd. Published 2020 by John Wiley & Sons Ltd.

- Two-thirds of the victims of recently recorded homicide from sharp force trauma in England and Wales were male and a substantial proportion of incidents resulted from brawls associated with alcohol. In urban areas many were related to gang disputes.

- Knife-related crimes relating to hospital admissions for assault with a sharp instrument showed little change over the past year following declines in previous years.

8.2   Characteristics of sharp force trauma scenes

8.2.1   Location

Domestic disputes are a common cause of fatal stabbings and in some, stabbing occurs in the victim's own home. In a series of 141 homicides from two Scandinavian capitals, Oslo and Copenhagen, Rogde et al. (2000) found that 78% of all females were killed in their own homes, while this was the case for 49% of males. This is hardly surprising as many of the victims are known to their assailants and knives in a household, particularly from the kitchen drawer, are close to hand to be used as weapons.

It is uncommon to find the knife lying at the scene. In a domestic situation it may be cleaned up and put back in the kitchen drawer or disposed of. In cases involving street violence, it is nearly always removed from the scene. In many cases it is found discarded within a short distance of the incident.

8.2.2   Blood distribution

The handling of the scene, the blood distribution, and the collection of trace evidence are, on the whole, tasks that are addressed by forensic scientists and police personnel, although with respect to blood distribution there are some areas of shared expertise between the biologist and the pathologist. The appearance of blood needs to be assessed in relation to the position of the body and in particular to any wounds that are found. The pattern of distribution of such blood stains may indicate whether they were produced during life or after death. Care must be taken to assess the distribution and quantity of blood with regard to whether or not movement of the body has taken place prior to carrying out scene examination, for example for resuscitation. Such movement may cause large quantities of blood to flow from major stab wounds. The blood in these cases originates from within the body cavity and, particularly with chest wounds, large quantities may spill out onto the floor on turning the body over. Examination of the blood stain patterns at the scene gives an insight into the actions and activities of victim and assailant, and may be of particular value in assessing the direction of travel of blood spots, their velocity on impact, and distance travelled. Forensic scientists, experienced in blood distribution patterns, will use their experience, together with experimental testing and published work, to interpret different patterns in order to estimate site of attack and number of impacts. The size and orientation of stains, from spots to splashes, is indicative of the type and location of the attack.

8.2.3   Homicide or suicide?

There are a number of considerations that the investigator must address when dealing with a stabbing where the possibility of suicide has been raised. Although it should be generally appreciated that in some cases this issue may never be resolved satisfactorily, there are a number of useful features of the scene, which, when considered together with other circumstances and autopsy examination, lead one to the opinion that the injuries were self-inflicted. Most suicidal stabbings occur in

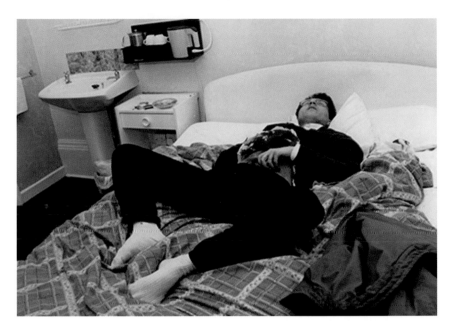

Figure 8.1 The clothing in this young adult male has been pulled up above stab wounds to the lower chest and abdomen.

private, and a substantial number in the bedroom of their own home (Start et al. 1992; Karlsson 1998). The weapon in nearly all cases is still at the scene and usually very close to the deceased, occasionally still in the hand or within the stab wound. One must be mindful of the possibility that a well-meaning relative has removed the implement in question from the scene. There is little disturbance of the scene, in marked contrast to the vast majority of homicidal scenes. Frequently a door is locked from the inside to ensure privacy. Careful examination of the clothing at the scene, before removal of the body to the mortuary, may reveal that garments have been lifted or moved aside to stab through the exposed skin rather than through clothing (Figure 8.1).

The presence of tentative wounds is another very helpful indicator of self-infliction (Vanezis and West 1983), but they should not be confused with signs of torture caused before killing a victim. In such cases there may be other signs at the scene to assist. The use of a mirror to view oneself just prior to death is also well recognised (Riddick et al. 1989) and was also observed by the author of this chapter in a middle-aged male who incised his own neck (Figure 8.2).

8.3 Incised (slash) wounds

Incised wounds that occur as part of the pattern of stabbing are described in section 8.4. There are a number of situations where the incised wounds are the major wounds to be considered both in living and deceased persons.

8.3.1 Incised wounds to the neck (cut throat wounds)

Such injuries are either homicidal or suicidal and occasionally accidental. Accidental wounds are seen particularly in vehicular accidents where such injuries are caused by fragments of glass. In the UK most deaths resulting from incised wounds to the neck are due to self-infliction but in other parts of the world at least as many or the majority of such deaths are homicidal (Bhattacharjee et al. 1997).

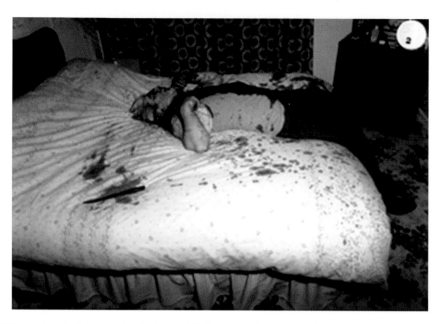

Figure 8.2   Middle-aged male lying on the bed with his feet near the ground after he had incised his neck. He appeared to have been facing the mirror on the dresser nearby.

The distinction between homicidal and suicidal wounds may be difficult if not impossible to make on post-mortem examination alone. It is essential before an opinion is given that account is taken of the circumstances surrounding the deceased's movements shortly before death, his/her personal history, and a thorough examination of the scene of discovery of the body. There are, however, a number of features in the character and distribution of such wounds that will frequently be of some assistance to the pathologist in making the distinction between self-infliction or attack by an assailant. Self-inflicted injuries when made by right-handed persons normally begin high on the left side of the neck and pass downwards across the front to end on the right side. They are deeper at their origin and then tail off on the right. Such wounds may also be horizontal, lying across the front of the neck. They are usually linear and clean cut, since the skin is likely to be put under tension. Separate shallow wounds – 'tentative' or 'hesitation' wounds – are strongly indicative of self-infliction. There are quite often accompanying incised wounds to the wrist or occasionally elsewhere. Some self-inflicted incised wounds may be extremely deep, leaving multiple pronounced score marks on the cervical vertebrae. It is also not unheard of for a victim to excise his own larynx (Giles 1956; Schuessler 1944).

Homicidal wounds as a rule do not have the regular planned appearance of those that are self-inflicted and they are unaccompanied by tentative injuries. Nevertheless, they are frequently accompanied by incised wounds that may be difficult to interpret without accompanying obvious self-inflicted injuries. As a rule, they are more haphazardly placed on the neck and, in some cases, have more irregular edges. In addition, such wounds tend to be deeper, although this is by no means invariably so. Accompanying stab wounds may also be present on the neck and other parts of the body, as well as defence cuts to the backs of the arms and hands. There may also be non-cutting injuries to the body which may have contributed to the cause of death.

Accidental incised wounds may be caused by glass in road traffic accidents. Such wounds are frequently accompanied by numerous small abrasions from glass fragments and particles of glass may be found in wounds if carefully searched for.

8.3.2 Incised wounds to the wrists

Multiple and commonly parallel incised wounds to the ventral aspect of the wrist and lower forearm are typical of self-inflicted injury. They frequently accompany other self-inflicted cutting wounds to other parts of the body. In a number of instances cutting the wrists is not an effective form of suicide and is seen in many cases as a cry for help. Although the victim is aiming to sever a major artery in the wrist, most frequently the radial artery, usually the resulting wounds are more superficial. Not unexpectedly, a substantial proportion of drug abusers have scars on wrists and forearms resulting from self-infliction. Incised wounds to the dorsal surface of the wrists are occasionally seen in cases of self-inflicted injury but, depending on their number and distribution, they may well be defensive injuries.

8.3.3 Incised wounds to other parts of the body

Planned incised wounds to various parts of the body, including the face and trunk, may well form part of a ritualistic torture. More commonly, however, they are deliberately self-inflicted to mislead or draw attention to oneself. Such wounds have a number of characteristic features in common. They are generally superficial and of approximately the same depth. They are arranged in parallel, and are in easily accessible parts of the body. In one case seen by the author, the subject, a young adult male, could not face sitting his final examinations therefore when he missed his sitting, he invented a story that he had been assaulted and knifed. The casualty surgeon suspected that this was not the case (Figure 8.3).

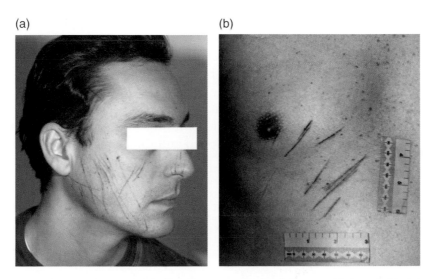

(a) (b)

Figure 8.3 Young male with multiple self-inflicted incised wounds: (a) right side of face and (b) right side of chest. The wounds are all superficial, have a regular parallel distribution, and are on accessible parts of his body.

8.4   Stab wounds and their assessment

Examination of the injuries should take into account the following:

- forces causing injury

- examination of clothing

- the number of wounds

- the position of wounds on the body

- the presence of defensive injuries

- the characteristic appearance (morphology) of defensive injuries

- the depth of defensive injuries and how they relate to internal findings

- the effect of the injuries on the victim

- activity after injury

- manner (category) of death.

8.4.1   Forces causing injury

The pathologist is frequently required to assess the amount of force used in stabbing, yet it is difficult to quantify, except in a relative way. Furthermore, its estimation may well not equate with the severity of the wound itself in terms of the length of its track or organs injured. It is evident that, all other conditions being equal, an impact with greater force is much more likely to produce severe injury than an impact of lesser force.

The various factors or conditions that need to be carefully assessed in the overall estimation of the severity of injury comprise those concerning the movement of the knife up to the point of impact with the skin and from the skin to the point of termination with the body. Furthermore, both these two phases must be considered in conjunction with the properties of the knife as well as the way the assailant delivers the blow, in terms of speed and direction. The various factors involved may be summarised thus:

- *Intrinsic properties of the knife*
    - Shape and sharpness of knife blade
    - Weight of knife

- *Delivery of blow by the assailant*
    - Velocity of the thrust, including follow through on impact
    - Type of thrust (whether over arm or under arm)

- *Movement of the knife up to the point of impact with the skin which is affected by*
  - Clothing worn
  - Movement of the victim

- *Movement of the knife from the skin to its point of termination in the body*
  - Skin resistance
  - Internal organs, muscle, soft tissue, bone

- *Movement of victim*
  - Force involved variable use of 'ran on to knife defence' occasionally used in court

Before means were available to accurately assess the dynamics of stabbing, observers were of the view that once the skin had been pierced, then unless the knife impacted against bone there was virtually no resistance offered by the internal soft tissues, including the major organs. (Knight 1975). Later work by a number of researchers has given us a more accurate assessment of the situation and indeed the appreciation that we are dealing with a more complex scenario than previously appreciated (Chadwick et al. 1999; Horsfall et al. 1999; O'Callaghan et al. 1999). It appears that once the skin has been pierced, significant resistance may be offered by the internal organs and other soft tissues. This is not merely of academic interest. Once the knife has impacted on the skin and even after piercing it, there still needs to be a firm hand on the knife to push the weapon further into the body because it has been slowed down by the resistance offered by the skin. In an accidental stabbing or where a knife has been thrown, one would expect there to be less penetration into the body. In the case of accidental stabbing, it is much more likely that once resistance is offered by the skin there would be not be a follow-through thrust as in a deliberate movement. To produce such a further deliberate movement, the weapon would need to be anchored or held firmly. To produce impalement onto a knife there would need to be enough momentum by the victim moving towards the knife and it would need to be fixed firmly in some way. When a knife is thrown at a person, the main resistance will be by the skin to cause significant loss of its kinetic energy. Because there would be no follow through, the penetration into the body may not be deep because of the further resistance of the internal tissue.

8.4.2 Examination of clothing

Part of the assessment of stab wounds must include examination of the deceased's clothing. The importance of the overlying garments has been discussed in relation to self-inflicted injuries. In homicide cases, careful examination of the defects of the garments produced by a sharp weapon such as a knife can be very instructive and frequently assist the pathologist in assessing the number of times the deceased has been stabbed (Figure 8.4). Although clothing will be submitted for examination by the forensic scientist, the pathologist must not miss the opportunity to examine the clothing and the various tears produced by a knife in conjunction with the wounds found on the body. In some instances, some or all of the clothing may have been removed or cut by paramedics at the scene to carry out resuscitation or removed and retained by the forensic scientists at the scene in order to avoid further contamination. In such cases it may not be possible to examine the clothing in the mortuary but it may still be possible to obtain photographs for comparison with the injuries found.

(a)   (b)

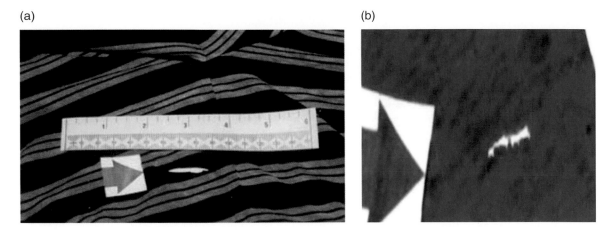

Figure 8.4   Tears in clothing resulting from stabbing (a) Shows a clean cut. (b) The cut is linear but irregular

Examination frequently demonstrates that the number of tears to garments does not always correspond to the number of wounds on the body. Such discrepancies may occur for a number of reasons:

- The weapon may impact on an outer garment but not reach the skin.

- Clothing may be folded and the knife may cause more than one tear from the same impact.

- Clothing at the point of impact may not be present, e.g. may have been pulled away from its normal position for various reasons.

8.4.3   Number of wounds

Single stab wounds in homicidal cases account for around a third to two-thirds of all stabbing cases (Ormstad et al. 1986; Thoresen and Rognum 1986; Murray and Green 1987; Levy and Rao 1988; Hunt and Cowling 1991; Rouse 1994). In the latter series, one or two wounds were most commonly seen in 58% of victims and it was also found by both the same authors as well as Hunt and Cowling (1991) that female assailants tended to cause fewer wounds than their male counterparts.

When a single stab wound is found to the body, it is most commonly seen on the chest or neck. The heart is the most commonly involved organ either solely or together with injuries to the lungs (Rouse 1994). Its singular nature lends itself to the possibility of being considered by the defence as accidental, i.e. that the deceased somehow ran onto a knife or at least came towards the implement, thus contributing to its speed of impact against the body.

8.4.4   Position on the body

The majority of stab wounds are found on the left side of the body and cluster around the main target area of the chest (Ormstad et al. 1986). This is hardly surprising, bearing in mind that most stabbings occur as a result of frontal confrontations between assailant and victim, and furthermore most people are right-handed. The locations of wounds from our own unpublished series of 87 stabbing homicides in and around Glasgow (1998–1999) are shown in Table 8.1.

Table 8.1 Location of stab wounds in 87 fatal stabbing homicides (Glasgow cases 1998–1999).

Site	Left	Right	Midline	Total
Chest	125	96	23	244
Abdomen	29	10	1	40
Neck	13	11	3	27
Head	24	16	2	42
Arms	22	17	–	39
Legs	19	11	–	30

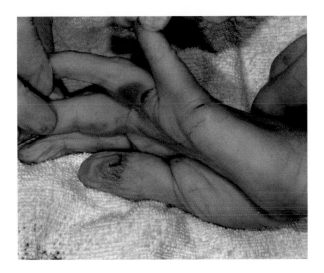

Figure 8.5 Defence cuts to left hand where the deceased tried to take hold of the knife which was being used by the assailant.

8.4.5 Defence wounds

We apply the term 'defence wounds' when we refer to injuries caused as a result of the victim attempting to defend themselves in some way from an assault. Most commonly, the arms and hands are used and these are the areas where we frequently see such injuries. When a person is on the ground or seated the legs may also be sometimes used in this way, although this is not commonly seen. The common sites where such injuries are found are on the upper limbs, including the dorsal and ulnar aspect of the forearms and hands, both back and palm (Figure 8.5). On the lower limbs, injuries to thighs may be seen where the leg is flexed at the knee to attempt to protect from a blow aimed at the chest or abdomen. The types of injuries that are seen depend very much on the implement used and its ability to leave a noticeable injury on the body.

Defence injuries resulting from sharp force trauma comprise cutting injuries principally to the hands and forearms. If the victim attempts to take hold of the weapon, usually a knife, then wounds are seen to the palm of the hand and pads of the fingers. In the latter situation care should be taken to differentiate between injuries caused by the knife slipping through the hand of the assailant, thus injuring his own hand, from a genuine defence injury suffered by the victim.

Superficial wounds may show the characteristics of the cutting edge of the implement, e.g. the serrated edge of a knife. The number of defence wounds tends to increase as the number of stab wounds to the body increases. The overall incidence in all stab wound cases in four series ranged from 39% to just over 45% (Table 8.2).

8.4.6   Characteristics (morphology) of surface wounds

Assessment of stab wound characteristics will frequently assist the pathologist in identifying the type of implement involved, its shape and size, and any possible individual features such as a broken or bent blade tip or anomalous serrations on the blade.

Stab wounds on the surface of the body may show a wide variety of morphological characteristics, depending on the type of implement used, cutting surface, sharpness, and width and shape of the blade. Most stab wounds seen in the UK result from knives with a single sharp-edged blade. Occasionally broken glass, screwdrivers, and other pointed objects are used. Most stab wounds caused by knives tend to have clean cut edges with one or both ends appearing pointed. The non-pointed end may be either squared off or split (fish tail) in appearance (Figure 8.6).

A wound overlying bone, especially over the skull, requires care in its interpretation. It is not unusual to find a laceration of the skin resulting from a blunt impact, having clean edges and a very similar superficial appearance to an incised or stab injury. The reason for this is that the skin, being close to a bony surface becomes easily stretched during impact thus tending to split it cleanly (see

Table 8.2 Incidence of defence wounds in fatal stabbings (%).

Series	Single wound	One to five wounds	Multiple wounds, >10	Multiple wounds, 20+	All cases
Hunt and Cowling (1991)	15.4	–	5.4	–	39
Katkici et al. (1994)	3	–	74	–	39
Karlsson (1998)	–	–	–	–	41
Rouse (1994)	–	42.1	56.1	62.5	45.2

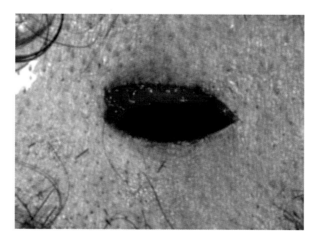

Figure 8.6 Stab wound caused by a knife with a single cutting edge. The right side of the wound is caused by the cutting side of the blade and the more ragged square/fishtail end is from the non-cutting side.

Chapter 5). A thorough exploration of the wound to detect bridging tissue as one would observe within a laceration is essential. With sharp force trauma one may see scoring by the weapon on the outer table of the skull (Figure 8.7a,b).

Bruising may surround the wound that is sometimes the result of impaction by the hilt of the knife. Sometimes the wound may show abraded edges. Frequently, wounds show a notch or change of direction along the margin on the skin (Figures 8.8 and 8.9). This is caused by relative movement of the knife and the body during the stabbing action causing the exit track of the wound to be slightly modified.

8.4.7 Assessment of wound tracts

Although the characteristics of a stab wound on the surface of the body give a great deal of information as discussed above, it is essential to examine the track of a particular wound (Figure 8.10) in order to assess a number of important factors, including:

(a)   (b)

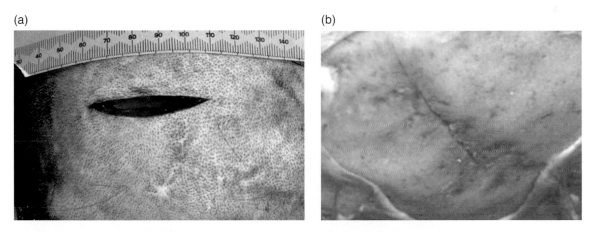

Figure 8.7   (a) Tangential stab wound to the crown of the head and underlying scoring of the cranium. (b) The mark on the skull assists in differentiating between a linear laceration and a cutting injury.

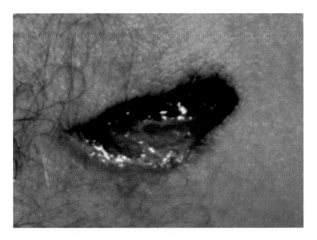

Figure 8.8   Stab wound showing a slight central notch on its upper margin. The lower margin shows 'shelving', with underlying tissue visible. Such wounds give the investigator an indication of the direction of the track of the wound.

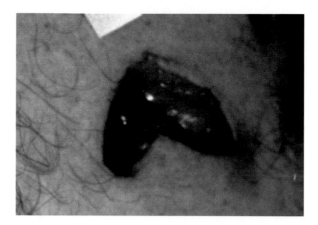

Figure 8.9   Stab wound with central notch giving the appearance of a V shape.

(a)   (b)

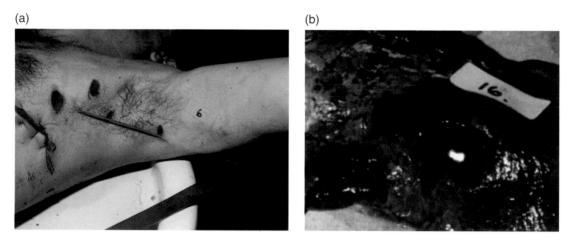

Figure 8.10   (a) Multiple stab wounds on the left side of the chest. The probe indicates the initial entry through the arm then to the chest wall. (b) The track of the wound continued into the upper lobe of the left lung.

- the direction of impact on to the body

- the depth of an injury resulting from stabbing

- the force used to inflict the injury, taking into account the various structures injured

- injured structures and their bearing on morbidity and mortality

- in cases of multiple stabbing, to assess which surface wounds are responsible for which internal injuries.

The depth, or more accurately the length, of the track of the wound may give some guidance as to how far the blade of the knife has penetrated into the body, although estimating the length of the blade of a knife from estimation of the track is notoriously unreliable. It should be appreciated that a number of factors affect the estimation of the length of the track, which is only an approximation. This is particularly the case with abdominal and neck wounds. In chest wounds one must allow for the elasticity of the ribs, especially in younger subjects.

8.4.8   Effects of injury

The pathologist is required to take into account the various possible effects of sharp force trauma as outlined below, including the impact of medical intervention on the overall outcome and possible contribution to morbidity and mortality. The list below is not meant to be exhaustive but includes the more recognised effects of sharp force trauma: acute, subacute, and chronic.

Acute effects include:

- hypovolaemic shock from blood loss

- tamponade

- direct effect of injury to organ function, e.g. heart, spinal cord

- air embolism

- asphyxia from airway obstruction from haematoma

- aspiration of blood

- pneumothorax

- haemothorax.

Subacute and chronic complications include:

- infection

- loss of or diminished function

- aneurysm

- dissection

- ischaemia

- fistula

- diaphragmatic hernia

- adhesions

- chronic inflammation.

8.4.9   Activity after stabbing injury

In many cases of fatal stabbing the victim may be capable of considerable activity before collapsing. It is important to consider the potential for such activity following an injury which ultimately proves to be fatal in order to understand the sequence and circumstances of events leading to death. Many factors are involved in the ability of the victim to continue with physical activity before death ensues and include the site and extent of internal injury to vital organs, rate and amount of blood loss, and the general fitness and state of health of the victim prior to the sustained injury. It is a question that is frequently posed in court when constructing the sequence of events and the pathologist must provide guidance based on autopsy findings together with consideration of the circumstances as related to him/her. Karger et al. (1999) investigated 65 consecutive witnessed suicides from sharp pointed weapons on the basis that suicide and homicide victims usually show similar injuries with regard to the critical organs wounded, and that witness accounts are more reliable in suicide cases. They found that with injuries to the chest (most to the heart) that the victims could walk and talk from minutes to over 2 hours.

An earlier study by Thoresen and Rognum (1986) on 109 victims of fatal injury from sharp weapons found the following with respect to survival time and physical activity. Of the 13 who died immediately, nine had penetrating lesions of the heart. This group also had the highest number of lesions. Sixty-four victims survived for some time. The survival time increased with decreasing number of lesions. The greatest blood loss and the highest blood alcohol concentrations were found in those who survived between 0.5 and 1 hour. Twenty-four victims were able to make physical efforts after the injury and the movements varied from a few steps to the running of several hundred metres. They found that decisive factors for decrease in survival time and acting capability were penetrating lesions to the heart and the great vessels, and multiplicity of injuries.

From my own experience I have encountered cases where the victim had run several metres in the street, climbed a flight of stairs or continued fighting for at least a number of minutes before becoming incapacitated.

8.4.10   Manner of death

The manner (category) of death, whether homicide, suicide or accident, is indicated by the site, number, and nature of the wounds, evaluated together with other circumstantial information relating to the injury. The indicators commonly seen in the different types are given in Table 8.3.

8.5   Glass injuries

Depending on its constitution, glass may be shattered or broken into sharp, jagged pieces or shards which can then cause injury.

8.5.1 Glass injuries from assaults

According to the 2009/10 British Crime Survey (BCS) (Home Office Statistical Bulletin 2010), glass and bottles were used as hitting instruments in 4% of violent incidents. The use of broken glass vessels of bottles to thrust onto a victim's face or other parts of the body is commonly referred to as 'glassing' and is seen frequently in public houses and other establishments where alcohol is served and the perpetrator and victim may be intoxicated.

The impact of glass can result in slash-type incised wounds, deeper stab wounds from shards or a combination of both sharp and blunt impact injuries (incised wound, Laceration, bruising). Sometimes, when someone is dragged through glass or the impact is tangential, the injury may appear as linear superficial incised wounds, sometimes parallel, reflecting the edges of the broken glass.

The pattern and distribution of the injuries may reveal whether the glass injuries are due to an assault or, as is sometimes claimed by defendants, that the victim fell onto or had been rolling on glass already broken on the ground.

In assessing glass injuries in both living and deceased individuals it should be appreciated that fragments of glass may be found in superficial and deeper wounds and indeed may be the only indication that a glass object was used when the type of implement causing the wound is not known (e.g. whether the implement was a knife or a glass shard). Glass fragments appear opaque on radiographs and these may assist in locating and retrieving fragments from wounds before treatment in the living victim and to retain them for evidential purposes.

8.5.2 Other types of glass injury

Glass injuries may also occur in many other situations, including the following:

- Domestic accidents such as falling/walking through glass doors, against and through windows are a common problem. Many such accidents occur in children and adolescents (Hashemi and

Table 8.3 Indicators seen between the three manners of death in sharp force trauma.

Homicide	Suicide	Accident
No tentative cuts	Tentative cuts common	No tentative wounds
Any number of wounds frequently seen	Single or very few deep wounds	Usually single
Wounds not regularly placed unless victim immobilised	Regularly placed wounds are common	Usually single wound
Target vital areas	Sites of election	Random location
Often repetition in 'frenzied' attack	Often repetition (each wound close to the others)	Usually single
May be injured anywhere	Accessible parts of the body	Random location
Deep	Deep	Variable depth
Defensive injuries	Self-mutilation	Absent
N/A	Usually in private	Either private or in the presence of others
Stab through clothing	Usually clothing lifted	Stab through clothing
Usually scene disturbance	No scene disturbance	May be scene disturbance
Weapon usually removed from scene	Weapon usually still at scene near deceased	May be at scene depending on type of incident

Subhedar 1986). Grieshaber and Stegmann (2006) reported in 100 consecutive patients, aged 16 years and under, with penetrating eye injuries, and found that 55% of injuries occurred at home, and all injuries to children under the age of 6 years occurred in a domestic location. Most children (66%) were injured during play. Most injuries occurred in the absence of a caregiver (85%). Sticks, wire, and glass caused half of all injuries (48%). Glass tables are the most common cause of domestic glass injuries when the victims are children.

• Road traffic collisions may produce injuries from glass windows of vehicles. Before safety regulations introduced in the 1980s, frontal impact collisions produced damage to the front windscreen leading to the release of numerous glass fragments. Since 1981, it has been mandatory for all vehicles in the UK (and Europe) to have laminated glass in the front windscreen with toughened glass in the side window (European National Car Assessment Programme (EuroNCAP 2016). This industry stipulation has made cars considerably safer and it is inferred that injuries directly attributable to such accidents have been reduced owing to the laminated windscreen, which prevents the escape of the glass fragments. Occasionally, however both laminated and toughened glass can become 'crazed', producing shards that penetrate soft tissues. The toughened glass of side windows has a different configuration to laminated glass from windscreens (typically breaking into small cubic fragments rather than slithers). In the clinical setting, both can produce a similar radiographic appearance and it is not always possible to be certain of the source, i.e. toughened side windows or a laminated windscreen (Ahmad et al. 2009).

• By handling broken glass in an accidental manner. Shards of glass may cause deep soft tissue injuries, including damage to blood and have the potential to be a health hazard if it is contaminated with toxic chemicals, blood, or infectious substances which may enter the body through a cut or puncture. This a particular hazard in a laboratory where glass containers are handled on a regular basis. If the injury involves potential exposure to infectious materials, then immediate medical attention is required. A further example of accidental injury relates to shards of glass lying on the street. This is a leading cause of glass injuries for children playing outside the home, with the feet being the most affected body part.

• Dispersed broken glass in explosions of all types (bombs, accidental as in industrial explosions and so on) can travel at high speeds, particularly from shattered windows as a result of the blast wave, and cause severe penetrating injuries.

8.5.3   Accidental glass injury: Case study

A 61-year-old male had been on holiday in Portugal when he apparently cut his right hand on broken glass from a champagne bottle whilst opening it. On his return to England he was admitted to the hospital a week after the incident with cellulitis and necrotising fasciitis caused by infection with ss – haemolytic group A streptococcus and required an urgent operation for debridement. During surgery he suffered a cardiac arrest for 2 minutes before resuscitation. Post-operatively he was taken to intensive care in multiorgan failure. He was reviewed 2 days later and he was taken back to the theatre because of aggressive fasciitis for further debridement, but unfortunately he died on the table. The medical notes revealed that he was in septic shock. He developed a coagulopathy and multiorgan failure.

8.6 Injuries from other sharp objects

It should also be appreciated that other objects that when fragmented may present sharp edges, such as ceramics (pottery), typically vases or plates, and can cause penetrating injuries or slash/incised wounds in a similar manner.

References

Ahmad, Z., Devaraj, V.S., Jenkins, J.P.R., and Silver, D.A.T. (2009). Penetrating injury from laminated glass – a trap for the unwary. Case report. *Br. J. Radiol.* 82: e114–e116.

Bhattacharjee, N., Arefin, S.M., Mazumder, S.M., and Khan, M.K. (1997). Cut throat injury: a retrospective study of 26 cases. *Bangladesh Med. Res. Council* 23 (3): 87–89.

Chadwick, E.K.J., Nicol, A.C., Lane, J.V., and Gray, T.G.F. (1999). Biomecchanics of knife stab attacks. *Forensic Sci. Int.* 105: 35–44.

EuroNCAP. Available from: www.euroncap.com (Accessed 20/04/2016).

Giles, C. (1956). Suicidal laryngectomy. *J. Forensic Med.* 3: 91–93.

Grieshaber, M.C. and Stegmann, R. (2006). Penetrating eye injuries in South African children: aetiology and visual outcome. *Eye (London)* 20: 7897–7895.

Hashemi, K. and Subhedar, V.Y. (1986). Accidents from glass. *BMJ* 292: 917–918.

Home Office Statistical Bulletin. Crime in England and Wales 2009/10. Edited by Flatley J., Smith K., Chaplin R. and Moon D. London, July 2010.

Horsfall, I., Prosser, P.D., Watson, C.H., and Champion, S.M. (1999). An assessment of human performance in stabbing. *Forensic Sci. Int.* 102: 79–89.

Hunt, A.C. and Cowling, R.J. (1991). Murder by stabbing. *Forensic Sci. Int.* 52: 107–112.

Karger, B., Niemeyer, J., and Brinkmann, B. (1999). Physical activity following fatal injury from sharp pointed weapons. *Int. J. Legal Med.* 112: 188–191.

Karlsson, T. (1998). Homicidal and suicidal sharp force fatalities in Stockholm, Sweden: orientation of entrance wounds in stabs gives information in the classification. *Forensic Sci. Int.* 93: 21–32.

Katkici, Ü., Özkök, M.S., and Örsal, M. (1994). An autopsy evaluation of defence wounds in 195 homicidal deaths due to stabbing. *J. Forensic Sci. Soc.* 34: 237–240.

Knight, B. (1975). The dynamics of stab wounds. *Forensic Sci.* 6: 249–255.

Levy, V. and Rao, V.J. (1988). Survival times in gunshot and stab wound victims. *Am. J. Forensic Med. Pathol.* 9: 215–217.

Murray, L.A. and Green, M.A. (1987). Hilts and knives: a survey of 10 years of fatal stabbings. *Med. Sci. Law* 27: 182–184.

O'Callaghan, P.T., Jones, M.D., James, D.S. et al. (1999). Dynamics of stab wounds: force required for penetration of various cadaveric human tissues. *Forensic Sci. Int.* 104: 173–178.

Office for National Statistics. Statistical bulletin: Crime in England and Wales: Year ending December 2017. 2018.

Ormstad, K., Karlsson, T., Enkler, L. et al. (1986). Patterns in sharp force fatalities – a comprehensive forensic medical study. *J. Forensic Sci.* 31: 529–542.

Riddick, L., Mussel, G., and Cumberland, G.D. (1989). The mirror's use in suicide. *Am. J. Forensic Med. Pathol.* 10: 14–16.

Rogde, S., Hougen, H.P., and Poulsen, K. (2000). Homicide by sharp force in two Scandinavian capitals. *Forensic Sci. Int.* 109: 135–145.

Rouse, D.A. (1994). Patterns of stab wounds: a six-year study. *Med. Sci. Law* 34: 67–71.

Schuessler, W.W. (1944). Self-inflicted excision of the larynx and thyroid and division of trachea and oesophagus with recovery. *J. Am. Med. Assoc.* 125: 551–552.

Start, R.D., Milroy, C.M., and Green, M.A. (1992). Suicide by self-stabbing. *Forensic Sci. Int.* 56: 89–94.

Thoresen, S.O. and Rognum, T.O. (1986). Survival time and acting capability after fatal injury by sharp weapons. *Forensic Sci. Int.* 31: 181–187.

Vanezis, P. and West, I.E. (1983). Tentative injuries in self-stabbing. *Forensic Sci. Int.* 21: 65–70.

9
Firearm and Explosion Injuries

Peter Vanezis
Queen Mary University of London, London, UK

9.1   Firearm injuries

When investigating deaths involving firearms and projectiles from other sources (explosions are dealt with in the next section), there are a number of basic questions that need to be addressed:

- Is the weapon causing the injury a firearm or has it come from some other source?

- If the injury has been caused by the discharge of a firearm:
  - What type of firearm fired the cartridge?
  - Did a particular firearm fire the cartridge?
  - Which are the entry and exit holes on the person and on other objects?
  - How far was the weapon from the victim?
  - Is death due to homicide, suicide or accident?

9.2   Types of firearms

Outside the military environment and the occasional politically motivated incident it is unusual to encounter weapons other than handguns, rifles and shotguns.

Handguns (pistols and revolvers) and rifles are known as rifled weapons from the spiral groves inside the barrel which are designed to cause the missile to spin as it goes through the barrel in

Essential Forensic Medicine, First Edition. Edited by Peter Vanezis.
© 2020 John Wiley & Sons Ltd. Published 2020 by John Wiley & Sons Ltd.

order to ensure that there is a steady flight produced by the gyroscopic effect. Shotguns which fire pellets or a single shot, by contrast have a smooth bore.

Rifles are designed to fire a missile at a high muzzle velocity of 1000–4000 ft/s, whereas short barrel weapons (pistols and revolvers) have a low muzzle velocity of 600–1000 ft/s.

9.3 Recoil

In the vast majority of weapons, the barrel will be situated above the grip and so when the gun discharges, the recoil force acting along the barrel sets up a turning moment along the grip, or butt-stock, the result being that the muzzle rises. As it rises in automatic fire, then this turning moment becomes increasingly larger, and unless in the hands of an experienced shooter, the gun will rapidly climb away out of control with potentially disastrous consequences. In the case of self-inflicted or accidental gunshot wounds with the weapon still at the scene, the violent recoil of a shotgun, particularly if sawn-off, can propel the weapon some distance from the body.

9.4 Handguns

There are two main types: pistol and revolver (Figure 9.1). Both are designed for firing with one hand but they have major differences which affect the evidence potentially retrievable at the scene. The important difference between the pistol and the revolver is that with the revolver the fired cartridge case remains within the chamber and is not ejected. Both pistols and revolvers discharge a single bullet. Although there are exceptions to every rule, generally speaking the pistol will fire a jacketed bullet whereas the revolver bullet is often plain lead. The jacket is a covering of a tough cupro-nickel, steel or brass over the lead core, designed to protect the soft lead from the violent actions of the loading cycle. While most bullets are designed to remain intact in the body, it is often the case that if bone is struck or the bullet exits from the body and goes on to strike a hard surface, the core and the jacket will separate and be separately located at the scene.

9.4.1 Pistols

Pistols are single-shot weapons which may be self-loading or semi-automatic. A popular configuration is a single-barrelled weapon, firing a single bullet through a rifled barrel. The magazine is

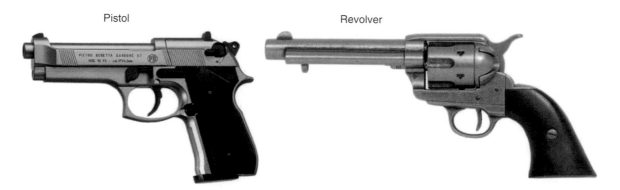

Pistol   Revolver

Figure 9.1 Handguns.

normally housed in the grip, which holds the rounds of ammunition. In a small pocket pistol of 0.22″, 0.25″ and 0.32″ calibres, the magazine capacity is seven to eight rounds, whereas in the larger calibres of 9 mm and 0.45″ and with modern designs, the magazine capacity may be as much as 18 rounds. The recoil force generated by the discharge of the cartridge will cycle the mechanism 'automatically' and eject the fired cartridge case clear of the gun. The action, however, does move backwards relative to the body of the pistol and takes the cartridge case with it, carried on the extractor. Towards the rear of its travel, this case is struck by the ejector and thrown clear. The return spring in the pistol will then exert itself and the action will run forward again, taking the next cartridge from the magazine, leaving the weapon cocked and ready for a further pull on the trigger to fire the next shot.

In the second type of pistol mechanism, the high-pressure gases generated within the cartridge and barrel are utilised to drive a piston rearward and cycle the action rather than just the recoil energy. This gas operation is far more common in modern military rifles and machine guns although a few pistols use it. The end result is the same, however, with a fired cartridge case ejected at the scene, sometimes several metres away from the gun.

9.4.2 Revolvers

A revolver is a repeating weapon, but with the rounds of ammunition held in separate chambers within a revolving cylinder. By far the most common configuration is six rounds, although with small calibres, capacities of up to 12 are sometimes seen.

Most revolvers can be fired in two ways. Either by a single action, where the exposed hammer is first cocked and a relatively light trigger pull applied, or by a double action, where a long heavy pull is applied to the trigger which both cocks the action and advances the cylinder one chamber prior to allowing the hammer to drop and fire the gun.

9.5 Rifles

A rifle (Figure 9.2) is designed to be fired from the shoulder. They are classified into *rimfire*, where the primer is to be found in the rim of the cartridge case, and *centrefire*, where it is in the centre. Rimfire rifles produce wounds similar to low-velocity handguns.

Rifles can be single-shot, lever action, pump action, bolt action or auto-loading. They can be sub-divided into semi-automatic and fully automatic. Automatic rifles are generally used by the military and by the police.

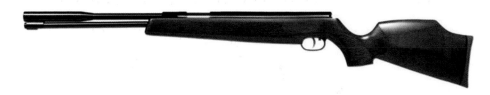

Figure 9.2 Rifle.

9.5.1   Machine guns and military rifles

Military weapons are seldom encountered in UK mainland crime outside politically motivated incidents and those involving military personnel. The modern military rifle, along with its close relation the submachine gun, differ in one major aspect from the shotguns and handguns referred to above. They are invariably selective-fire weapons; that is to say they will fire in a single-shot fashion in just the same way as a self-loading pistol but they have the additional capacity to discharge in a fully automatic fashion where missiles continue to be discharged until the trigger is released or the magazine is empty. A typical modern military weapon will have a magazine capacity of 25–30 rounds and a cyclic rate in the region of 400–600 rounds per minute, so will empty in approximately 3 seconds on continuous fire. As with ejected cases from the self-loading pistol and shotgun, the careful analysis of the distribution of the cases is very important. Of particular significance will be the distribution of the bullet impacts, the position of which will, if the gun is in automatic mode, alter as the recoil angle increases.

9.5.2   Ammunition used in rifled firearms

There is a wide variety of ammunition used in rifled firearms. A detailed description is beyond the scope of this text, hence for further information the reader is directed to the bibliography section at the end of this chapter. Three examples are shown in Figure 9.3.

9.6   Shotguns

The shotgun (Figure 9.4) in its unmodified state is a large weapon, designed to be fired from the shoulder and typically with a barrel of some 26–30 in. in length. It differs fundamentally from the handgun in that it has a smooth bored barrel and it fires a charge of pellets (shot) propelled by wadding (Figure 9.5) which will travel with the shot for a few feet before falling away. It is common for the wadding to be retrieved at post-mortem together with pellets when the range

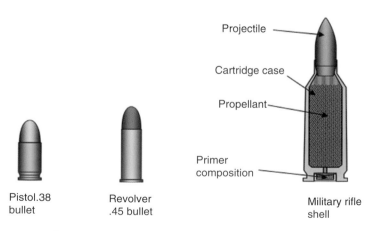

Figure 9.3   Examples of ammunition in rifled firearms.

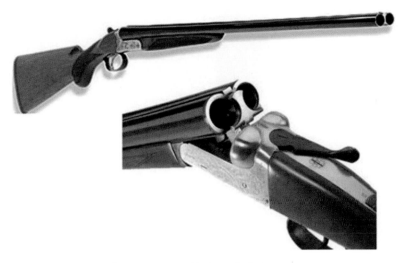

Figure 9.4 Double-barrelled shotgun.

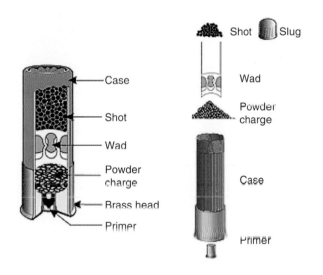

Figure 9.5 Shotgun ammunition.

of firing is short. In a typical 12-bore cartridge there will be around 300 pellets, which are potentially retrievable at the scene of a shooting. A shotgun may fire a few large projectiles or even a single slug, but these are rarely met with in forensic practice. The constriction (choke) at the end of the barrel is designed to control the amount of spread of the pellets. The shotgun may be illegally modified by sawing off part of the barrel for ease of concealment and wider spread of pellets.

The historical term 'gauge' is used to describe the calibre of a shotgun and refers to the number of lead balls of the given bore diameter that make up a pound (Figure 9.6). In 12-gauge, for

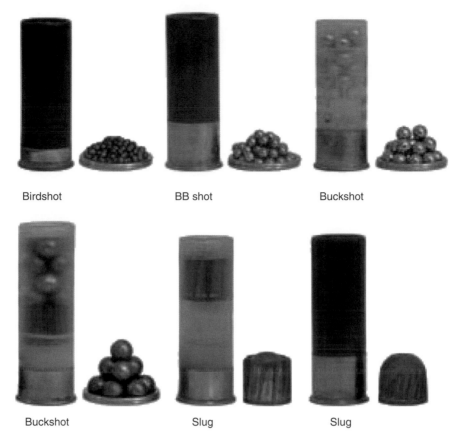

Figure 9.6   Shotgun loading – showing different shot sizes and slugs.

example, it would take 12 of the lead balls to make 1 lb. This is the most popular shotgun bore size used in the USA.

Shotguns come in all shapes and sizes, from single- and double-barrelled sporting guns through to pump action and other repeating designs with magazine capacities of up to nine cartridges.

9.7   Wounds from firearms and other missile injuries

With regard to firearms, the appearance and extent of injury will depend on the transfer of kinetic energy (KE) of the missile or missiles. Gunshots inflict damage by disrupting tissues, causing haemorrhage and permitting the entrance of infection. Generally, three factors determine the severity of a gunshot injury: the amount of KE transferred by the bullet to the surrounding tissues, the internal organs and structures damaged by the bullet, and the bullet's final disposition. The formula KE = $\frac{1}{2}mv^2$ expresses the amount of energy transferred to the body by a bullet. KE is the amount of tissue damage delivered to the surrounding organs and is the product of the mass of the bullet times the square of the bullet's velocity, divided by 2. Increasing the velocity of the bullet is more significant than increasing its mass because an increase in velocity is exponential, whereas an increase in mass is linear.

Missiles may be especially designed or altered (hollow point and soft point types) so that they slow down or stop within the body, thus ensuring that more energy is employed for tissue displacement with the aim of causing maximum damage. The 'dumdum' bullet, which has a scored nose with an air-cavity within the tip, is intended to splay open and expand on impact to increase the deceleration effect. It was invented in the Dum Dum Arsenal near Calcutta for the 0.303 British cartridge in 1896 by Lt Cl Neville Bertie-Clay.

The extent of injury caused, as stated above, will depend on the mass and speed of the bullet as well as its area of contact and resistance of tissues. When the skin is penetrated, the tissues are separated and the track becomes wider than the missile, resulting in soft tissue damage along the track, with cavitation. Permanent cavitation is a particular feature of high-velocity projectiles, with solid organs such as the brain and liver being more affected than the lung, which is a spongy organ.

9.8 Investigation of firearm injuries

9.8.1 The scene

The investigation of firearm injuries involves a thorough examination of the scene of the shooting in the first instance and ideally involves the pathologist and specialist firearms expert in addition to the usual scene investigation team. It is well documented that some considerable physical activity can follow after shooting, which makes accurate recording of the scene essential.

A necessary part of scene investigation is the accurate reconstruction of events, which aims to provide valuable information about trajectories (Roberts and Hanby 1985), position of victim(s), and firing position of gunman (Nennstiel 1985) and their various movements. For example, a thorough scene examination should be carried out to ascertain the number, location, and damage produced by missiles, the distribution of spent cartridge cases and wadding, the scattered debris produced by damage from impacts to structures such as walls, glass and wood, the position of blood spattering, and the position of body tissues found at the scene. All such findings when considered in the light of information provided by the pathologist such as position of entry and exit wounds and their positions on the body, ricochet injuries and approximate estimation of range, should allow a reasonable attempt to be made at reconstructing events.

Reay et al (1986) describe how they were able to reconstruct a shooting scene in which 13 people were killed because they were immobilised before being shot. The victims were patrons of an oriental gambling club and were murdered systematically during a robbery. Each of the victims was tied with a ligature, with their hands and feet behind their back (hog tied), robbed then shot. The investigators were able to assess the trajectories of the gunshot wounds and the approximate position of the weapon at the time of firing. They found that initially shots were fired from a distance of some 5–7 m away from the victims, from a slightly elevated platform. Furthermore, by assessing the location of ejected casings they were also able to say that shots were fired as the perpetrators walked amongst the victims. The one survivor was able to corroborate this reconstruction.

Crime scenes where bullets have ricocheted will generally leave traces of metal from the projectile, whether bullet or pellet, which can be readily identified in the laboratory (Burke and Rowe 1992). In addition, the surface may be damaged by the projectile, producing a crater in the wall or gouging out part of the surface. The nature of the damage sustained will depend to a great extent on the type of surface. For example, elongated gouge marks, extending in the long axis of the direction of the projectile, will appear elongated in a soft metal surface (Mitosinka 1971; Janssen and

Levine 1982) or plasterboard (Jordan et al. 1988). The width of the gouge marks will indicate the diameter of the projectile. On the other hand, ricochet marks in soil or sand will be less well defined (Haag 1975). Projectiles may pick up trace evidence from surfaces and a scanning electron microscope can be used to identify particles. In the case described by Di Maio et al. (1987), limestone was detected, which had originated from a stone surface from which the bullet had ricocheted.

In terms of whether death is due to homicide, suicide or an accident, in the vast majority of cases there is little doubt. At the scene, consideration should be given to the presence or absence of a weapon and its position in relation to the body, position of blood stains, signs of a disturbance, accessibility to the scene, position of spent cartridge cases, trajectory of missiles, and impact marks on objects or surfaces from missiles and their distribution. However, in some cases the distinction is not so clear and one must therefore always approach each case with an open and enquiring mind. Pathological factors which need to be taken into account include the site of the wound or wounds, their multiplicity, range, signs of a struggle on the body, dexterity of the victim (left or right-handedness), residues on hands, and injuries on hands from the firing weapon. The site of the wound in most suicide cases conforms to well-recognised selected sites such the temple, centre of the forehead, mouth, under the chin, centre of the chest, and other midline structures to the front of the body. The direction of the wound track from the site is a further good indication of the aim of the deceased towards a particular vital structure such as the heart or brain. The range of discharge of the firearm is also another useful factor which may help confirm or negate death as being self-inflicted. Unless there is some mechanism to discharge a firearm from a distance further than arm's reach, then such a discharge is extremely unlikely to have been self-inflicted. Suicide notes are only occasionally found. There may also be evidence of recent or older self-harm injuries or known psychiatric history.

9.8.2 Radiological examination

It is mandatory in cases involving firearm injuries that the body is subjected to radiological examination (Figure 9.7), ideally of the whole body. The examination may either be in the form of conventional radiography in which posterior-anterior, lateral, and oblique views should be taken. Wherever possible a whole-body computerised tomography (CT) scan is desirable and with modern scanning equipment and software post-processing to view injuries and missiles in three dimensions as well as cross-sectional two-dimensional images renders assessment of injuries and retrieval of missiles much easier (Figure 9.8).

9.8.3 Gross autopsy examination

The post-mortem examination in the mortuary will be carried out in the conventional manner of any forensic investigation with full description of injuries and clear and appropriate photography. The findings at the scene will be carefully considered in conjunction with the autopsy room findings. The pathologist will, with the aid of pre-post-mortem imaging, retrieve missiles, wadding, and any fragments. The sequence of wounds, trajectory as well as range of discharge will be considered from the character and position of wounds. At this stage it should also be appreciated that careful examination of the clothing worn should be carried out to assess tears caused by a firearm and the direction of the fibres to indicate entry or exit as well as the possibility of missiles and fragments lying loose in clothing. Recovery of firearm residues from the body (principally primer and

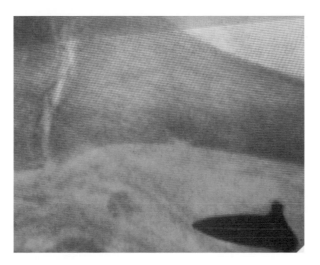

Figure 9.7 Fluoroscope used to find missiles in victims of genocide found in mass graves. Note the bullet from a high-velocity firearm in the bottom right-hand corner.

propellant) is also important, although soiling from firearm residues may be present on interposed clothing rather than on the skin.

In order to understand the extent of injury that can be produced by different firearms and to enable a satisfactory investigation to be carried out, it is essential to consider and assess the physical characteristics of the wounds (whether entry or exit), their effects on internal organs, location, number, range where possible, as well as other injuries on the body.

The characteristics of a gunshot wound will be affected by a number of factors, including range and trajectory of discharge, the type of firearm which has been used, whether a smooth bore weapon (e.g. shot gun) or rifled weapon (e.g. pistol), as well as the type of projectile(s) discharged. The type of propellant, muzzle velocity, and choke if present are also important.

9.9 Wounds and range of discharge from rifled firearms

9.9.1 Contact wounds

9.9.1.1 Close contact and loose contact The appearance of a close-contact wound will be governed by whether the skin is supported by underlying bone such as the skull or mainly underlying soft tissue. Where there is underlying bone, a close-contact wound will cause tissue expansion with discharge of gases and typically gives rise to a ragged stellate defect in the skin with soot soiling within the wound margins and in the underlying soft tissue (Figure 9.9). With such tight impact of skin against the gun and with underlying bone, a muzzle imprint is also commonly seen. Where there is close contact over soft tissues without underlying bone support, a muzzle imprint is still possible. There will be soot soiling within the wound and margins, and the wound will have a circular appearance and a collar abrasion (Figure 9.10). Occasionally, patterned burns from contact with a rifle which has a flash eliminator may be seen (Figure 9.11).

There will also be bruising of the skin in both types of wound as well as some reddening associated with the release of carbon monoxide. Soiling externally from the propellant in both types of

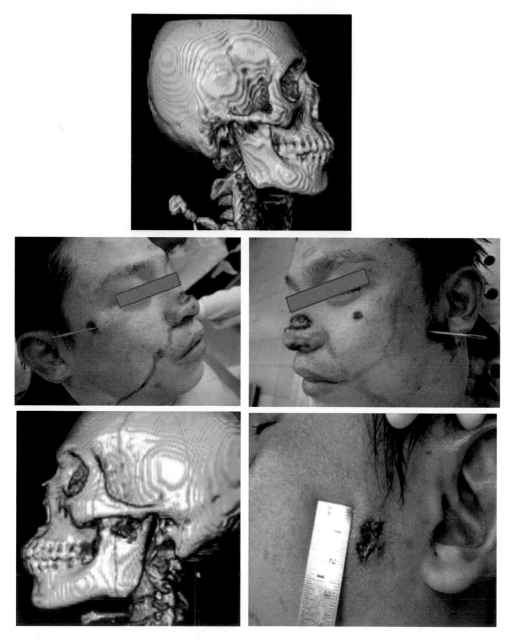

Figure 9.8 Gunshot entry wound on right upper cheek exiting at left mid-cheek adjacent to the ear. Reconstructed CT scan at top showing entry wound and bottom left showing exit wound.

wound will be absent or very little. In addition to the above, the effect of missiles passing through clothing should also be taken into account.

A loose-contact wound is produced when the muzzle of the weapon is held in very light contact with the skin at the time of discharge and the skin is not indented by the muzzle. Gas from the propellant preceding the bullet and the bullet itself can indent the skin, creating a temporary gap between the skin and the muzzle through which gas can escape. Soot carried by the gas is deposited in a band around the entrance. This soot can be easily wiped away (bullet wipe).

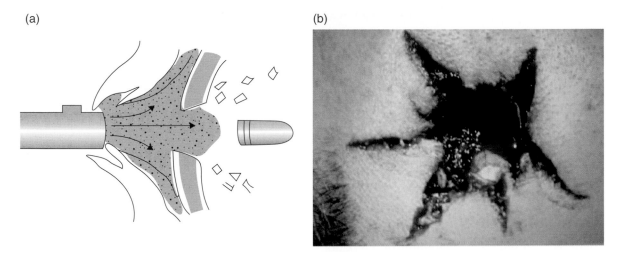

Figure 9.9 (a) Cross-section of skin overlying the skull showing the effects of discharge at close contact. There is tearing of the skin from the underlying explosive expansion of gases in the soft tissue with soot soiling of the underlying soft tissue. (b) Homicide case: close contact wound of the head, which shows a typical stellate appearance.

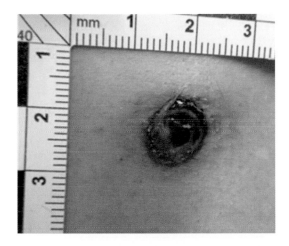

Figure 9.10 Contact entry wound. There is abraded skin around the wound together with some bruising.

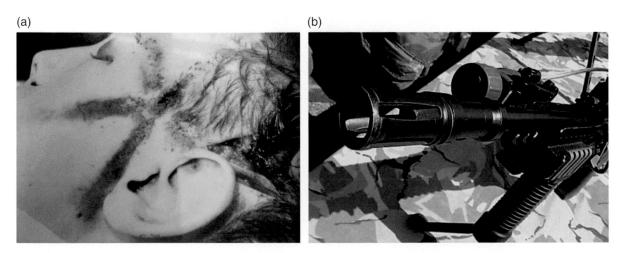

Figure 9.11 Contact wound from suicide case. Patterned burning (a) is caused by flash eliminator from British military rifle (b).

9.9.2 Near contact

Near contact is when the muzzle is close to but not touching the skin, and up to the intermediate range.

There is frequently an overlap between the appearance of near- and loose-contact wounds, making it difficult to differentiate the two. In near-contact wounds, because the muzzle of the weapon is not in contact with the skin but the distance is very small, powder grains emerging from the muzzle do not have a chance to disperse and mark the skin, as is the case with intermediate-range wounds. In near-contact wounds there is an entrance wound surrounded by a wide zone of powder soot overlying seared, blackened skin. The zone of searing is wider than that seen in a loose-contact wound. The soot in the seared zone is baked into the skin and cannot be completely wiped away. Small clumps of unburned powder may be present in the seared zones.

9.9.3 Intermediate range

An intermediate-range gunshot wound is one in which the muzzle of the weapon is away from the body at the time of discharge yet is sufficiently close so that powder grains emerging from the muzzle strike the skin, producing powder tattooing (Figure 9.12). This is the characteristic finding of intermediate-range gunshot wounds. In addition to the powder tattooing, there may be blackening of the skin or material around the entrance site from soot produced by combustion of the propellant.

The size and density of the area of powder blackening varies with the calibre of the weapon, the barrel length, the type of propellant powder, and the distance from muzzle to target. As the range increases, the intensity of powder blackening decreases and the size of the soot pattern area increases. For virtually all handgun cartridges, soot is absent beyond 30 cm (12 in.).

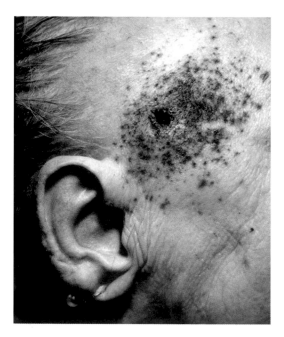

Figure 9.12 Powder tattooing in an intermediate range gunshot wound.

Although soot usually can be wiped away, powder tattooing cannot. Tattooing consists of numerous reddish-brown to orange-red punctate lesions surrounding the entry wound and is due to the impact of unburned, partially burned, or burning powder grains onto and into the skin. The distance up to which powder tattooing is seen varies with the calibre and type of the weapon but is generally up to about 60 cm (2 ft.).

9.9.4 Distant gunshot wounds

In distant gunshot wounds, the muzzle of the weapon is sufficiently far from the body so that there is neither deposition of soot nor powder tattooing. For centrefire handguns, distant gunshot wounds begin beyond 60 cm (2 ft.). The exact range depends on the particular weapon and ammunition, and can be determined exactly only by test firing with the specific weapon and ammunition. These wounds usually demonstrate none of the characteristics described above, although irregular, cruciform, or stellate entrance wounds can occur in individuals shot at distant range, where gas plays no role in the production of a wound. These occur when the bullet perforates the skin over a bony prominence or curved area of bone covered by a thin layer of tightly stretched skin. The head is the most common site for such wounds. The forehead as it slopes back at the hairline, the top and back of the head, the supraorbital ridges, and the cheek bone are common sites.

9.10 Entry and exit wounds from single bullets

9.10.1 Entry wounds

Entry wounds are generally circular in configuration apart from those that are close contact over bone, as discussed above, and wounds resulting from the projectile impacting on the body at an angle rather than the bullet nose striking perpendicular to the skin. There is a ring of scuffed skin around the wound (collar abrasion) (Figure 9.13). This is said to be produced by the bullet as it pushes inward. When the abrasion collar is eccentric from an angled impact, it is generally thicker on one side thus enabling an assessment of the direction of fire in relation to the position of the body.

Entry wounds may also have an irregular shape with tears at the margins. This may happen when a bullet loses the spin produced by the rifling in the barrel of the gun and 'wobbles' as it strikes the skin. Atypical entry wounds can also be caused by a weapon that malfunctions, defective ammunition, from ricochets or from the passage of a bullet through an intermediate target, such as a car window, before it strikes the body. With intermediate targets, there may be fragments from the intervening material, for example glass from a window, around the entry wound.

9.10.2 Exit wounds

Exit wounds can have a variety of appearances. They may be round, oval, slit-like (Figure 9.14), stellate, or crescent shaped. Furthermore, it is not true to say that an exit wound is larger than its corresponding entry wound. Size does not determine whether a gunshot wound is an exit wound; rather, it is the lack of a margin of abrasion that makes the distinction between them. Exit wounds may have small marginal tears caused by the bullet pushing the skin outward and may also have an associated margin of abrasion if they have been shored. This occurs when the skin is supported by a firm surface, such as a wall or floor, as the bullet exits. Articles of clothing, such as leather belts,

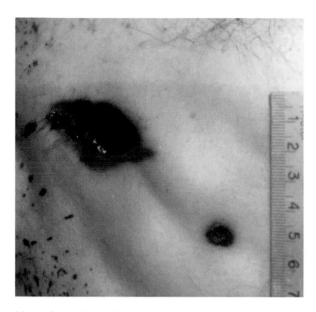

Figure 9.13   Entry wound and large funnelled exit wound from a high-velocity rifle on the back of the right shoulder. Note the collar abrasion of the entry wound below and the irregular abraded edges of the larger corresponding funnelled exit wound.

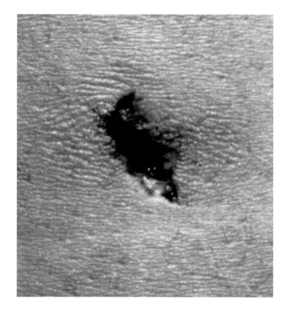

Figure 9.14   Exit wound with 'slit' appearance.

may also provide sufficient firmness to produce shored exit wounds. Exit wounds from high-powered rifles may be large because of the high velocity and KE of rifle ammunition. Stellate-shaped exit wounds, which in rifle wounds occur over soft tissue as well as over bony surfaces, are common and may resemble contact entrance wounds. Even though an exit wound from a rifle may be larger and may cause more damage than an exit wound from a handgun, an exit wound from a rifle will still lack a margin of abrasion.

9.10.3 Entry or exit?

Bevelling of bone allows determination of the direction of the wound by examining the bone. It is caused by the forward moving force of the bullet, which creates a cone-shaped deformity as it pushes through the layers of bone. The tip of the cone points in the direction from which the bullet came. In an exit wound involving the skull, the pattern is reversed and is referred to as external or outward bevelling. However, when a bullet strikes the skull at a very shallow angle, giving rise to the so-called 'keyhole defect', it may produce an entry wound with both internal and external bevelling.

9.10.4 Graze wounds

These occur when a bullet strikes at an angle and grazes the skin rather than entering deeply into the body (Figure 9.15). The appearance of such wounds is usually elongated and may give a good indication to the pathologist of the direction of fire.

9.10.5 Ricochet wounds

A ricochet wound is produced by a projectile such as a bullet which strikes and rebounds off an intervening object and strikes an individual. The bullet may still maintain sufficient kinetic energy to cause serious or fatal wounding. The shape of the wound on the skin surface may vary from round, elliptical to large and irregular.

9.11 Shotgun Wounds

9.11.1 Contact wounds

Contact shotgun wounds of the head are amongst the most mutilating of firearm wounds. Extensive destruction of bone and soft tissue structures with bursting ruptures of the head are typical. The severity of the injuries in contact wounds of the head is due to two factors: the charge of shot

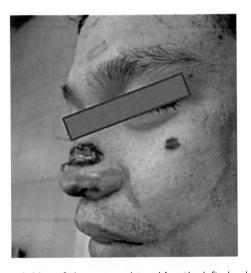

Figure 9.15 Graze wound across bridge of the nose and touching the left cheek from a high-velocity weapon.

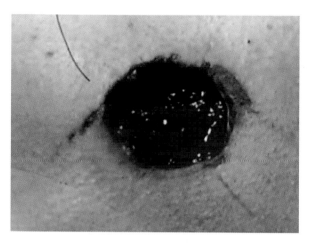

Figure 9.16   Shotgun contact wound on the abdomen. Searing from emission of hot gases is seen around the wound.

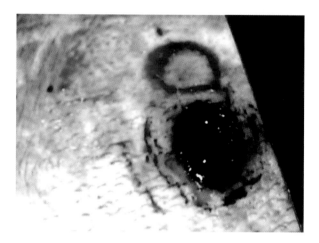

Figure 9.17   Contact wound with imprint of front sight and muzzle of shotgun.

entering the skull and the gas from combustion of the propellant. Most contact shotgun wounds of the head are suicidal in origin. Intermediate-range and close-range shotgun wounds of the head are almost as mutilating as contact wounds because the pellets are still travelling in a single mass.

Contact wounds of the trunk appear relatively innocuous when compared with the massive destruction produced by such wounds in the head. The entrance wound will be circular in shape and will have a diameter approximately equal to that of the bore of the weapon. In hard-contact wounds, no soot surrounds the entrance site, but the edges of the wound will be seared and blackened by the hot gases (Figure 9.16). A muzzle imprint may also be seen with contact wounds (Figure 9.17).

9.11.2   Near-range wounds

As the range increases beyond 1–2 cm from the muzzle to the target, powder tattooing will occur. The maximum range out to which powder tattooing occurs from a shotgun depends to a great degree on the type of powder, i.e. ball (up to 125 cm) or flake (60 cm).

9.11.3 Intermediate-range wounds

As the muzzle of the shotgun is moved farther from the body, tattooing disappears and the diameter of the circular entrance wound increases in size until a point is reached where individual pellets begin to separate from the main mass. By 90 cm the wound widens and the edges of the wounds will have scalloped margins. By 120 cm, scattered satellite pellet holes are present around the main entrance. By 180–210 cm there is a definite cuff of satellite pellet holes around a slightly irregular wound of entrance (Figure 9.18).

Beyond 300 cm, there is great variation in the size of the pellet pattern depending on the ammunition used, the choke of the gun, and, most important, the range. At the same range, the pattern for different guns and brands of ammunition may vary from a central irregular perforation with numerous satellite wounds to a pattern of multiple individual pellet wounds. In all deaths from shotgun wounds the size of the shot pattern on the body should be measured so that the range can be estimated. However, it should be appreciated that the size and appearance of the pattern should be used only as a rough guide in determining the range. The only reliable method of determining range is to obtain the actual weapon and the same brand of ammunition used and then conduct a series of test shots to reproduce on paper the pattern of the fatal wound on the body.

9.11.4 Location of wadding

At close range, when there is only a single large entrance wound, the wad from a shotgun shell will be found inside the body. Depending upon the range of fire, as the wad enters the body, the individual arms or petals that have peeled back in flight may produce a patterned abrasion around the entrance wound. These petal marks can occur even if the entrance site is covered with clothing. Petal marks are seen at ranges between 30 and 90 cm. After 90 cm they are generally flush with the sides of the wad base and no petal marks are produced.

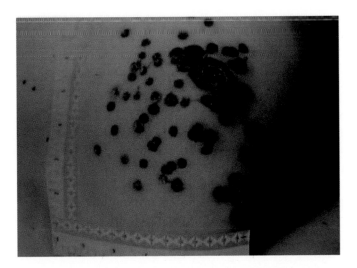

Figure 9.18 Intermediate-range shotgun wound. There is a spread of pellets with only a small central hole. The distance in this case was over 5 metres.

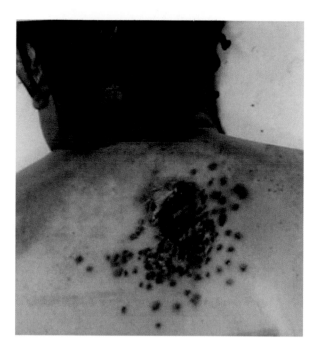

Figure 9.19 Taxi driver shot through the glass partition between the driver and passenger compartments.

9.11.5 Intermediate target

Shot charges may strike an intermediary target, e.g. glass, with a resultant increase in the dispersion of the shot. The effects of the dispersion will need to be taken into account in estimating range (Figure 9.19).

9.12 High-velocity rifle wounds

The muzzle velocities of modern high-velocity centerfire rifles range between 2400 and 4000 ft/s and the muzzle kinetic energy is never less than 1000 ft-lb. With discharge from firearms with low muzzle velocity and kinetic energy, injuries from bullets are confined to tissues directly in the wound path. On the other hand, high muzzle velocity weapons bullets can injure structures well away from the wound path. The size of the temporary wound cavitation, resulting in the radial stretching of tissues around a bullet track, is caused by the high pressure surrounding the projectile, which accelerates material away from its path. The other factors affecting the degree of wound trauma are related to the bullet itself. Apart from bullet placement, the shape, construction, mass, and terminal velocity all determine how much tissue is actually disrupted.

In head wounds the skull may be particularly severely disrupted from skull fractures, skin laceration, and brain disruption due to the high on impact, and cavitation and the release of gas into tissues produced by combustion of the propellant. Elsewhere the external entry and exit wounds may not appear as dramatic as the injuries to the head, but this appearance belies the production of severe internal organ and musculo-skeletal damage.

9.13 Modified projectiles

Modified projectiles produce more irregular entry wounds and there is greater damage to initial structures. The internal track is more liable to deviate. Such projectiles penetrate to a lesser depth.

9.14 Air-gun injuries

Wounds from air guns have some of the characteristics of firearm injuries. A small single missile which resembles a shotgun pellet is fired through a rifled barrel.

Air guns have relatively low muzzle velocity and may be either 0.177 or 22 in. calibre. Both can penetrate the thin temporal bone of a child or adult, the eye, and in children into the chest cavity and elsewhere to cause fatal injury (Milroy et al. 1998; Ceylan et al. 2002).

9.15 Injuries from humane veterinary killers, industrial stud guns, and blank cartridge guns

Powder-actuated tools are used in abattoirs and by veterinary surgeons to stun large animals. They may be of the captive-bolt type, which consists of a metal rod, the distal end of which is propelled for several centimetres from the muzzle of the weapon by a blank cartridge inserted in a chamber behind the proximal end. The captive bolt inflicts a clean, penetrating injury. Humane killers may cause injuries on humans.

Blank cartridge firing guns are used in military training, theatrical events, as starter pistols in sports events, and also to threaten a potential assailant, particularly when loaded with tear gas cartridges. Often these guns are replicas of real weapons and are, due to easier access, also frequently used in criminal activities. In contact shots, or even when fired at close range, blank firing guns are capable of causing extensive damage to soft tissues as the expelled gas can penetrate the thoracic wall, the neck and the inguinal region or cause fractures to the skull and cause fatal injuries. The presence of a muzzle imprint, powder tattooing, and soot soiling depend on the firing distance and the type of propellant.

Stud-guns and similar devices used in industry for driving a hardened metal pin or threaded stud into masonry or other wood or metal structures as a rapid and convenient means of attachment, and may result in accidents, with the occasional suicide also seen.

9.16 Injuries from rubber and plastic bullets

The 'rubber bullet' was first introduced in 1970 in Northern Ireland. It was specifically designed to be 'less-lethal' and intended for use to control riots. Six years later they were replaced by plastic bullets. They are not meant to be fired at a distance closer than 20 m from the intended target and in order to avoid head and neck injuries police were instructed to aim at the lower half of the body. As well as non-fatal injuries, some deaths were reported with their use.

9.17 The effects of being shot

Contrary to popular media portrayal, the shot individual is not thrown over or backwards. The wounded person usually carries on forward, and even when shot through the heart may carry on fighting. Instant death will only occur with brain stem/upper cervical spinal cord injury.

9.18 Explosions

Explosions can be divided into three categories: those where high explosives have been used, those involving dispersed phase explosives, and those which have been damaged by mechanical explosions. Most of the procedures for recovering the body and investigating such incidents are the same as for any other sudden death, with the proviso that in industrial premises or at large-scale incidents the Health and Safety Executive, or a nominated body such as British Gas, may have a statutory duty to investigate the cause.

Incidents arising from the use of *high explosives* are usually related to terrorist offences. At scenes where a high explosive device has operated, the only action to be taken by other services should be to contain and secure the ground pending the arrival of the proper authorities. No entry or search should be conducted as there is a possibility that further devices or booby-traps could be present.

Dispersed phase explosions are those which have been caused by gas, flammable vapours or combustible dusts.

Mechanical explosions arise from the sudden release of pressure when a sealed container such as a gas cylinder ruptures.

In *industrial* concerns, explosions may arise from such items as compressed air tanks, equipment using steam under pressure, furnaces, boilers, finely pulverised coal dust in mine shafts, flour dust in mills and granaries or pulverised sawdust. In the industrial situation safety-directed engineering devices are often built into such potentially explosive loci and will ensure that the effects of any such explosions are limited and localised, and loss of life and casualties are often on a small scale.

In the *domestic* situation the ignition of vapours of flammable substances, e.g. gasoline, and the escape of gases, e.g. butane cylinders and domestic 'natural gas' supplies, may also cause very serious explosions; a mixture of 'natural gas' in a one in 10 mixture with air in a confined space can be readily ignited by a spark from an electrical appliance.

Meteorological phenomena such as lightning strikes may also produce explosions.

9.19 Effects of an explosion

It is essential to understand the effects of an explosion, which may be summarised as follows:

a. A direct blast force (i.e. pressure or mechanical waves) is generated, lasting a few milliseconds and moving out concentrically from the explosion epicentre, followed by a negative pressure suction-type wave. The semi-vacuum formed by the initial blast wave is refilled with air rushing back in.
b. Hot gases are generated, which may cause fires in the vicinity and flash burns in victims.
c. There is fragmentation of the components of the explosive device and other items in the vicinity, causing missile injuries in victims. Some terrorist devices are packed with metal nails and similar objects.
d. There is frequently destruction of buildings or other nearby structures causing injuries to victims, particularly from falling masonry.

The severity of an explosion can vary considerably and the damage may range from the loss of a few window panes to the complete destruction of a multi-storey structure. Most dispersed phase explosions are deflagrations – extremely rapid fires – and the damage they cause is due to the pressure rise induced in the building when large amounts of hot combustion gases are produced. Similar structural damage is caused by mechanical explosions, but the cylinder or other container may also be propelled a considerable distance when its pressurised contents are released.

Due to the likelihood of structural damage the same care should be exercised at scenes of explosions as at fires and the premises should be assessed for safety before work begins. Body recovery will be made more difficult if large amounts of collapsed masonry have to be removed and it may be necessary to organise site teams and obtain mechanical assistance to remove heavy objects.

In large explosions bodies as well as survivors are likely to be uncovered during rescue work and it is advisable that any recovery and identification procedures developed for major incidents be implemented as part of the rescue services operation.

9.20 Explosion injuries

The type and severity of injuries seen in explosions will vary greatly depending on a number of different factors, including the type of detonation, the severity of the blast, and the position and distance of the victim from the epicentre of the explosion (Figures 9.20–9.23)

Death and injury in explosions are caused by the following:

- The effects of the blast wave from the bomb. The velocity of the wave causing compression depends on the distance from the epicentre of the explosion, starting at many times above the speed of sound and decreasing as the distance increases. The compression wave is followed by a transient below-atmospheric pressure zone, thus there is a double effect on the body. The lung suffers the most damage and the gastrointestinal tract is also vulnerable, as most of the damage occurs at the interface between tissues in contact with the atmosphere. On the other hand, solid organs such as the liver and muscle suffer little or no injury.

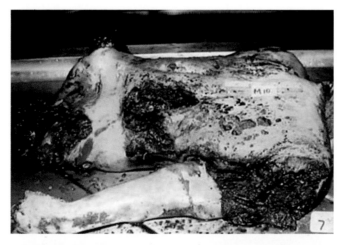

Figure 9.20 Dismemberment and multiple punctate and larger lacerations.

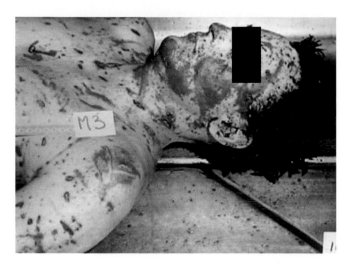

Figure 9.21   Grazes, lacerations, and burns to the trunk and face.

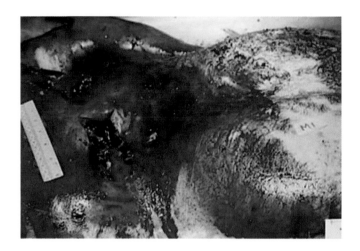

Figure 9.22   Penetrating wounds to the back from shrapnel.

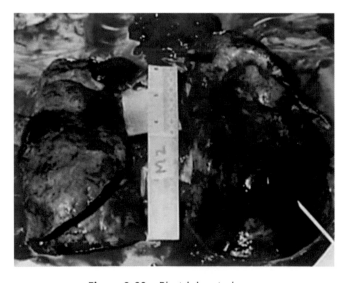

Figure 9.23   Blast injury to lungs.

- Projectiles impacting on the body derived from the explosive device. The body may well suffer high-speed impact from fragments from the bomb, including metals such as nails packed into it as well as from other associated fragmented material.

- Impact from surrounding objects and debris projected by the explosion, giving rise to 'peppering' of the body and discolouration from dust blasting. The peppering effect described by Marshall is caused by bruising, lacerations and punctate wounds and is known as Marshall's triad (Marshall 1976).

- Burns from hot gas and incandescent objects. Flash burns occur when a victim is near the explosive device. Singeing of the hair, occasionally giving a swept-back appearance, is commonly seen in victims.

- Secondary injuries from falling masonry, beams and furnishings dislodged by the explosion. This is a common hazard when there has been collapse of building structures.

As a general rule, and particularly when dealing with multiple deaths, many parts of bodies can be expected to be strewn over a very wide area and it is not unusual to find the disrupted remains of the person nearest to the explosive device further away from those of others fatally injured.

The type, extent, and distribution of injuries, together with associated debris, either on the surface or within the body, will assist the scene investigators in locating the position of each person at the moment the explosion took place. Bodies within 1 or 2 metres of the explosion will frequently be severely disrupted. Injuries in bodies which are lying over 2 metres from the explosion show a picture consisting of punctate and speckled lacerations and abrasions, often circular and oval bruises which are scattered throughout the exposed parts of the body. Their concentration on the surface of the body is variable, but may be very extensive. These are caused by debris and shrapnel from the blast coming into forceful contact with the skin to produce wounding and may even become embedded in the tissues or penetrate deeply into muscle compartments and body cavities.

Frequently, flying debris from the centre of an explosion causes wounding which has an orientation in the direction of the blast. This is also assisted by the position of any flash burns which are present. Hair may also have a 'swept-back' appearance where the deceased was facing the blast.

Radiography (including CT and magnetic resonance imaging where available) is an essential procedure to be carried out in each case prior to autopsy) to enable identification of foreign bodies which have come from an explosive device, as well as to assist in identification of the body.

Furthermore, it should be appreciated that, especially when dealing with a perpetrator who was carrying an explosive device and has died as a result of its accidental or deliberate detonation, the distribution of injuries and fragments found in the deceased, his/her position at the scene, as well as identification of his/her remains, will enable an accurate assessment to be made of his/her role in the incident.

Bodies found away from the immediate area where the explosion has occurred will frequently have suffered mechanical injuries due to falling masonry from collapse of a building.

Dispersed phase explosions do not produce the high-velocity penetration wounds typical of high explosives but if the victim was within the burning gas or vapour then flash-burns will be present on the body and clothing.

9.21   Investigating the cause of the explosion

Investigating the cause of a major explosion is very time-consuming as it requires the recovery and inspection of much of the contents of the structure.

With minor explosions it may be possible to identify the origin by plotting a displacement diagram showing direction of movement of walls, doors, and windows during the incident. The diagram may indicate a single room of origin which can then be excavated and inspected in order to establish whether a dispersed phase or a mechanical explosion has occurred. Dispersed phase explosions, involving as they do the combustion of a fuel/air mixture, leave evidence of heat damage from the passage of the flame front through the premises. Mechanical explosions are not always caused by a combustion-related process, although most arise from the rupture of a sealed container which has been heated in a fire. Distinguishing between the two types of explosion is possible if it can be established whether there was a fire within the premises before the explosion occurred or whether there were sealed or pressurised gas or water systems present. The most common fuels encountered in dispersed phase explosions are methane (natural gas from the mains), propane (Calor gas), butane (camping gas), and the vapours from volatile flammable liquids such as petrol. Of these, only methane is less dense than air in the vapour phase and as a result it tends to accumulate in a layer above the point of release, while propane, butane, and petrol vapour will all form layers at low level unless disturbed by draughts. When the gas or vapour is ignited this stratification leads to an uneven pattern of burning or scorching of exposed surfaces which can aid the identification of the explosive material. This burning is very superficial and should not be confused with the damage caused by a fire after the explosion or flaring from a broken gas supply pipe. If the presence of a vapour or gas denser than air is indicated, then a search must be made for flammable liquid residues or cylinders. Most gas explosions are the result of accidental release but appliances and pipework should be examined for evidence of tampering or attempts to bypass the meter. The presence of flammable liquid should be regarded as cause for suspicion unless there is good reason for such material to be present. Containers in the vicinity of the body may indicate that the victim was caught in a vapour explosion after having distributed a flammable liquid around the premises.

For a detailed treatment of explosion investigation techniques the reader is referred to Harris (1983) and Yallop (1980).

References

Firearms

Burke, T.W. and Rowe, W.F. (1992). Bullet ricochet: a comprehensive review. *J. Forensic Sci.* 37: 1254–1260.

Ceylan, H., McGowan, A., and Stringer, M.D. (2002). Air weapon injuries: a serious and persistent problem. *Arch. Dis. Child.* 86: 234–235.

Di Maio, V.J.M., Dana, S.E., Taylor, W.E., and Ondrusek, J. (1987). Use of scanning electron microscope and energy dispersive x-ray analysis (SEM-EDXA) in identification of foreign material on bullets. *J. Forensic Sci.* 32: 38–47.

Haag, L.C. (1975). Bullet ricochet: an empirical study and a device for measuring ricochet angle. *AFTE J.* 7: 44–51.

Janssen, D.W. and Levine, R.T. (1982). Bullet ricochet from automobile ceilings. *J. Forensic Sci.* 27: 209–212.

Jordan, G.E., Bratton, D.D., Donahue, H.C.H., and Rowe, W.F. (1988). Bullet ricochet from gypsum wallboard. *J. Forensic Sci.* 33: 1477–1482.

Milroy, C.M., Clark, J.C., Carter, N. et al. (1998). Air weapon fatalities. *J. Clin. Pathol.* 51: 525–529.

Mitosinka, G.T. (1971). Technique for determining and illustrating the trajectory of bullets. *J. Forensic Sci. Soc.* 11: 55–61.

Nennstiel, R. (1985). Accuracy in determining long-range firing position of gunman. *AFTE* 17: 47–54.

Reay, D.T., Haglund, W.D., and Bonnell, H.J. (1986). Wah Mee massacre. *Am. J. Forensic Med. Pathol.* 7: 330–336.

Roberts, J. and Hanby, J. (1985). Reconstuction of a shooting to prove/disprove trajectory. *AFTE* 17: 53–55.

Further reading

Firearms

Di Maio, V.J.M. (1999). *Gunshot Wounds: Practical Aspects of Firearms, Ballistics and Forensic Techniques*, 2e. CRC Press.

Harris, R.J. (1983). *The Investigation and Control of Gas Explosions in Buildings and Heating Plants*. Midlands, England, UK: British Gas Corporation.

Hcard, B.J. (2008). *Handbook of Firearms & Ballistics*, 2c. Wilcy.

Explosions

Marshall, T.K. (1976). Death from explosive devices. *Med. Sci. Law* 16: 235–239.

Marshall, T.K. (1978). The investigation of bombings. In: *Legal Medicine Annual* (ed. C. Wecht). New York: Appleton Century Crofts.

Marshall, T.K. (1988). A pathologist's view of terrorist violence. *Forensic Sci. Int.* 36: 57–67.

Yallop, H.J. (1980). *Explosion Investigation*. The Forensic Science Society. Scottish Academic Press.

10

Forensic Aspects of Asphyxia and Drowning

Peter Vanezis

Queen Mary University of London, London, UK

Asphyxia (Greek 'Ασφυξια', which means 'without a pulse') in terms of its usage in forensic medical practice may be defined broadly as deprivation of oxygen to the tissues. There are many types of deaths which have asphyxia as the main mechanism and some where it is a contributory secondary outcome. This chapter will deal with those that are in the former category and are of forensic interest. Within the asphyxia category it should also be appreciated that some deaths which are categorised as such are related more to initial cardiovascular or neurogenic effects rather than direct interference with oxygen intake from the environment. A good example is the application of pressure on the neck in non-judicial hanging.

Asphyxia can occur as a result of defects in any part of the process of breathing and respiration from the initial intake of oxygen from the environment to the lungs, followed by gas exchange in the alveoli and oxygen diffusion into the blood in exchange for carbon dioxide, to delivery to the cells for energy production and the production of carbon dioxide to be exhaled as a waste product.

For the purposes of description of asphyxia cases of forensic interest, they can be categorised into two broad groups:

- *Non-mechanical asphyxia (chemical asphyxia):* This type of asphyxia may result from the effects of a vitiated atmosphere or the presence of irrespirable or toxic gases. It also refers to any other conditions, including natural disease, which may cause low oxygen uptake by the tissues.

- *Mechanical asphyxia*: This term applies to the diminution of oxygen uptake from any mechanical (physical) means, including compression and/or obstruction of the airways at any level both internally and externally. Some authorities regard breathing in an oxygen-deficient atmosphere as a type of mechanical asphyxia, although for the purposes of this chapter mechanical asphyxia will be confined to a physical defect impeding the act of breathing.

10.1   Non-mechanical asphyxia

Causes of non-mechanical asphyxia include:

- reduced atmospheric pressure in aircraft cabin failure or at high altitude
- inert gases, e.g. carbon dioxide – an oxygen-depleted atmosphere may be associated with very rapid death
- carbon monoxide
- cyanide poisoning.

10.1.1   Reduced atmospheric pressure in aircraft cabin failure or at high altitude

Exposure to high altitude and other situations of reduced atmospheric pressure is characterised by the reduced availability of oxygen and therefore hypoxia. Its effect depends on the level and the duration of hypoxia, individual susceptibility as well as the presence of pre-existing diseases, particularly of a respiratory, cardiovascular or haematological nature.

Pressurisation in an aircraft becomes necessary at altitudes above 12 500 ft (3800 m) to 14 000 ft (4300 m) above sea level. If for some reason there is a reduction in the supply of oxygen, this will lead to hypoxia. The body's most common response to this condition is to hyperventilate, which does assist in partially restoring the partial pressure of oxygen in the blood, but at the same time it also increases the level of carbon dioxide, causing a metabolic alkalosis leading to altitude sickness. In such a situation, passengers may experience general symptoms such as fatigue, drowsiness, nausea, and headaches, and occasionally on long-haul flights, pulmonary oedema. Mountaineers may also experience similar symptoms. The effects of short-term hypoxia in various activities is explored further by Burtscher et al. (2012).

10.1.2   Asphyxia from other gases

Methane, which is component of natural gas, is not toxic but may cause asphyxia if the oxygen concentration is reduced by displacement to below 16%. It can penetrate buildings and landfill. Deaths from asphyxiation can also occur in coal mines. It is well known that miners used to carry caged canaries into coal mines to detect methane or carbon monoxide. This practice began in 1911 and the birds were made redundant in 1986 with the advent of modern technology. The canary is particularly sensitive to toxic gases such as carbon monoxide and methane. Following a mine fire or explosion, mine rescuers would descend into the mine carrying a canary in a small wooden or metal cage. Any sign of distress from the canary was a clear signal that the conditions underground were unsafe and miners should be evacuated from the pit and the mine shafts made safer.

Byard and Wilson (1992) describe two cases of methane asphyxia occurring in two boys of 11 and 12 years who were found at the bottom of a 37 ft (11.1 m) deep sewer shaft. Analysis of gas in the shaft revealed 21% oxygen at the surface, 14.3% at a depth of 5 ft (1.5 m), and only 4.8% at depths of 10 ft (3 m) and below. Other gases detected at lower levels were methane, nitrogen, and carbon dioxide (4.3%). These cases demonstrate the value of atmospheric gas analysis in cases of possible methane asphyxia in confirming the presence of methane and in demonstrating levels of oxygen below that necessary to support life.

Manning et al. (1981) discuss the importance of proper scene investigation in order to determine the correct cause of death. They describe the deaths of three men who descended into an open drainage pit to recover a fallen grate lid. Each man in turn was immediately overcome and died within minutes of his descent. Initial analysis of the pit's air indicated a methane level of 15%. It was therefore initially assumed that death was due to methane poisoning. Post-mortem analysis of the victim's tissues, however, yielded methane levels in only faint trace quantities (0–100 mcg/100 g range). Analysis of the air samples taken at various pit levels revealed that going down the pit, there was a decrease in oxygen levels from 20% at the top to 3% at the bottom. Carbon dioxide levels, however, increased on going down the pit and reached a level of 22% at a depth of 6 ft. The accepted lethal level of carbon dioxide is only 10%. The cause originally attributed to these deaths was shown to be incorrect.

Downs et al. (1994) describe two suicides, one resulting from *carbon dioxide* in the form of dry ice and the other from the use of *propane* gas. They emphasise the importance of environmental sampling. As with all cases where the atmosphere is potentially hazardous, appropriate protective clothing, including full breathing apparatus, will need to be worn.

More recently, asphyxiation from the use of *helium* gas has become more prevalent and has been used as a method of suicide as an alternative to the use of car exhausts. There was a rapid rise in deaths due to helium inhalation from five in the period 2001–2002 to 89 in 2010–2011, a 17-fold increase (Gunnell et al. 2015).

Carbon monoxide, which is an odourless, colourless gas, has 200–300 times greater affinity for haemoglobin than oxygen, producing carboxyhaemoglobin. The binding of carbon monoxide competitively inhibits the ability of the red blood cell to bind with oxygen and thereby reduces the transport of oxygen, which results in histotoxic hypoxia. The signs and symptoms from different levels of carbon monoxide in the atmosphere (parts per million [ppm]) and percentage of carboxyhaemoglobin are shown in the Table 10.1. The level at which death occurs will also depend on the prior state of health of the subject. Carbon monoxide poisoning is commonly seen in house fire deaths and where there has been incomplete combustion from other causes.

When investigating the cause of a carbon monoxide poisoning potential sources of the gas must be identified and tested to find out which is responsible for its production: whether doors and windows were open or closed, the status of the appliances, which should be tested, the location and last reported movements of the victims, and the length of time over which exposure to fumes could have taken place.

Exhaust fumes from internal combustion engines contain very high concentrations of carbon monoxide which can rapidly cause death if inhaled within an enclosed space. The deliberate introduction of fumes into the interior of a car by means of a pipe attached to the exhaust or by running the engine in a closed garage was a common method of suicide but its incidence as declined dramatically with the introduction of catalytic converters in the last two decades or so in many countries (Mott et al. 2002; Studdert et al. 2010). Accidental death can also occur in the latter circumstances if the victim is unaware of the toxic nature of exhaust gases or fails to make adequate provision for ventilation when working on a vehicle.

Table 10.1 Carbon monoxide concentration (CO), carboxyhaemoglobin (COHb) level, and associated symptoms.

CO concentration	COHb level (%)	Signs and symptoms
35 ppm	<10	Headache and dizziness within 6–8 hours of constant exposure
100 ppm	>10	Slight headache in 2–3 hours
200 ppm	20	Slight headache within 2–3 hours; loss of judgement
400 ppm	25	Frontal headache within 1–2 hours
800 ppm	30	Dizziness, nausea, and convulsions within 45 minutes; insensible within 2 hours
1 600 ppm	40	Headache, tachycardia, dizziness, and nausea within 20 minutes; death in less than 2 hours
3 200 ppm	50	Headache, dizziness, and nausea in 5–10 minutes; death within 30 minutes
6 400 ppm	60	Headache and dizziness in 1–2 minutes; convulsions, respiratory arrest, and death in less than 20 minutes
12 800 ppm	>70	Death in less than 3 minutes

Source: Data from Struttmann et al. (1998).

Inhalation of carbon monoxide from charcoal burners has become a widely practised method of suicide in South-East Asia over the last 15 years, notably in Hong Kong (Leung et al. 2002), Taiwan, and Japan. Occasional cases are also now seen in Western countries, as information about methods of suicide becomes more easily accessible on the Internet (Chen et al. 2013).

10.1.3 Cyanide poisoning

Cyanide exists in gas, liquid, and solid forms and it can cause human toxicity via multiple routes, including inhalation, ingestion, parenteral administration, and dermal or conjunctival contact (Nelson 2006). It is encountered in smoke from fires. It is used as a method of suicide, murder, and terrorism, and is also an industrial and occupational hazard. It is one of the most rapidly acting and deadly of poisons, which can kill within seconds or minutes to hours of exposure, depending on the dose, route, and length of exposure.

Cyanide prevents cells from using oxygen by inhibiting the oxidative function of mitochondrial cytochrome oxidase, an enzyme in the electron transport chain that is integral to production of aerobic energy for cellular function. Cyanide, which has a chemical structure similar to that of oxygen, binds to the ferric iron portion of cytochrome oxidase. By doing so, it inhibits the ability of cytochrome oxidase to use oxygen, thereby reducing production of adenosine triphosphate (ATP) and preventing the proper functioning of the mitochondria. The reduced availability of ATP results in cellular dysfunction and death.

10.2 Mechanical asphyxias

10.2.1 Introduction

The term mechanical asphyxia, as used in this context, is a general term taken to mean that the flow of air into the body is physically compromised in some way, e.g. by strangulation, traumatic asphyxia or choking, whereas non-mechanical asphyxia relates to a physiological impediment in the uptake of oxygen by the body, as discussed in the previous section.

Certain types of deaths which involve compression of the neck although not predominantly asphyxial in nature, are also included in mechanical asphyxia. These are cases where death does not result predominantly from deprivation of oxygen but rather from some form of cardio-inhibitory mechanism well recognised to be produced by hyperstimulation of the vagus nerve, which supplies parasympathetic innervation to the heart and can thus cause bradyarrhythmias, including atrioventricular conduction block.

10.2.2 Signs of mechanical asphyxia

Leaving aside external and internal injuries, the signs which have been attributed to mechanical asphyxia are by no means diagnostic. In combination, however, and considered together with injuries and other marks found on the body, they may allow a confident conclusion to be drawn that there has been mechanical asphyxia.

10.2.2.1 Petechial haemorrhages Where there is compression of the neck, petechial haemorrhages (Figure 10.1) are seen typically in the eyes, face, and neck, and over the upper chest where there is compression of the chest region. Tardieu was one of the first to describe petechial haemorrhages in the skin, eyes, and viscera, and they are still referred to as Tardieu's spots (Tardieu 1855, 1859). Christison (1829) found petechial haemorrhages in the conjunctivae of the last of Burke and Hare's victims. He nevertheless emphasised the need for caution when examining asphyxia deaths, particularly those due to suffocation, where petechial haemorrhages are frequently absent. Although petechial haemorrhages are not pathognomonic of suffocation or strangulation, as Tardieu thought, if they are above the level of compression on the neck or chest they are very much a strong indication that pressure has occurred in the region directly below the lower point at which they are found. Internally, they are seen in mucous membranes within the mouth, epiglottis, and scalp. They are also seen in many viscera elsewhere, especially on subepicardial and subpleural surfaces. They occur as a result of blood escaping from the capillaries and may either have the appearance on the skin of a fine rash or may form larger aggregates if sufficient in number.

10.2.2.2 Cyanosis The blue shade of the skin referred to as cyanosis (Figure 10.2) has to be interpreted with great caution in cases of mechanical asphyxia. Its appearance on the skin and mucous membranes is due to the presence of reduced haemoglobin in the blood of the superficial capillaries. It depends on the absolute amount of reduced haemoglobin in the capillary blood and not the relative proportions of reduced haemoglobin and oxyhaemoglobin. The presence of cyanosis means that the tissues are hypoxic, although its absence does not necessarily indicate no hypoxia, as, for example, in an anaemic subject.

10.2.2.3 Congestion of organs Congestion of organs with blood is a non-specific sign seen in many types of deaths and cannot therefore be regarded as a reliable sign in asphyxia.

10.2.2.4 Pulmonary oedema Pulmonary oedema is commonly seen in asphyxia deaths, but its severity varies and indeed it may be entirely absent. It is also regularly seen in many other types of deaths. Its pathogenesis following acute airway obstruction is thought to be due to alveolar and capillary damage induced by the negative pressure generated to inspire against the closed upper airway (Oswalt et al. 1977).

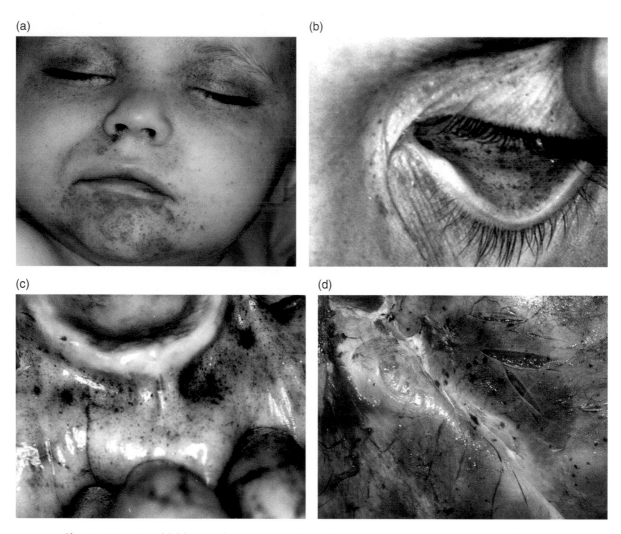

Figure 10.1 Petechial haemorrhages seen on the (a) face, (b) conjunctivae, (c)gums and (d) scalp.

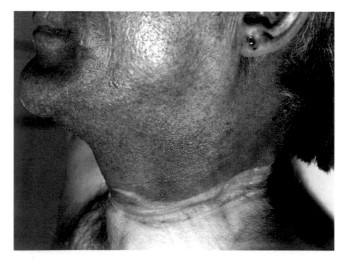

Figure 10.2 Cyanosis of the face in a case of suicidal strangulation (see also Figure 10.12). Note that the cyanosis is present above the level of compression by a ligature, with relative pallor below.

10.2.2.5   Fluidity of blood   Up until a few years ago it was thought that blood maintained its fluidity in asphyxia and was a diagnostic sign. Mole (1948), however, concluded that fluid blood with no evidence of clotting can occur in any death where there has been sudden collapse or 'shock'. In fact, the fluidity of blood results from an imbalance between clotting and fibrinolytic factors.

10.3   Types of mechanical asphyxias and related conditions

10.3.1   Smothering (external airway obstruction)

With *homicidal smothering*, careful examination of a scene is essential, especially where death may involve the elderly, infirmed or very young and there are very few signs of disturbance. Any items which may have been used for smothering, such as a pillow or bedding, need to be collected and examined for saliva, blood, hair, and other trace evidence that could have been transferred from the deceased. A pillow, for example, may also show an obvious indentation where it has been pressed over the face. This must be photographed before removal. In very young children the bedding in the cot needs to be carefully examined.

Suicidal smothering by means of a pillow is very unusual but has been described by Hicks et al. (1990) in a chronically mentally ill patient. The death scene in this case was a major part of the investigation which enabled homicide to be ruled out.

In cases of *plastic bag suffocation*, unless the bag is still in position over the face it will be extremely difficult to reach the conclusion that death has resulted from this method. If the bag had been recently removed prior to discovery, there may be an inappropriate degree of condensation found on the face. In addition, in cases where the bag had been covering the face for some time, the degree of putrefactive change to the face may be accelerated in relation to other exposed parts of the body. Occasionally, if the bag had been placed tightly around the neck, a ligature mark may be found. The use of a plastic bag together with drugs and/or a gas (helium has frequently been used in combination with a plastic bag) is a method favoured in assisted suicide cases. A careful search of the scene in such cases may reveal tablets and/or containers, tubing, and a gas cylinder, as well as literature on assisted suicide. A computer at the scene may also show a history of visits to websites containing similar material.

10.3.2   Choking (internal airway obstruction)

Choking occurs when there is a mechanical obstruction of the flow of air to the lungs by an internal obstruction within the air passages. Gagging, by placing an object to obstruct the airway from the mouth, should not be confused with choking, which refers to objects causing obstruction within the airway at a lower level. However, when an object is thrust into the mouth, there may well be involvement of the pharyngeal/laryngeal area and thus overlap between the two entities. Occasionally death may be very rapid with no visible asphyxia signs and one must consider whether *laryngeal spasm* may have occurred or *vagal stimulation* leading to cardiac arrest. However, such a conclusion should not be arrived at lightly, but only after careful consideration of all the circumstances surrounding death. It should also be appreciated that where findings at autopsy are negative, apart from regurgitated food particles in the airways, that the latter should not be assumed to have caused death. It is not unusual for regurgitation to occur during the process of dying, including during attempts at resuscitation, from an unrelated cause.

(a)   (b)   (c)

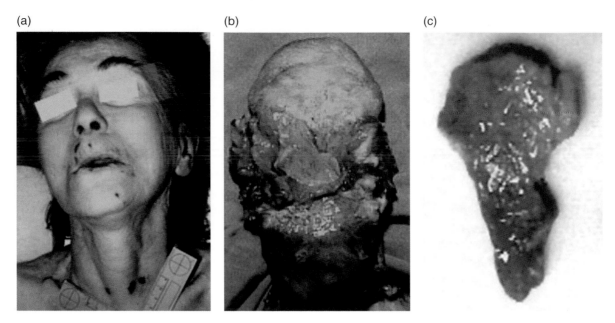

Figure 10.3   (a) Elderly woman with a piece of meat obstructing her laryngeal airway. Note self-inflicted fingernail marks around the face and neck, resembling a case of manual strangulation. Excisesd larynx (b) with food bolus (c) lodged within it.

Accidental choking is the most common type seen and typically results from objects lodged in the throat (Figure 10.3). It is most commonly seen in the very young, the elderly, psychiatric patients or in the infirm and particularly when their ability to chew or swallow is impaired. The first few years of life, when young children are learning to eat solid food and experimenting by putting all manner of objects into their mouths, are clearly the most hazardous years (Sturner et al. 1976; Mittleman 1984). The vast majority of such deaths occur between the ages of 2 months and 4 years.

Homicidal choking and *suicidal choking* are both very rare. There are a few cases of homicide by this method reported in the literature. Littlejohn (1855–1856) reported a case in which a cork was forcibly thrust into the victim's throat. In another of his cases he describes how a mother thrust dough into a baby's mouth and it lodged in the larynx. Most reported cases of suicidal choking are in mental patients or persons in custody. Renton (1908) reported on a middle-aged man who had forced three pieces of flannel firmly into his larynx with the lowest piece packed firmly into his supraglottic region.

10.3.3   Aspiration

Aspiration of foreign material (not as a bolus) or blood into the airways for various reasons, including regurgitation of stomach contents, water in drowning (see below), or blood from trauma or natural disease, can lead to asphyxia acutely or complicated by aspiration pneumonitis.

10.3.4   Postural (positional) asphyxia

In cases of postural (positional) asphyxia it is essential to appreciate that asphyxia has resulted from the position of the body causing some form of restriction of the airway. Almost invariably there are predisposing factors such as alcohol, drug abuse or some form of infirmity. Careful assessment of the scene in relation to body position is essential in order to allow correct interpretation of the autopsy findings. In a study by Bell et al. (1992), 30 cases were assessed. They found chronic alcoholism or acute alcohol intoxication to be a significant factor in 75%, with an average blood alcohol of 240 mg/100 ml. Victims were commonly found in a restrictive position producing hyperflexion of the head and neck.

It is important to differentiate such cases from those due to other causes in which the deceased is found face down with florid hypostasis in the dependent areas accompanied by coarse petechial haemorrhages within these areas. The petechial haemorrhages in such circumstances are produced after death. The most difficult cases to assess are those where the head is found at a lower level than the trunk and there is gross congestion to the upper part of the chest, head, and neck.

10.3.5 Traumatic (compression) asphyxia

Traumatic (compression) asphyxia involves compression of the chest and/or abdomen preventing movement of the chest and preventing respiration. The rapid increase in intrathoracic pressure in such cases results in extensive petechiae and cyanosis from consequent vascular pressure effects. An example of traumatic asphyxia is the Hillsborough football disaster in 1989 in which 96 people died, most from the effects of crushing causing traumatic asphyxia. There have been two inquiries, the Taylor Report in 1990 and the Hillsborough Independent Panel Inquiry published in 2012 as well as two inquests, the last concluding in 2016. In 2018 six people were charged with criminal offences, including the former match Police Commander, who was charged with gross negligence manslaughter. At the time of writing the trial is ongoing at Preston Crown Court.

10.3.6 Manual strangulation

Compression of the neck with one or both hands is one of the most common methods of homicide. Victims may include young children, the elderly, and possibly infirm individuals and females, who may also show some evidence of sexual assault. It is not uncommon to see such deaths in a domestic environment where after an altercation it is the female (generally having lesser strength than a male) who is usually the victim. In a series of 26 cases Vanezis (1989a) found 23 female victims of whom 14 (61%) were between 21 and 60 years of age (peak 31–40 years).

There are a variety of *external injuries* in strangulation cases that may be found on the neck and frequently also over the face and elsewhere. One of the most common injuries is *bruising caused by fingertips*. The bruises may be separately placed or merge into each other and tend to be rounded. They vary in shape and intensity depending on how the hands are applied and the force used. *Grazes (abrasions or scratches) from fingernails* accompany bruising or may be seen separately (Figure 10.4). Classically they appear as crescentic marks although they may be straight linear grazes. Occasionally one sees deeper lacerations caused by nails.

Occasionally marks are seen which have been produced by the victim in an attempt to remove the constricting hands. In such cases it is unlikely that surface marks will be accompanied by subcutaneous fingertip bruises.

The effect of manual strangulation in a person who has not died virtually instantaneously, as can occur with pressure on the carotid sinus, is to leave *internal injuries* in the form of *bruising to the underlying soft tissues and fractures to the hyoid and/or laryngeal structures* (Figures 10.5 and 10.6).

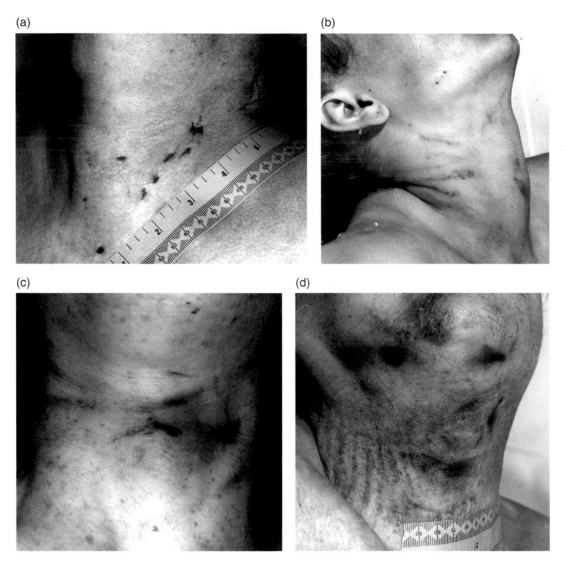

Figure 10.4   Bruises and grazes on the neck in manual strangulation: (a) fingernail abrasions, (b) linear grazes from fingernails, (c) fingertip bruising with intervening clothing pattern, and (d) combination of pulled clothing around neck with fingernail marks.

In many cases there is appreciable bruising to the sternomastoid muscle corresponding with any external skin bruising. The muscles surrounding the larynx both anteriorly and posteriorly also frequently show well-marked bruising.

There is also frequently bruising of the laryngeal mucosa and in some cases this is accompanied by severe laryngeal swelling (Figure 10.5).

Carotid artery tears may also occasionally be seen. Fractures to the laryngeal cartilages and hyoid bone are more likely to occur with increasing age with increasing calcification of the cartilages compared to a young person. Typically, fractures are seen in one or both superior thyroid horns and less commonly in the hyoid bone. With substantial force, one may also see fractures to

(a) (b)

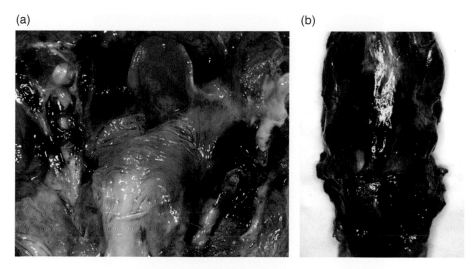

Figure 10.5 (a) Fractures to superior thyroid cartilage horns. (b) Bruising into strap muscles surrounding the larynx.

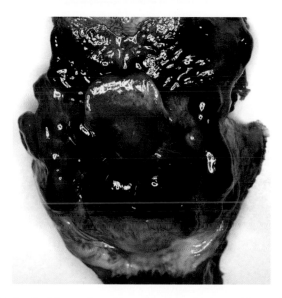

Figure 10.6 Bruising and swelling of laryngeal inlet and base of tongue.

the thyroid laminae and even the cricoid cartilage. In all forms of neck compression, particularly manual and ligature strangulation, radiographic or computerised tomography (CT) scan imaging may be useful prior to the autopsy and also after excision of the larynx and hyoid to look for undisplaced hairline fractures as well as more obvious damage (Kempter et al. 2009) (Figure 10.7).

Associated injuries in other regions are commonly seen. These include *fingertip bruising to the face* where the face may have been immobilised. Frequently, associated bruising to the mouth is seen externally and over the inner lips, formed when the lips are pressed against the teeth or gum margins (Figure 10.8) by a hand obstructing the mouth to prevent breathing or to stop the person from shouting out.

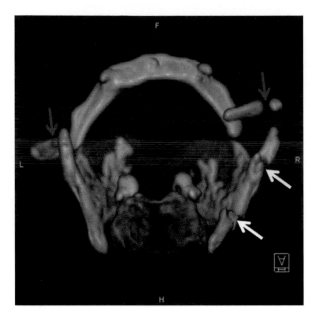

Figure 10.7 Three-dimensional CT reconstruction in a case of homicidal ligature strangulation, postero-anterior view. Besides a fracture of the right inferior horn (white arrow), a fracture of the right superior horn (yellow arrow) and fractures of the distal thirds of the greater horns on both sides of the hyoid bone (red arrows) are visible. Source: Reproduced with permission of Elsevier.

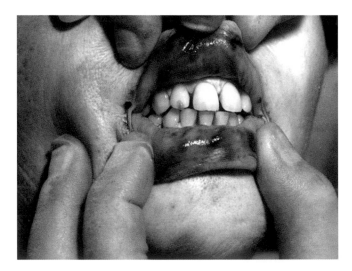

Figure 10.8 Bruising on the inside of the upper and lower lips from pressure against teeth when the mouth was forcibly closed.

Occasionally bruising to the head and elsewhere may be seen caused by direct assaults or by the person impacting against surfaces in a confined space, particularly if held down against a wall or the ground (Figure 10.9).

The assessment at the autopsy of the *degree of violence and force used* relies partly on the extent of bruising and, more importantly, the type and location of laryngeal and hyoid fractures, given the

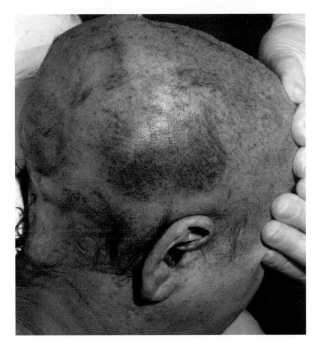

Figure 10.9 Bruising to head from movement during a struggle.

degree of calcification in each case. Occasionally, if death is rapid, bruising will not have had time to develop and the degree of violence may be impossible to assess. Some indication of the type of pressure and force used is also given by the degree of development of congestive changes which are as a rule well marked if considerable force has been used. Victims of attempted strangulation may well show petechial haemorrhages in their eyes for some time after the assault. The question of *how long the assailant's grip needs to be maintained to cause death* is a complex one. There are a number of essential factors which need to be carefully considered before an opinion is given, including the mechanism of death, extent of bruising, other marks present, extent of laryngeal injuries, intensity of signs associated with asphyxia, and other associated injuries to the body.

10.3.7 Neck holds in law enforcement

In view of the number of deaths that have been associated with neck holds over the years, they are now actively discouraged as a means of restraint to subdue suspects resisting arrest or prisoners who are combative and unmanageable. Two types of holds are recognised: the bar arm choke control and the carotid sleeper (Figure 10.10a,b).

The *carotid sleeper hold* (Figure 10.10b) is designed to compress the common carotid arteries and produce transient cerebral ischaemia. When the person has become incapacitated in this manner, the hold is released and full recovery is expected. The forearm and upper arm are placed around the upper neck in the form of a pincer, providing pressure to the lateral aspects of the neck in order to impede blood flow within the carotid arteries. Transient cerebral ischaemia can also be caused with this hold by carotid sinus stimulation, which can produce bradycardia and, occasionally, cardiac arrest.

(a) Bar (choke) hold   (b) Carotid sleeper

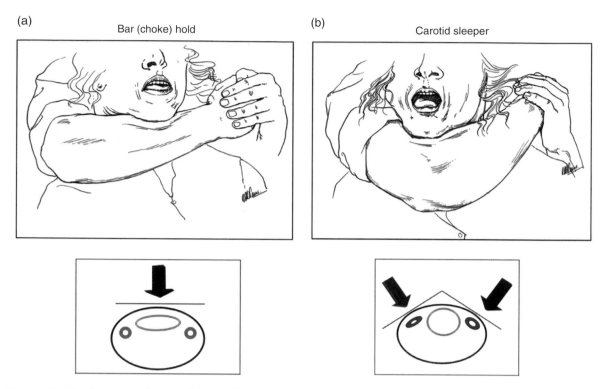

Figure 10.10   (a) Bar choke and (b) carotid sleeper holds. The front of the neck and the two carotid arteries are compressed as shown.

The *bar arm* or *choke hold* (Figure 10.10a) occludes the airway by forearm compression of the exposed anterior aspect of the neck. The thyroid cartilage is compressed and may be fractured. The base of the tongue may also be moved backwards to occlude the hypopharynx.

Fatal consequences of neck holds can be anticipated because of their physiological effects. Pre-existing natural disease increases the likelihood of a fatal outcome, even when a hold such as the carotid sleeper is applied correctly. Underlying cardiac disease is particularly vulnerable to reflex carotid artery stimulation and hypoxia. The carotid arteries may be atherosclerotic and narrowed. The pressure applied may dislodge atherosclerotic plaque and produce a fatal stroke.

Despite the well-known dangers of both these holds, they are still occasionally used by some police agencies throughout the world. The Metropolitan Police (London), with only rare exceptions, do not currently teach neck restraints within their recently updated officer safety programme (Metropolitan Police: The Current Officer Safety Manual 2013).

10.3.8   Ligature strangulation

The vast majority of cases of ligature strangulation are homicidal. It is commonly seen in women and is frequently associated with sexual assault (Figure 10.11).

Suicidal ligature strangulation is only occasionally seen (Figure 10.12) and must always be treated with great caution, taking careful account of the circumstances surrounding the death, including scene examination.

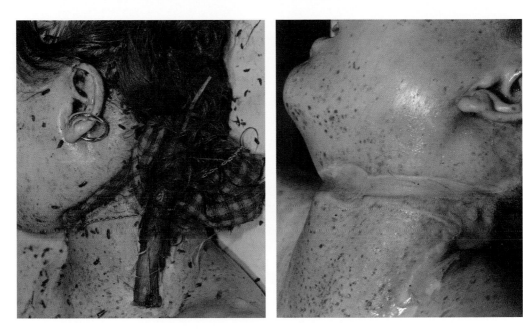

Figure 10.11 Young woman strangled with part of her torn blouse. The branch was used as a tourniquet to tighten the ligature and a knot was fashioned at the front to cause further pressure to the front of the neck at the larynx. She had been raped prior to the strangulation. The image on the right shows the neck after removal of the ligature.

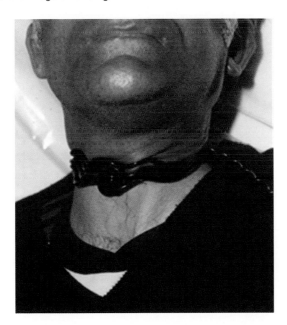

Figure 10.12 Case of suicidal ligature strangulation in a middle-aged male. Note congestion above the black cable.

Accidental cases are few and are seen mainly in children. They may become entangled in curtain cords or flexes from electrical equipment at home, for example. An unsafe or modified cot may be another source of danger. In the case shown in (Figure 10.13), the lining of the bedding had become loose, forming a noose around the child's neck.

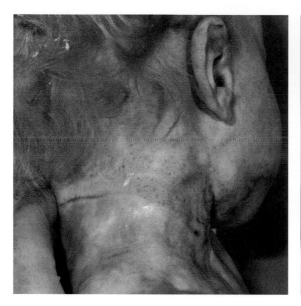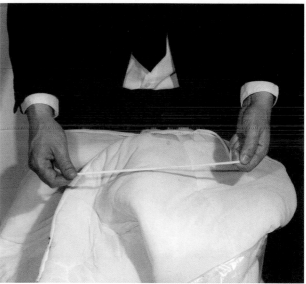

Figure 10.13   Accidental ligature strangulation in a young infant. His neck became trapped in a partially detached lining of his duvet which was found wrapped around his neck.

10.3.9   Ligature marks

Certain features on the skin may resemble ligature marks, such as normal skin creases, especially in infants where they may be quite deep due to generous folds of fat in young necks. Collars and similar clothing or chains may also leave suspicious marks. Gaseous swelling in decomposing bodies may not only obscure ligature marks, but may accentuate crease marks by clothes tightening against the skin.

The ligature mark may have a pattern which can be matched with a particular ligature. If a knot has been used to secure the ligature, it may leave a mark which could assist in reconstructing how the ligature was secured around the neck. In addition to the position of a knot, the position of the ligature mark itself in strangulation is approximately horizontal, in contrast to hanging, where in most cases it slopes up towards the point of suspension.

As with manual strangulation, the length of time from application of the ligature to death cannot be reliably estimated. Some assistance to the length of a physical altercation can be given from the assessment of all local injuries to the face and neck as well as other injuries to the body.

Internally the injuries are similar to manual strangulation except that bruising of the muscles surrounding the larynx may be distributed in a broad band rather than along most of the vertical length of the hyoid and laryngeal region.

10.3.10   Hanging

The vast majority of hangings are suicidal in nature. From time to time accidental cases are seen, especially in children, as well as other categories include auto-erotic, homicidal, and simulated hanging. Judicial execution by hanging is still encountered in many countries although in the UK the death penalty was abolished in 1965. Constriction of the neck is caused by the weight of the body as opposed to direct compression in manual and ligature strangulation.

In contrast to ligature strangulation, in hanging the *slope of the ligature mark* is upwards towards the back of the neck, although occasionally this may be reversed. An impression of a knot may be found, usually to either side or to the back of the neck. Depending on the degree of constriction, congestion which is due to obstruction of the venous return, is seen without complete occlusion of the carotid system. In such cases petechial haemorrhages may also be seen above the level of the ligature and particularly in the conjunctivae. It should be appreciated, however, that in the majority of hangings the face appears normal or pale; the ligature mark and protrusion of the tongue are frequently the only external signs of hanging.

The *internal signs* of hanging, such as soft tissue injuries, are more likely to be found if the body is fully suspended or just touching the ground. In the majority of cases bruising of the laryngeal/hyoid strap muscle or other nearby soft tissue structures is not seen. The reason for this may be due to occlusion of both the carotid and jugular vessels, thus creating a 'bloodless' field in the vicinity of the ligature. On the other hand, fractures of the larynx and hyoid bone are common. Some of the older literature reports that fractures are rarely seen. In all probability, the reason for this view is that such damage is accompanied by very little haemorrhage, thus not drawing attention to the possibility of injury. Carotid artery intimal tears below the level of the bifurcation and vertebral artery tears resulting from stretching are occasionally seen in suicidal hanging but are much more frequent in judicial hanging.

Leaving aside judicial hanging, which is discussed in section 10.3.11, it should be noted that the *mechanism of death* in hanging may be complex. It should be borne in mind that there may be obstruction of the airway, occlusion of the cerebral circulation or stimulation of the vagus nerve. The first two factors appear to be more important, as they can be related to circumstantial and physical findings whereas vagal effects are impossible to quantify at autopsy. The degree of suspension appears to play the most important role in influencing the type of mechanism involved. When the body is either fully or partially suspended, with the most substantial weight of the body causing constriction of the ligature and with the point of suspension at the back, the main force is to the sides and front of the neck, producing an upward and backward movement of the base of the tongue, thus obstructing the upper airway. Nevertheless, it is felt that occlusion of the vessels plays the primary role in such positions. Compromise of the cerebral circulation is severe or total and leads to rapid unconsciousness followed by death, which usually supervenes in minutes. In cases where the body is substantially supported by a surface, e.g. by the knees or sitting, it is much more likely that vessel occlusion will be incomplete. Usually the venous circulation is obstructed with consequent congestion and the production of petechial haemorrhages. Obstruction to the airway is more likely in such circumstances.

The *scene of the hanging* in most instances is at the person's home (Bowen 1982; Davison and Marshall 1986). Other frequently encountered locations include custodial environments such as police cells and prisons, places of work, hospitals, and secluded outdoor environments. In the latter situation the person may not be found for a considerable length of time after death. Examination of the scene will assist the examiner to appreciate the ease with which death from hanging may occur from easily accessible and low points of attachment. One must also look for any objects or items of furniture which may facilitate hanging, such as a chair, which may be pushed away to effect suspension. The point of attachment of the rope should be examined as well as the surrounding area. There may be disturbance of dust caused by the ligature being attached, particularly on a high point such as a beam. Corresponding dirt marks may be found on the hands or clothing of the deceased.

In cases where the deceased has been killed by a third party, the body may be suspended in order to mimic a suicidal hanging. Such cases of *simulated hanging* may be problematical unless meticulous attention is paid to the post-mortem examination, particularly to the type and distribution of injuries to the neck region. The scene may at first give no cause for concern and indeed there may be signs which are suggestive of suicide until the autopsy is carried out.

Cases of homicidal hanging are quite rare. Puschel et al. (1984) describe six cases of homicidal hanging and point out that distinction between murder and suicide may be impossible by examination of the body alone. It is essential to carry out a detailed investigation of the scene, reconstruction of the position of the suspended body, and examination of the rope, the knots, and the direction of the fibres on the rope. The body may have been incapacitated in some way, e.g. through drink or drugs, in order to effect hanging. Furthermore, it may be relatively easy to achieve if the assailant is a fit healthy person and the victim is very young, infirm, and/or elderly.

10.3.11 Judicial hanging

Although judicial hanging was recorded as early as the fifth century in the British Isles, in England it was established as a form of capital punishment by the time of Henry II (1133–1189) and hanging was carried out in public until 1868. In the early days of hanging, the condemned person would be hoisted up from the ground and then allowed to dangle so that death was caused by the effects of slow strangulation. Assistance from the hangman was occasionally needed to effect the eventual demise by pulling at the feet or hanging on the condemned person's back to provide the necessary extra weight. The long drop became standard only in the late eighteenth century and was probably first introduced at Newgate Prison in London.

The cause of death in judicial hanging is controversial and often attributed to 'hangman's fracture' of the second cervical vertebra. However, the cause of death may involve a number of different mechanisms, particularly as a consequence of compression or rupture of the vertebral and carotid arteries leading to cerebral ischaemia. Furthermore, the rapidity of loss of consciousness and death is highly dependent upon knot positioning and the length of drop. In a series of 19 executions from Pentonville Prison, London from 1932 to 1959 (Vanezis 1989b) in nearly all the cases the point of suspension was near the angle of the left side of the mandible. In all cases there was cervical dislocation and occasionally cervical fractures were described together with spinal cord or brain stem injury. The most common level of cervical spine injury was C2/C3 (seven cases) and in two cases there were signs of asphyxia.

10.3.12 Auto-erotic asphyxia

The vast majority of auto-erotic deaths result from the use of asphyxia to obtain sexual gratification. In most cases this is achieved by producing partial asphyxia from the application of pressure on the neck. Other methods of sexual asphyxia include obstructing the mouth by a plastic bag, pillow or some such similar device.

Sauvageau and Racette (2006), in a review of the literature on autoerotic deaths, found that studies showed a male predominance, with 390 male victims compared to 18 females (22 : 1 male–female ratio). Victims are of all ages and most are solitary acts. Persons within this group are thought to be happy, well adjusted, and with no suicidal tendencies (Figure 10.14). A second group comprises mainly adult males, usually with homosexual preferences. They tend to carry out the procedure in pairs as a means of protection from accidental death.

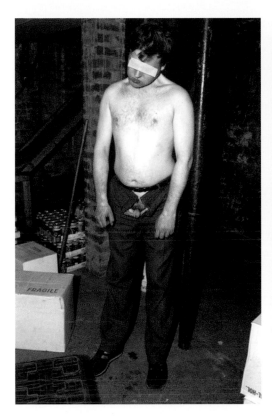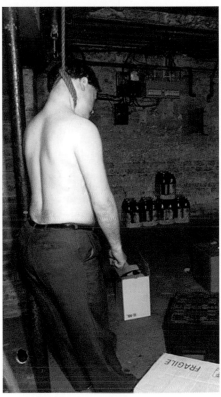

Figure 10.14 Young male, hanging in the basement of a wine shop. His feet are just touching the ground so that he can control the degree of asphyxia delivered. He is naked from the waist up and his trouser zip is undone.

When examining the scene, in the first instance it is essential to assess whether the asphyxia was in fact auto-erotic or whether there is some other explanation. It is important to establish that death was due to the deceased's own actions or whether a third party was involved, and if a third party was involved whether there was any intention to harm the victim. Resnick (1972) was one of the first to enumerate the features which are typical of this category of asphyxial death, which he called 'eroticized repetitive hanging syndrome'. The features he observed are listed below and should be borne in mind when the scene is examined.

- Involvement of adolescent or young men (not exclusively and occasionally such deaths are also seen in females).

- Ropes, belts, or other binding material are found and so arranged that compression of the neck may be produced and controlled voluntarily.

- Evidence of masturbation.

- Partial or complete nudity.

- A solitary act.

- Repetitive behaviour with attempt by the deceased to ensure that no visible marks are left on his person.

- No apparent wish to die.

- Binding of the body and/or extremities and/or genitals with ropes, chains, or leather (less frequently).

- Female attire may be present.

One should also add to Resnick's list the frequent finding of sexual aids such as pornographic material.

10.4   Drowning

10.4.1   The scope of the problem

World Health Organization statistics (WHO 2014) show that there are 372 000 annual deaths by drowning worldwide, over 9% of global mortality. Figure 10.15 shows a painting by Vasily Perov of a woman who had committed suicide by drowning. This work is not untypical of the Russian nineteenth century realist painters depicting the tragic circumstances of ordinary people.

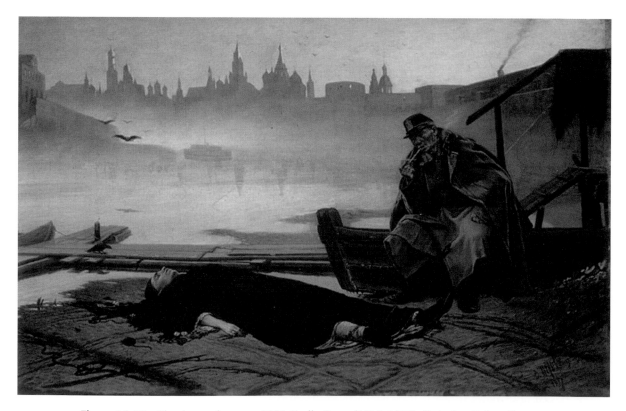

Figure 10.15   The drowned woman 1867, Vasily Perov (1834–1882). Tretyakov Gallery Moscow.

Children, males, and individuals with increased access to water are most at risk from drowning. More recently the plight of migrants or asylum seekers has been highlighted. They often travel illegally in overcrowded unsafe vessels lacking in equipment and operated by personnel untrained in dealing with transport incidents or in navigation.

10.4.2 Initial considerations and approach

There are a number of important considerations in bodies that are recovered from or found near to water:

- Was death due to the effects of immersion (most are cases are of typical drowning) in water?
- Was the person dead prior to entry into water? The presence of silt and water within the upper airways and mouth is an indication of immersion but not indicative of drowning and may have been caused by the passive movement of water and other material in a person deceased prior to entry.
- Was the person injured in the water when alive? Occasionally when entering water a person may become injured from objects such as rocks or other surfaces, depending on the environment, or may be struck by a vessel within the water.
- Was death due to natural causes before entry or within the water? This assessment may be quite challenging. Natural disease may well contribute to drowning and it is sometimes not possible to differentiate with certainty which was the cause of death.
- How long was the person in the water? Assessment will require consideration of a number of factors, including:
    o cooling of the body, which will depend on the temperature of the water
    o rigor mortis may be retarded due to rapid cooling
    o hypostasis may be pink, faint, and variably distributed due to a floating body and changes in its position
    o decomposition is generally slower in water than in the open air unless the water is heavily polluted, in which case it may be accelerated; decomposition is also accelerated when the body is recovered from water into a warmer environment
    o maceration of skin – 'washerwoman' hands and feet, imbibition of water into skin, which becomes sodden, thickened, wrinkled, and white. There may be also degloving of skin of the hands and feet. These are common features of immersion (but not necessarily drowning). It is not possible to state with accuracy how long the individual has been submerged from an assessment of the skin. It should be appreciated that wrinkling of digits can start in hot water after a few minutes.
    o formation of adipocere is also seen in immersion and in other situations where a body has been lying in a damp environment. The time for its development is variable and cannot be accurately assessed.
- Who was the deceased? Identification of a body which has been immersed in water, particularly if some time has passed from entry to recovery, may prove challenging. It is not unusual for facial tissues to be decomposed and/or destroyed by carnivorous fish and crustaceans.
- Where did the deceased enter the water in relation to where the body was recovered? It must be borne in mind that where a body is found is not necessarily where the body entered the water.

In assessing whether death is due to typical (classical/wet) drowning the pathologist will need to carry out a thorough post-mortem examination, including imaging (CT and/or conventional radiology) prior to the autopsy.

If the body is in a fresh state, the post-mortem in cases of typical drowning will demonstrate a number of findings which will assist in arriving at the cause of death. The common findings seen are frothy fluid at the mouth and in the airways further down. The lungs are waterlogged and very heavy. There is typically over-inflation of the lungs (emphysema aquosum) and they are held in an inspired position. The stomach sometimes contains watery fluid or foreign material. However, in many cases of recovered bodies from water, there are significant post-mortem changes that make an assessment difficult if not impossible.

10.5   Mechanism and pathophysiology of drowning

Deaths involving immersion in water present a challenge to the pathologist. In order to understand and interpret autopsy findings, it is important to understand the mechanisms and pathophysiology of the effects of immersion of a live person in water.

10.5.1   Mechanisms of drowning

Drowning may be what is described as 'true' or 'wet' drowning or 'dry' drowning, when there are no signs of inhalation of water into the lungs and in essence very few findings to indicate a cause of death.

10.5.1.1   Dry drowning   Dry drowning is associated with rapid death where entry into the water is witnessed and retrieval of the body occurs within a few minutes. There are no features typical of drowning and it is important to exclude all other reasonable causes. There are a number of possible mechanisms, although one is not able to confirm them at autopsy, such as reflex cardiac inhibition caused by sudden immersion in cold water or sudden impact of cold water into the nose, mouth, and voice box.

10.5.1.2   Wet drowning   The mechanism of death in wet drowning involves a combination of hypoxia from water and obstruction of airways. There is progressive entry of water into the lungs causing dilution of blood and resulting in relative anaemia and reduction of oxygen in the blood. Red blood cells are ruptured, with release of potassium into the blood. In addition, there may be an element of reflex cardiac arrest.

10.5.2   Pathophysiology of drowning

The alveolar lining behaves as semi-permeable membrane and will exchange water if introduced. As well as the direct effect of oxygen deprivation, there are also dangerous effects on blood chemistry if water is taken into the lungs. The mechanism for this is different for fresh and sea water. The extent and direction depends on the osmotic pressure gradient between water and blood.

Fresh water taken into the lungs will be pulled into the pulmonary circulation by osmosis. The dilution of blood leads to hemolysis (bursting of red blood cells). The resulting elevation of the plasma K+ (potassium) level and depression of the Na+ (sodium) level alter the electrical activity of the heart, often causing ventricular fibrillation. Acute renal failure can also result from haemoglobin from the burst blood cells accumulating in the kidneys, and cardiac arrest can result if cold freshwater taken into the bloodstream sufficiently cools the heart.

Sea water is hypertonic (more salty) than blood. It poses the opposite danger. Osmosis will instead pull water from the bloodstream into the lungs, thickening the blood. In animal experiments the thicker blood requires more work from the heart, leading to cardiac arrest in 8–10 minutes.

Autopsies on human drowning victims show no indications of these effects and there appears to be little difference between drownings in salt water and fresh water. After death, the ability of live cell membranes to separate fluid and electrolytes is rapidly lost and one cannot rely on electrolyte estimations post-mortem to differentiate between sea and fresh water drowning, as was demonstrated by the work of Durlacher et al. (1953), who found no reliable changes in sodium, potassium, and chloride concentration, as did Fuller (1963).

10.6 Diatoms and their use in the investigation of drowning

Diatoms are unicellular algae enclosed within a silica cell wall called a frustule (Figure 10.16). They show wide diversity in form and are bilaterally symmetrical (hence their name).

The diatom test has been used to diagnose drowning for many years. Essentially the principle is that if a live person enters into and inhales water which contains diatoms, they then enter the lungs, pass into the blood from the alveolar membrane, and enter peripheral organs such as the kidney and bone marrow, thus supporting live entry and death from drowning.

Samples of lung and a peripheral organ or organs can be digested with strong acid to dissolve the soft tissue, thus leaving the highly resistant diatom skeletons to be identified under the microscope.

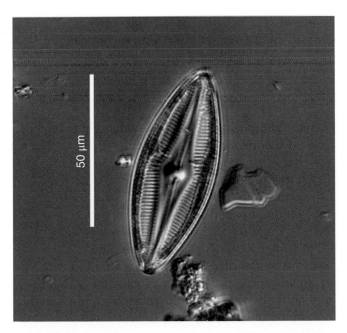

Figure 10.16 *Navicula* spp. one of the most common type of diatoms seen. Source: Phyto'pedia – The Phytoplankton Encyclopaedia Project, University of British Columbia, www.eoas.ubc.ca/research/phytoplankton.

A control sample of water is also taken from the area where the deceased was recovered as well as from other locations where the deceased may be thought to have entered the water, if the entry point is not known.

If the person had been dead on entry then one may find diatoms in the lungs from passive movement of water, but not in peripheral organs as there will have been no circulation to have carried them away from the lungs.

The diatom test, if reliable, could be extremely useful as a positive diagnosis of drowning, particularly where putrefaction is present and the usual findings that one sees in the fresh body are not present.

One should also appreciate that the lack of diatoms in a victim does not negate a cause of drowning. It all depends on the population numbers and presence of diatoms in the water when and where entry occurred.

However, there is a great deal of controversy over the reliability of the test, particularly if only a few or no diatoms are found. Because of their ubiquitous nature in water, in the atmosphere, and in some foods, one must be scrupulous in sample collection and in the use of techniques for their extraction in order minimise contamination. Bortolotti et al. (2011) found that false-positive results were not significant in cases where victims did not die of drowning and indeed supported the validity of the diatoms test as a proof of drowning. Pollanen et al. (1997) from a retrospective study of 738 freshwater drownings and 33 cases of drownings in bathtubs, pools, or toilets found that the diatom test will identify approximately one in three victims of freshwater drowning and may be useful in the assessment of deaths occurring in bathtubs, thus providing further evidence for the reliability of the test. Pollanen (1997), analysing of the diatom content of samples of the putative drowning medium by month, revealed that winter months had the highest frequency of samples devoid of diatoms. The data indicated that the true positive rate of the diatom test for drowning was at least 90% and that small pennate frustules (siliceous diatom walls) are most commonly associated with drowning, particular in non-winter months.

It seems reasonable to conclude that drowning has occurred if similar types of diatoms are found in the water sample known to be the entry location and in the lungs and peripheral organs of the deceased.

References

Bell, M.D., Rao, V.J., Wetli, C.V., and Rodriguez, R.N. (1992). Positional asphyxiation in adults: a series of 30 cases from the Dade and Broward County Florida medical examiner offices from 1982 to 1990. *Am. J. Forensic Med. Pathol.* 13: 101–107.

Bortolotti, F., Del Balzo, G., Calza, R. et al. (2011). Testing the specificity of the diatom test: search for false-positives. *Med. Sci. Law.* 51 (Suppl 1): S7–S10.

Bowen, D.A.L. (1982). Hanging – a review. *Forensic Sci. Int.* 20: 247–249.

Burtscher, M., Mairer, K., Wille, M. et al. (2012). Short-term exposure to hypoxia for work and leisure activities in health and disease: which level of hypoxia is safe? *Sleep Breath.* 16: 435–442.

Byard, R.W. and Wilson, G.W. (1992). Death scene gas analysis in suspected methane asphyxia. *Am. J. Forensic Med. Pathol.* 13: 69–71.

Chen, Y.Y., Bennewith, O., Hawton, K. et al. (2013). Suicide by burning barbecue charcoal in England. *J. Public Health (Oxford)* 35: 223–227.

Christison, R. (1829). Case lv. Murder by suffocation. Injury of the spine after death imitating injury during life – experiments on the effects of blows soon after death. *Edinb. Med. J.* 31: 236–250.

Davison, A. and Marshall, T.K. (1986). Hanging in Northern Ireland – a survey. *Med. Sci. Law* 26: 23–28.

Downs, J.C., Conradi, S.E., and Nichols, C.A. (1994). Suicide by environmental hypoxia (forced depletion of oxygen). *Am. J. Forensic Med. Pathol.* 15: 216–223.

Durlacher, S.H., Freimuth, H.C., and Swan, H.E. Jr. (1953). Blood changes in man following death due to drowning, with comments on tests for drowning. *AMA Arch. Pathol.* 56: 454–461.

Fuller, R.H. (1963). The clinical pathology of human near-drowning. *Proc. R. Soc. Med.* 56: 33–38.

Gunnell, D., Coope, C., Fearn, V. et al. (2015). Suicide by gases in England and Wales 2001–2011: evidence of the emergence of new methods of suicide. *J. Affect. Disord.* 170: 190–195.

Hicks, L.J., Scanlon, M.J., Bostwick, T.C., and Batten, P.J. (1990). Death by smothering and its investigation. *Am. J. Forensic Med. Pathol.* 11: 291–293.

Hillsborough Independent Panel (12 September 2012). The Report of the Hillsborough Independent Panel (Report). London: The Stationery Office.

Kempter, M., Ross, S., Spendlove, D. et al. (2009). Post-mortem imaging of laryngohyoid fractures in strangulation incidents: first results. *Leg. Med. (Tokyo)* 11: 267–271.

Leung, C.M., Chung, W.S., and So, E.P. (2002). Burning charcoal: an indigenous method of committing suicide in Hong Kong. *J. Clin. Psychiatry* 63: 447–450.

Littlejohn, H.D. (1855–1856). Cases of homicidal and accidental suffocation with remarks. *Edinb. Med. J.* 1: 511–524.

Manning, T.J., Ziminnki, K., Hyman, A. et al. (1981). Methane deaths? Was it the cause? *Am. J. Forensic Med. Pathol.* 2: 333–336.

Metropolitan Police: The Current Officer Safety Manual 2013 at: www.met.police.uk/foi/pdfs/disclosure_2013/october_2013/2013010000744.pdf.

Mittleman, R.E. (1984). Fatal choking in infants and children. *Am. J. Forensic Med. Pathol.* 5: 201–210.

Mole, R.H. (1948). Fibrinolysin and fluidity of the blood post mortem. *J. Pathol. Bacteriol.* 60: 413–427.

Mott, J.A., Wolfe, M.I., Alveson, C.J. et al. (2002). National vehicle emissions policies and practices and declining US carbon monoxide – related mortality. *JAMA* 288: 988–995.

Nelson, L. (2006). Acute cyanide toxicity: mechanisms and manifestations. *J. Emerg. Nurs.* 32 (4): S8—S11.

Oswalt, C.E., Gates, G.A., and Holmstrom, M.G. (1977). Pulmonary edema as a complication of acute airway obstruction. *JAMA* 238: 1833–1835.

Pollanen, M.S. (1997). The diagnostic value of the diatom test for drowning, II. Validity: analysis of diatoms in bone marrow and drowning medium. *J. Forensic Sci.* 42: 286–290.

Pollanen, M.S., Cheung, C., and Chiasson, D.A. (1997). The diagnostic value of the diatom test for drowning, I. Utility: a retrospective analysis of 771 cases of drowning in Ontario, Canada. *J. Forensic Sci.* 42: 281–285.

Puschel, K., Holtz, W., Hidebrand, E. et al. (1984). Hanging, suicide or homicide? *Arch Kriminol.* 174: 141–153.

Renton, J.M. (1908). An unusual case of suicide by suffocation. *BMJ* 1: 493.

Resnick, H. (1972). Eroticized repetitive hanging: a form of self-destructive behavior. *Am. J. Psychother.* 26: 4–21.

Sauvageau, A. and Racette, S. (2006). Autoerotic deaths in the literature from 1954 to 2004: a review. *J. Forensic Sci.* 51: 140–146.

Struttmann, T., Scheerer, A., Prince, S., and Goldstein, L. (1998). Unintentional carbon monoxide poisoning from an unlikely source. *J. Am. Board Fam. Pract.* 11: 481–484.

Studdert, D.M., Gurrin, L.C., Jatkar, U., and Pirkis, J. (2010). Relationship between vehicle emissions laws and incidence of suicide by motor vehicle exhaust gas in Australia, 2001–06: an ecological analysis. *PLoS Med.* 7 (1): e1000210.

Sturner, W.Q., Spruill, F.G., Smith, R.A., and Lene, W.J. (1976). Accidental asphyxia deaths involving infants and young children. *J. Forensic Sci.* 21: 483–487.

Tardieu A (1855). Memoire sur la mort par suffocation. Annales d'Hygeine Publique et de Medecine Legale. 2e serie T. IV.

Tardieu (1859). Etude medico-legale sur la strangulation. Annales d'Hygeine Publique et de Medecine Legale. 2e serie T. eXl.

Taylor, Lord Justice. (January 1990). Final report on the Hillsborough stadium disaster. Her Majesty's Stationery Office.

Vanezis, P. (1989a). *Pathology of Neck Injury*, 51. Butterworth Chapter 6.

Vanezis, P. (1989b). *Pathology of Neck Injury*, 79–80. Butterworth Chapter 8.

World Health Organization (2014). Drowning. Fact sheet No. 347 accessed at http://www.who.int/mediacentre/factsheets/fs347/en.

11
Forensic Medical Aspects of Human Rights Issues

Peter Vanezis
Queen Mary University of London, London, UK

Human rights are rights inherent to all human beings, whatever our nationality, place of residence, sex, national or ethnic origin, colour, religion, language, or any other status. We are all equally entitled to our human rights without discrimination. These rights are all interrelated, interdependent, and indivisible.

Universal human rights are often expressed and guaranteed by law, in the forms of treaties, customary international law, general principles, and other sources of international law. International human rights law lays down obligations of Governments to act in certain ways or to refrain from certain acts, in order to promote and protect human rights and fundamental freedoms of individuals or groups.

The Office of the United Nations High Commissioner for Human Rights (OHCHR) (2016).

11.1 Torture

Torture is defined by the United Nations (1984) as any act by which severe pain or suffering, whether physical or mental, is intentionally inflicted on a person for such purposes as:

- obtaining information or a confession from an individual or a third person

- punishing an individual for an act he/she or a third person has committed or is suspected of having committed

Essential Forensic Medicine, First Edition. Edited by Peter Vanezis.
© 2020 John Wiley & Sons Ltd. Published 2020 by John Wiley & Sons Ltd.

- intimidating or coercing an individual or a third person, or for any reason based on discrimination of any kind, when such pain or suffering is inflicted by or at the instigation of or with the consent or acquiescence of a public official or other person acting in an official capacity

It does not include pain or suffering arising only from, inherent in or incidental to lawful sanctions.

11.1.1   The use of torture throughout history

Until the last century, most forms of torture that were recognised as such were mainly physical in nature. However, psychological torture also took place. A good example of this was the Spanish Inquisition, where the inquisitors would show the implements of torture to potential victims to scare them into submission.

Early torture developed mainly out of the need for survival and maintaining group or tribal entities. Primitive humans used laws for exile and punishment of major offences.

With the passage of time and the growth of civilisation, codes of laws evolved. Any actual tortures inflicted would only be committed against enemy tribes and animals. In many cultures, religious sacrifices preceded the use of torture. The early European codes were usually based on the principle of *lex talionis*, the idea of an eye for an eye, i.e. the punishment for crime should be similar to the offence. This was the Law of Hammurabi, written around 2000 BCE. This civil code was expanded to include other crimes in the Mosaic Code 1000 years later that would form the basis of Hebrew, Greek, and Roman legal systems. At the time, torture was mainly used as a means of extracting vengeance for real or imagined wrongs. Public displays such as stoning and crucifixion were used mainly to deter other criminals.

From the fall of Rome till the thirteenth century, torture was used mainly as a weapon of private citizens and eventually the State. Torture was adopted by rulers that realised that their citizens respected such a display of force. And as one form of torture would become commonplace, the next generation of people would adopt more harsh forms of punishment. Some torture was used for religious persecution. Christian leaders forced conversion of others with the application of torture. Burning at the stake, drowning, and suffocation were common tortures. As the Church used torture in its proceedings, this would prompt civil authorities to adopt the practice as well.

In the sixth century, Pope Gregory I made statements given under torture inadmissible, which meant that torture was then not used as a legal device, only as a punishment. However, the use of the ordeals of fire and water were still used to prove guilt and remained in fairly common use until their abolition in 1215 by the Papacy.

One of the most infamous chapters in the history of torture involved the role of the various mediaeval inquisitions, with the first papal inquisition instituted by Pope Gregory IX in 1231. Its purpose was to purge the apparent threat to the Catholic Church. The movement against heretics spread rapidly to Germany, Holland, Spain, Portugal, and eventually to most of Europe. The procedure adopted by the Inquisition, which would be used later in the witch trials, reintroduced torture to Europe. It was in 1808 that Napoleon's capture of Almanza and other cities in Spain that ended the Spanish Inquisition. A revision of the history of the Inquisition was made by Henry Kamen (2014), who takes the position that the Inquisition in Spain was motivated more by political considerations than religion, with the monarchs routinely protecting those close to the crown.

Eventually, the focus of persecution would shift from religious sects, to the purging of supposed witches and sorcerers. An early example of burning at the stake for witchcraft and heresy was Joan of Arc, who led France to victory over its long-running war with England in the besieged city of Orléans. She was captured by the Anglo-Burgundians, held captive for a year, then burned at the stake in 1431 at the age of 19 years (Figure 11.1).

This purge was carried into the British Isles, and eventually out of Europe. In Scotland and Ireland in the sixteenth and seventeenth centuries torture was commonly used to get the accused to confess their crimes.

Harsh forms of torture persisted in the twentieth century and were particularly associated with wars and revolutions. The atrocities of World War II had inmates of concentration camps forced to live in lice-infested barracks, where they lived in a constant atmosphere of death and cruelty. In Dachau alone, it is estimated that around 200 000 people were killed.

Despite man's prevailing cruelty to their fellow man, since the earliest times, there have been a few notable individuals who voiced their objections to torture in its many forms. Seneca, Cicero, and St Augustine all recognised that torture may result in the unjust conviction of innocents. Frederick the Great in Prussia abolished it in 1740. Italy followed suit in 1786, followed by France

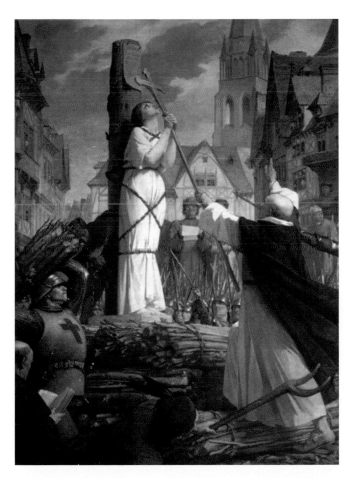

Figure 11.1 Joan of Arc burning at the stake. Jules-Eugène Lenepveu (1819–1898) (Panthéon, Paris, France).

in 1789 and Russia in 1801. Eventually, nearly every nation of Europe would abolish most forms of torture. Whilst occasional aberrations would arise over the years, there were few government-sanctioned tortures besides incarceration after this time.

11.1.2   Modern methods of torture and its investigation

Despite the lessons of the past, countries still practice what is defined as torture by the United Nations Convention (see above) to varying degrees and forms. Indeed, there are many torture methods. Those listed in Table 11.1 are not exhaustive but demonstrate the wide range used.

The greatest risk of torture is in the first phase of arrest and detention, before the individual has access to a lawyer or court. This risk persists as long as the investigation lasts, irrespective of where a suspect is being held. The place of detention where the torture is inflicted may be a police station, interrogation centre, prison, labour camp, or military or paramilitary facility.

Table 11.1   Methods of torture.

Blunt trauma, such as a punch, kick, slap, whipping, beating with wires or truncheons or falling down; falanga, beating of the feet (Figure 11.12); systematic and violent beating (Figure 11.13).

Positional torture, using suspension, stretching limbs apart, prolonged constraint of movement, forced positioning, 'Palestinian hanging' (a form of suspension that involves the victim being suspended with the arms bent backwards for hours or days on end).

Burns with cigarettes, heated instruments, scalding with liquid or a caustic substance (Figure 11.1).

Electric shocks

Asphyxiation, such as wet and dry methods, drowning, smothering, choking or use of chemicals.

Crush injuries, such as smashing fingers or traumatic removal of digits or limbs, or using a heavy roller to injure the thighs or back.

Penetrating injuries, such as stab and gunshot wounds, wires under nails.

Chemical exposure to salt, chilli pepper, gasoline, etc. (in wounds or body cavities).

Sexual violence to genitals, molestation, instrumentation, rape.

Medical amputation of digits or limbs, surgical removal of organs.

Pharmacological torture using toxic doses of sedatives, neuroleptics, paralytics, etc.

Conditions of detention, such as a small or overcrowded cell, solitary confinement, unhygienic conditions, no access to toilet facilities, irregular or contaminated food and water, exposure to extremes of temperature, denial of privacy and forced nakedness.

Deprivation of normal sensory stimulation and abuse of physiological needs such as sound, light, sense of time, isolation, manipulation of brightness of the cell, restriction of sleep, food, water, toilet facilities, bathing, motor activities, medical care, social contacts, isolation within prison, loss of contact with the outside world (victims are often kept in isolation in order to prevent bonding and mutual identification, and to encourage traumatic bonding with the torturer).

Humiliation, such as verbal abuse, performance of humiliating acts.

Threats of death, harm to family, further torture, imprisonment, mock execution, threats of attack by animals, such as dogs, cats, rats or scorpions.

Psychological techniques to break down the individual, including forced betrayals, accentuating feelings of helplessness, exposure to ambiguous situations or contradictory messages.

Violation of taboos

Behavioural coercion, e.g. forced practices against the religion of the victim (e.g. forcing Muslims to eat pork), forced harm to others through torture or other abuses, forced destruction of property, forced betrayal of someone placing them at risk of harm, forcing the victim to witness torture or atrocities being inflicted.

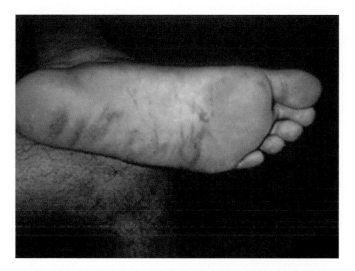

Figure 11.2 Example of falanga – beating on the soles of the feet.

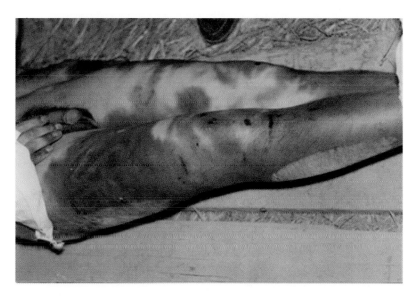

Figure 11.3 Systematic and violent beating. There were also multiple bruises to the upper limbs and trunk.

11.1.2.1 Investigation of cases of torture The *Manual on Effective Investigation and Documentation of Torture and Other Cruel, Inhuman or Degrading Treatment or Punishment,* commonly known as the *Istanbul Protocol,* is the first and the most important set of international guidelines for documentation of torture and its consequences. It became an official United Nations document in 1999 (Office of the United Nations High Commissioner for Human Rights 2004).

Its intention is to serve as a set of comprehensive international guidelines for doctors, lawyers, and others for the assessment of persons who allege torture and ill-treatment, for investigating cases of alleged torture, and for reporting such findings to the judiciary and any other investigative bodies.

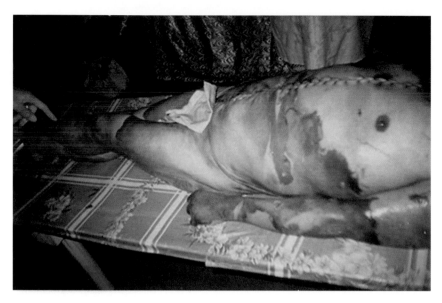

Figure 11.4   The pattern of the scalding noted shows a well-demarcated line on the lower chest/abdomen, indicating the forceful application of hot water whilst the person was within some kind of bath or similar vessel. Such scalding does not have the splash pattern that is associated with random application as one would expect with accidental scalding.

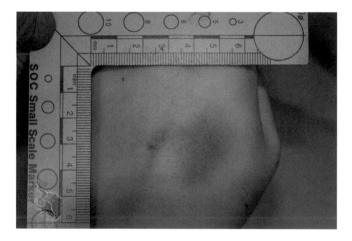

Figure 11.5   Photograph of bruise with a scale.

Investigations are carried out during the course of an examination which aims specifically to produce medical evidence that may corroborate or rebut allegations of torture. Initially, a detailed history needs to be obtained from the victim and an in-depth psychological assessment should be made to assist in determining whether the allegations of torture are genuine and to direct further investigations.

The investigations will depend on whether resources are available; if resources are limited it would be unethical to divert valuable clinical resources for medico-legal purposes. Which investigations are needed will depend on the level of proof necessary. Some survivors will have been tortured using, for example, electric shock devices, and being examined using medical equipment might trigger intrusive memories.

Where investigations are indicated, and the individual consents, there are a wide range of possible investigations which can be carried out.

Radiological imaging provides important visual evidence of recent or old trauma or its effects and includes:

- routine radiography

- radioisotopic scintigraphy

- computerised tomography (CT),

- magnetic resonance imaging (MRI)

- ultrasonography.

All injured areas should have routine radiographs as the initial examination. Whilst routine radiographs will demonstrate facial fractures, CT is a superior examination as it demonstrates more fractures, fragment displacement, and associated soft tissue injury and complications. It is possible for a fracture to heal, leaving no radiographic evidence of previous injury. This is especially true in children. When periosteal damage or minimal fractures are suspected, bone scintigraphy should be used in addition to X-rays. A percentage of X-rays will be negative even when there is an acute fracture or early osteomyelitis. Scintigraphy can also be used to detect testicular torsion and to assess falanga.

Ultrasound can be used to evaluate acute abdominal trauma, injuries to tendons as well as testicular abnormalities. It is also useful in the evaluation of the shoulder in the acute and chronic period following suspension. In the acute period, oedema, i.e. fluid collection on and around the shoulder joint, lacerations, and haematomas of the rotator cuffs can be observed.

CT, if available, is an excellent method of visualising bone and soft tissue, although MRI is preferable for soft tissue. CT enables the alignment and displacement of fractures to be assessed. When considering the time since injury, MRI can give a better correlation with time than CT.

Occasionally a skin biopsy may be necessary to examine for histological features specific to electric shock and studies have demonstrated pathognomonic changes in skin biopsies for several months following electric shocks. Negative findings, however, cannot be construed as evidence that the alleged torture did not occur, and the diagnosis is better made from elucidating a detailed history of electric shock injury.

There are also various toxicological and biochemical tests that can be carried out which may throw light on any short- or long-term effects of torture. For example, rhabdomyolysis due to muscle trauma will require the testing of blood and urine for its assessment.

Accurate documentation of findings, which can be reviewed by other personnel, is an essential part of the overall assessment of torture cases. Imaging as described above and the use of video, dictaphone, and sketches are all essential means of documentation in the examination of torture victims. The general requirements for documentation of injuries and other associated findings include:

- morphological description

- measurement of injury

- position on the body

- use of scales in imagery (Figure 11.55).

When handwritten notes or recorded findings are made they should be contemporaneous and retrospective. Handwritten notes should be legible and need to be signed and dated. Written and dictated material should be kept as permanent record and will form the basis of a report (statement) suitable for use in court.

In order to maintain the integrity of any documentation it must be free of any interference or tampering. Documentation must be signed and dated by the originator and, wherever possible, witnessed, be kept safe and secure, and be retrieved only by parties with authority to do so.

11.1.3 Torture and International Law

Systematic or widespread torture belongs to a special group of crimes recognised by international law as 'crimes against humanity'. This category further includes the practice of systematic or widespread murder, forced disappearances, deportation and forcible transfers, arbitrary detention, and persecutions on political or other grounds.

As discussed above, the law did not always define and prohibit torture. Instead, it was used to exercise formal, effective control over others, and as an instrument to implement official social control. Cultural, religious or ideological perspectives of the powerful elite often covertly sanctioned it. Thus validated, torture was understood as being in the interest of the community. In other words, in order for torture to be effective, it has to be used on public enemies with a religious, cultural or ideological mechanism of overt or implied justification that it is in the community interest (usually public order, security or law and order).

In common law torture was part of the legal process. The methods by which oaths and proofs could be established were invariably linked to the judicial infliction of pain for the establishment of a 'legal' truth – as in trial by ordeal. In certain situations, where the torturer exhibited a certain masochistic impulse that could influence operational behaviour, the torturer rationalised the infliction of pain and suffering as a form of moral cleansing or a moral purgative. It is a tribute to human progress that the judiciary were able to reform their procedural methods to conform to ideas of practical reason and operational moral sensibility. Religion and law generated a complex moral paradox. Torture was often deemed indispensable for the discovery of truth. The pain and suffering experienced in the practice of torture were also seen as providing the socially redeeming benefits of moral and spiritual cleansing.

11.1.4 The use of torture by the State

Torture is a powerful institutional expression of state craft, power, and social control. The official use of torture functionally means that the state uses these powers as critical components of security to intimidate or sometimes even eliminate its enemies, or indeed non-enemies. When torture becomes routine practice the state does not represent the moral order of the community, but instead is recognised as dispensing authorised violence and coercion, ensuring that power is achieved through the use of brute force. However, when power is maintained by practices of torture and ill-treatment, the claim to state legitimacy is illusory or weakened. The state also seeks to validate its use of violence and coercion by appeals to its authority. The use of torture by the state indicates insecurity in the processes of governance. Thus, the state tries to elevate the morality of its use of violence by appeals to notions of self-defence, the protection of security interests at all levels, and the morality of the survival of the state.

11.2 Development of Humanitarian Law and the Geneva Conventions

Humanitarian law came into being between 1864 and 1949 as a result of efforts by Henry Dunant, the founder of the International Committee of the Red Cross (ICRC). The conventions safeguard the human rights of individuals involved in armed conflict, and build on the 1899 and 1907 Hague Conventions, the international community's first attempt to formalise the laws of war and war crimes within secular international law. The conventions were revised as a result of the Second World War and readopted by the international community in 1949.

11.2.1 Humanitarian and Human Rights Law

International humanitarian law (IHL) and international human rights law (human rights) are complementary. Both strive to protect the lives, health, and dignity of individuals, albeit from different perspectives.

Humanitarian law applies in situations of armed conflict whereas human rights law protects the individual at all times, in war and peace alike. However, some human rights treaties permit governments to derogate from certain rights in situations of public emergency. No derogations are permitted under IHL because it was conceived for emergency situations, namely armed conflict.

Humanitarian law aims to protect people who do not or are no longer taking part in hostilities. The rules embodied in IHL impose duties on all parties to a conflict. Human rights law, being tailored primarily for peacetime, apply to everyone. Their principal goal is to protect individuals from arbitrary behaviour by their own governments. Human rights law does not deal with the conduct of hostilities.

Since humanitarian law applies precisely to the exceptional situations which constitute armed conflicts, the content of human rights law that states must respect in all circumstances tends to converge with the fundamental and legal guarantees provided by humanitarian law, e.g. the prohibition of torture and summary executions.

11.2.2 Recent international conventions or instruments

A number of international conventions or instruments recognise these crimes as crimes against humanity. Although humanitarian law had its roots in the nineteenth century with the founding of the ICRC, it was not until the end of the Second World War that a concerted effort was made to uphold human rights in all respects with the Universal Declaration of Human Rights.

11.2.2.1 Universal Declaration of Human Rights On 10 December 1948, the General Assembly of the United Nations adopted and proclaimed the Universal Declaration of Human Rights. Following this historic act, the Assembly called upon all member countries to publicise the text of the Declaration and to 'cause it to be disseminated, displayed, read and expounded principally in schools and other educational institutions, without distinction based on political status of countries or territories'.

Some of the relevant articles to forensic medical practitioners include:

- Article 3: Everyone has a right to life, liberty and security of person.

- Article 5: No one shall be subject to torture or to cruel, inhuman or degrading treatment or punishment.

- Article 11(1): Everyone charged with a penal offence has the right to be presumed innocent until proved guilty according to law in a public trial at which he has had all the guarantees necessary for his defence.

Since the Universal Declaration of Human Rights in 1948, the right to be free from torture has been taken up in major international and regional treaties and instruments. A chronology some of these is shown in Figure 11.6.

1949	The Four Geneva Conventions
1950	The European Convention on Human Rights
1966	UN Standard Minimum Rules for the Treatment of Prisoners
1966	International Covenant on Civil and Political Rights
1979	The American Convention on Human Rights
1979	UN Code of Conduct for Law Enforcement Officials
1981	The African Charter on Human and People's Rights
1982	Principles of Medical Ethics Relevant to the Role of Health Personnel, Particularly Physicians, in the Protection of Prisoners and Detainees against Torture and Other Cruel, Inhuman or Degrading Treatment or Punishment
1984	UN Convention against Torture and Other Cruel, Inhuman or Degrading Treatment or Punishment
1987	The European Convention for the Prevention of Torture and Inhuman or Degrading Treatment or Punishment entry into force
1989	Council of Europe Committee for the Prevention of Torture
1990	UN Rules for the Protection of Juveniles Deprived of their Liberty
1998	Statute of the International Criminal Court
1999	Istanbul Protocol: Manual on the effective investigation and documentation of torture and other cruel, inhuman or degrading treatment or punishment. Submitted to the United Nations Commission for Human Rights.
2002	Optional Protocol to the UN Committee against Torture establishing a universal visiting scheme

Figure 11.6 Chronology of major international and regional treaties and instruments after the Universal Declaration of Human Rights.

11.2.3 Global support for human security

The International Criminal Court, in force and active since 2002, represents a tool to end impunity for genocide, crimes against humanity, and war crimes at the global level. Torture is recognised by its statute as a crime against humanity. A crime against humanity can be committed in times of armed conflict, but also in times of 'peace'. The prerequisite is that torture is conducted in a widespread or systematic attack against any civilian population.

11.3 Responses to torture and its eradication

In order to combat and eradicate torture there needs to be an effective legal framework assuring its full implementation. There must be appropriate safeguards applied for prevention and combating impunity. Control mechanisms need to be established, including national visiting mechanisms to places of detention and independent monitoring and reporting by civil organisations. It is also vital that ongoing training should be in place for police officers, prison guards, lawyers, judges, and medical doctors.

11.4 Physician participation in torture

The medical establishment's involvement in torture dates back to ancient Greece, although the first official reference to medical activity in the practice is in the Constitutio Criminalis Carolina of 1532 in the time of Charles V, emperor of the Holy Roman Empire, which established the European legal roots of the physician's presence during torture.

Torture was thought of as necessary to prevent criminal activity, so it was enshrined in the legal system and widely acknowledged. As representatives of the state, physicians were expected to carry out the law. Their cooperation was not a consequence of coercion or fear of reprisal. Surprisingly, in light of this legal situation, much of the criticism of torture beginning in the sixteenth century came from the very physicians who participated in it. Doctors did not at first argue on moral or ethical grounds, condemning the cruelty of torment or the infliction of pain, rather, they questioned the reliability of the testimony given under torture by those who were persecuted. Physicians provided medical certificates that documented the defendant's state of health and mind and his or her ability to survive torture. If the accused was weak or ill, doctors recommended different methods of torment that could be endured. Physicians also determined when the pain had to be stopped in order to prevent sudden death. They assessed whether the accused was truly unconscious or not and treated injuries to allow the persecution to continue.

As modern torture became progressively more scientific, physicians became actively involved by inventing new technical possibilities and by administering, for example, psychiatric, pharmacological, and psychological forms of torture.

Miles (2015) goes as far as to state that doctors are integral to the practice of modern torture. Some devise torture techniques (like rectal water infusions) in order to minimise incriminating scars. Some monitor and treat prisoners undergoing torture in order to prevent them from unintentionally dying. Some falsify medical records and death certificates to assist regimes in concealing injuries or deaths from torture. Many claim to act under duress, but the example set by the majority of their national colleagues who either fight against torture or refuse to collaborate with the practice belies such claims.

International declarations condemning medical personnel's participation in torture began to appear. Amongst the most important of these are the Declaration of Geneva and the Declaration of Tokyo, which were adopted by the World Medical Association in 1968 and 1975, respectively. These declarations state that physicians must maintain 'the utmost respect for human life' even under threat, and any medical participation in torture is forbidden. Similarly, the United Nations' resolution on Principles of Medical Ethics (1983) forbids physician abuse of the patient–doctor relationship to aid in torture or interrogation of suspects.

11.5 Physician participation in Capital punishment

Despite objections by many professional organisations, the participation of physicians and nurses in capital punishment continues and is likely to become more common in the years ahead. This participation raises important questions about the ethical standards of the medical profession and how they should be enforced (Boehnlein 2013). The majority of Americans favour capital punishment and many physicians believe that medical participation in executions is not only ethical but a civic duty. Simply requiring that physicians not be forced to participate against their conscience would not put an end to medical involvement in capital punishment.

During the French Revolution, the physician Joseph Ignace Guillotin developed the guillotine as a more humane and efficient method of execution. In recent years, lethal injection has become increasingly popular as a method of execution. It is less expensive than the alternatives, it is more acceptable to those who must witness the execution, it may increase the willingness of judges and juries to apply the death penalty, and it is generally seen, as the guillotine was in its day, as more humane and less painful than other methods.

11.5.1 Stages of participation in an execution

Stage 1   The first stage of participation is the provision of medical care for prisoners on death row. As part of this care, physicians may prescribe sedatives and tranquillisers at the request of inmates who are anxious about their impending execution. This form of medical involvement represents the *appropriate and humane care* that physicians have traditionally provided for all their patients.

Stage 2   This stage involves activities that are necessary to prepare for the execution. Physicians have helped design the protocols for execution by lethal injection and have given advice on the execution of particular convicts.

Stage 3   This may include participation in the execution itself. Although some claim that it is not necessary for physicians to participate in executions by lethal injection, several well-documented mishaps underscore the advantages of medical participation. For example, the execution of Ricky Ray Rector in Arkansas in January 1992 was delayed for 45 minutes whilst the prison staff, under the supervision of a former military medic, attempted to insert an intravenous catheter, both percutaneously and by surgical cut down.

Stage 4   Declaring or pronouncing death may place the physician in the same role as that of a physician who participates in torture – that is, directing and regulating the administration of the punishment until the desired end is achieved. When Alpha Otis Stephens was electrocuted in

Georgia in 1984, the first two-minute charge of electricity failed to kill him. His body had to cool for six minutes before doctors could examine him, during which time Stephens appeared to be struggling to breathe. After two doctors had determined that he was still alive, a fatal charge of electricity was applied.

Stage 5 Stage 5 is the certification of death. The AMA guidelines distinguish between 'pronouncing' death, which is claimed to be unethical, and 'certifying' death, which is said to be acceptable. Pronouncing death involves 'monitoring the condition of the condemned during the execution and determining the point at which the individual has actually died'. Certifying death, on the other hand, is 'confirming that the individual is dead after another person has pronounced or determined that the individual is dead'. This distinction is rejected and it is agreed that physicians should not be permitted either to pronounce or to certify death. Certification of death occurs after the execution has been completed, does not require medical expertise, and in fact may be performed by non-medical civic officials in some jurisdictions.

Stage 6 Stage 6, which follows certification of death, is the retrieval of organs for donation – a common practice in some countries. An unsuccessful attempt was made to retrieve organs after the execution of Margie Barfield by lethal injection in North Carolina in 1984. This practice should be prohibited.

11.5.2 Ethical considerations

Objections to physicians' participation in the death penalty are usually based on the Hippocratic dictum *Primum non nocere*, 'First, do no harm'. This reasoning is reasonable, provided that the harms involved are adequately described. Some have argued, for example, that the involvement of physicians in executions is ethically equivalent to their participation in torture. This argument misses an essential point, however, since some level of medical involvement (e.g. during stages 1 to 3) would probably minimise the torturous aspect of the death penalty. The death-row inmate may be seen as a terminally ill 'patient' whose death is unavoidable and imminent. The prisoner may request that a physician attend the execution to minimise the likelihood of suffering. In such circumstances, it can be argued that the participation of the physician is consistent with the professional norms of beneficence and consent.

Similarly, if the participation of physicians in capital punishment is harmful simply because such punishment is killing, then their involvement in euthanasia should be equally problematic. Yet it can be argued that euthanasia may be an ethical option for physicians in at least some instances. The paradox is that medical participation in euthanasia is nearly always illegal, even when it may be ethical, whereas medical participation in capital punishment is generally legal but widely viewed as unethical. Thus, the harm of participation by physicians in capital punishment is not entirely represented by the fact that capital punishment involves killing. The execution of a condemned criminal lies far outside the medical sphere. A physician's participation in that execution does nothing to promote the moral community of medicine. Indeed, such participation offends the sense of community by prostituting medical knowledge and skills to serve the purposes of the state and its criminal justice system. Similarly, much concern about the participation of physicians in euthanasia centres on the place of euthanasia, or its lack of place, in the community of medicine. The role of physicians in executions is even further removed from the legitimate sphere of medicine, subverting the profession for the non-beneficent goals of the state. Medicine is at heart a profession of care, compassion, and healing. Physician-assisted capital punishment does not encompass these virtues.

11.6   The investigation of mass graves/multiple deaths related to armed conflict

The pathologist will be involved in the three essential stages of any mission involving the investigation of mass graves (Vanezis 1999):

– planning and organisation the mission before deployment of a team
– execution of the mission
– documentation of the mission and presentation of evidence.

11.6.1   Planning

It is essential to appreciate that there is no substitute for meticulous planning and organisation before the first team member actually leaves the home base on a mission. However, situations which require such expertise may erupt suddenly and then there may be little time to prepare for every eventuality. It should also be borne in mind that it is the responsibility of the international scientific and investigative community to learn from the successes and failures of the past, to allow them to prepare adequately for the uncertainties of the future.

The team will comprise multidisciplinary members from different relevant fields and will also depend on the type of scenario involved. The following are included in mass grave investigations:

pathologist	police team leader
anthropologist	support manager
archaeologist	logistics
mortuary technician	exhibit officers
radiographer/radiologist	recovery officers
safety officer	photographers.
other experts as necessary	

Before any mission can be started, there needs to be a preliminary assessment which involves a visit by a small group comprising the team leader and other appropriate personnel to assess the feasibility of the mission There should be meetings with key personnel and hosts of the country in question to address the issues that need to be resolved. Once this has been carried out, then the organisers of the mission are in a position to decide how to plan and execute the mission.

The timing of a mission may be influenced by a number of factors, including the political situation and security, funding, and climate/season. There may also be other priorities dictated nationally or by the international community.

It is essential to understand that the pathologist is not just on a fact-finding, evidence-gathering mission, but must also fully understand the importance of having a humanitarian and compassionate approach to his/her task. Victims and their families are central in the search for truth and justice, and ultimately to find closure in their grief.

In mass grave investigations carried out in the Balkans, my experience and that of other colleagues has been that it is important to involve the local population if the political situation allows. Many who have lost relatives, friends or compatriots in the conflict are more than willing to assist the exhumation team in appropriate ways. This has been helpful to mission teams. On their part members of the team, where appropriate, have also attended some of the funerals of the deceased whilst maintaining their professional objectivity (Figure 11.7).

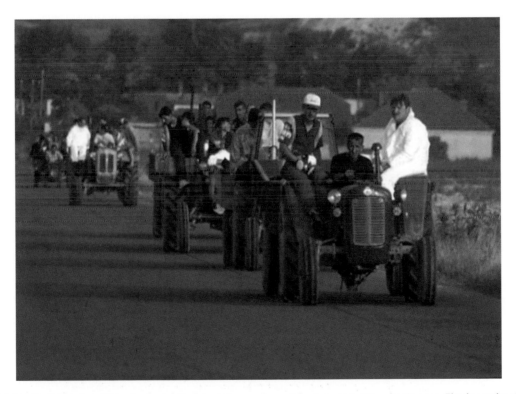

Figure 11.7 Victims being taken for burial that had been exhumed from a mass grave in Kosovo. The investigating team were also present at the burials.

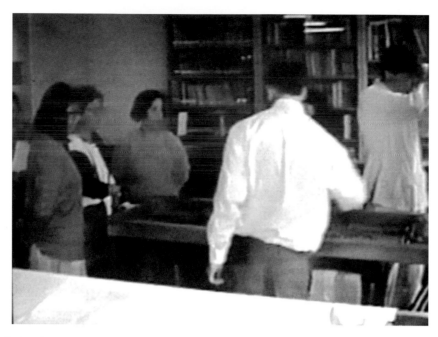

Figure 11.8   Relatives being shown skeletal remains of a victim who had 'disappeared' in Santiago Chile during the 1973 coup d'etat. (Source: Medico-Legal Institute, Santiago, Chile.)

The needs of relatives are paramount in all investigations involving their loved ones and they should be kept informed of progress on a regular basis. With regard to identification, once it has been confirmed, then if the relatives wish they should be permitted to view the remains of their loved ones and to have one of the members of the investigation explain the findings to them (Figure 11.8). On the other hand, it is not acceptable to request them to view bodies that are compromised in some way by injury or decomposition for the purpose of assisting in the initial stages as a means of identification. Identification should be confirmed first by the investigation team, using recognised scientific primary methods and corroborated with secondary means as necessary.

An example where humanitarian action was the purpose of an investigation concerns the exhumations carried out in Chile in 1991 of 126 bodies which were buried in 1973 in one of the largest cemeteries of the capital city, Santiago. They were killed between September and December 1973 by the new military junta following the coup d'etat in the same year, headed by the regime of Augusto Pinochet which ousted the democratically elected president Salvador Allende. Most of the victims had been shot, mainly in the head. According to existing records, post-mortem examinations were carried out on all of the deceased before burial but no identifications were made. The main reason for not being able to identify the victims, according to the forensic specialists who carried out the autopsies, was that the bodies were too decomposed. The bodies remained buried for 18 years until a judicial investigation was opened and an exhumation was ordered. A general amnesty in 1978 ensured that the exhumations in Santiago were purely for humanitarian reasons.

In all situations the attitude of professionals involved in the investigation of human rights abuses should be one of objectivity, but this does not mean one has to be neutral. The pathologist would be wise to consider the words of CNN's Christiane Amanpour 1997, a very respected news correspondent, who reported on the conflict in the Balkans, in her defence of her style of journalism. She had outspokenly accused some Bosnian Serbs of vicious, unspeakable war crimes and refuted any suggestion that she lacked balance or objectivity. When interviewed Amanpour stated:

> It depends on what you mean by balance. If you want to balance the victim and the aggressor, be my guest. It's not the kind of thing that is accurate and therefore I cannot report that way. In certain instances it is very clear who is the victim and who is the aggressor and what is the result. Bosnia was one of those.

She would also be the first to agree, however, that both sides should receive a fair hearing. Although there are two sides to any argument, if one is looking for motives, citing history, race or religion to list but a few, does not provide any form of justification for the slaughter that had been witnessed over the last few years and is currently being witnessed in the Middle East. From the pathologist's point of view, where there is unequivocal evidence of abuse his/her position should be clear. The truth must come out and there should be no fence-sitting or attempts to bend over backwards to see both sides' point of view.

References

Amanpour C. (1997). On top of a troubled world. *Highlife*, British Airways magazine June 1997.

Boehnlein, J.K. (2013). Should physicians participate in state-ordered executions? *AMA J. Ethics* 15: 240–243.

Kamen, H. (2014). *The Spanish Inquisition: A Historical Revision*. New Haven: Yale University Press.

Miles, S.H. (2015). Policy forum: medical associations and accountability for physician participation in torture. *AMA J. Ethics* 17: 945–951.

Office of the United Nations High Commissioner for Human Rights (2004). Professional Training Series No. 8/Rev.1 Istanbul Protocol. Manual on the Effective Investigation and Documentation of Torture and Other Cruel, Inhuman or Degrading Treatment or Punishment. United Nations, New York and Geneva.

Office of the United Nations High Commissioner for Human Rights (OHCHR) (2016). Palais des Nations, Geneva.

United Nations Convention against Torture and Other Cruel, Inhuman or Degrading Treatment or Punishment (1984)

United Nations (1983). United Nations' resolution on the Principles of Medical Ethics. A/RES/38/118.

Vanezis, P. (1999). Investigation of clandestine graves resulting from human rights abuses. *J. Clin. Forensic Med.* 6: 238–242.

World Medical Association Declaration of Tokyo (1975). Guidelines for physicians concerning torture and other cruel, inhuman or degrading treatment or punishment in relation to detention and imprisonment adopted by the 29th World Medical Assembly, Tokyo, Japan.

12
Sexual Offences

Philip Beh
Department of Pathology, University of Hong Kong, Hong Kong, PRC

12.1   Introduction

The evolution of society and in particular the acceptance of sexual equality has driven many changes in how society views sexual offences and hence how the criminal justice system responds to victims of sexual offences and sexual offenders. Readers would benefit greatly if they invest some time in reading about the history of rape laws (Dunn 2013). It is also important to remember that, as the world gets more connected and events in a particular region become widely known the world over, sexual offences during wars and conflicts now draw international outrage and condemnation. Rape during or as an aftermath of conflicts was commonplace and viewed as collateral from the times of the ancient world (Heineman 2013), but is now regarded as a crime against humanity and instigators can be prosecuted by the International Criminal Court.

12.2   Sexual offences

Every jurisdiction will have a variety of laws that cover what that community deems to be a sexual offence. Generically speaking legislation will aim to protect individuals against sexual acts that are deemed abhorrent to the community. It is therefore impossible to list all the possible different laws that exist around the world. However, Table 12.1 helps to illustrate the commonly found categories of sexual offences and also highlights some of the changes seen in recent decades (Table 12.1).

Essential Forensic Medicine, First Edition. Edited by Peter Vanezis.
© 2020 John Wiley & Sons Ltd. Published 2020 by John Wiley & Sons Ltd.

Table 12.1 Spectrum of laws on sexual offences.

Offence	Coverage	Law reform
Indecent assault	This covers a wide range of sexual assaults. It is often mistakenly thought that it involves only minor offences of inappropriate unwelcome touching of an individual. In reality it is often a catch-all for behaviours not covered by other specific laws. For example, in many jurisdictions forced oral sex and penetration of genitalia or anus with objects other than the male penis fall under this offence.	In some jurisdictions unauthorised photography of the private parts of individuals even when 'clothed' is an offence. Exposure of children to adult sexual content is another developing area.
Unlawful sexual intercourse	This covers a whole class of offences originally meant for the protection of young females. Hence, even with consent, children under a certain age (16) are deemed incapable of consent. Most jurisdictions consider that it is an even more serious form of assault at age 13. It is also common for the law to include individuals deemed to be mentally incompetent.	Changes here have seen the law apply also to male children. The sentencing for such offences now also reflects the moral norms of the community. In communities where teenagers are more likely to engage in sex, offences involving males who are also teenagers are dealt with much more leniently.
Rape	The definition of rape traditionally looks at the presence of consent as well as evidence of penetration of a female victim's genitalia by a male penis.	Reforms have looked at moving towards a requirement of 'positive consent' and not accepting an 'absence of dissent'. Reforms are also looking to apply the penetration to include all objects and to include oral and anal intercourse. Some have described this as making rape a non-gender specific crime. Increasingly, rape is also an offence within marriage, hence recognising the right of the wife to refuse.
Male homosexual intercourse	This was meant to protect young boys as well as non-consenting adults. Even consenting adults were technically in breach of the law and could be prosecuted.	Reform has allowed consenting acts in private. Ages of consent have also been aligned with those for the protection of young females in unlawful sexual intercourse legislation
Incest	This is an offence in most societies with a Christian influence. It is not always found in laws but may still be socially taboo in many communities.	Some jurisdictions are looking at expanding the coverage of this offence to include members of a step-family and also members of an adopted family.
Bestiality	This is a reflection of social morality. It is not always found in laws and may or may not be a social taboo in some communities	None
Public indecency	In some communities, strict controls on dress and behaviour apply to females and close proximity of an unmarried female to a male is considered an offence.	

12.3 Responding to sexual offences

The care and management of survivors of sexual offences have seen much improvement and changes in emphasis in the last half century. In a nutshell, the emphasis is now clearly on the provision of a variety of services from a team of multidisciplinary specialists in a way that best meets the needs of the 'individual survivor' (victim). It is widely promoted now that such services should best be integrated and delivered as a 'one-stop service' (WHO 2003). This approach was first proposed by Burgess and Holmstrom (1973). Typically, the team will consist of social workers, crisis counsellors, nurses, doctors, psychologists, and in some settings even police officers and prosecutors. The availability of these individuals can be a challenge in locations where resources are limited; however, the concept of a multidisciplinary approach to care can still occur with an individual adopting several roles. It is quite common therefore to see social workers adopting the role of counsellors and advocates, nurses taking the roles of doctors and counsellors, and police officers the role of prosecutors.

A state-of-the-art response also recommends a self-contained dedicated facility for survivors of sexual assaults where the victim can feel safe and receive all the services required. Such a facility must include reception, interview rooms, counselling rooms, medical examination room, shower facilities and changing room, evidence storage, and in some a video-recording room for recording statements (see Figures 12.1–12.4). Routine cleaning of the surfaces at least of the medical examination room must be carried out in order to prevent cross-contamination of trace evidence in between cases. A shower facility may appear a luxury for administrators but is a very important

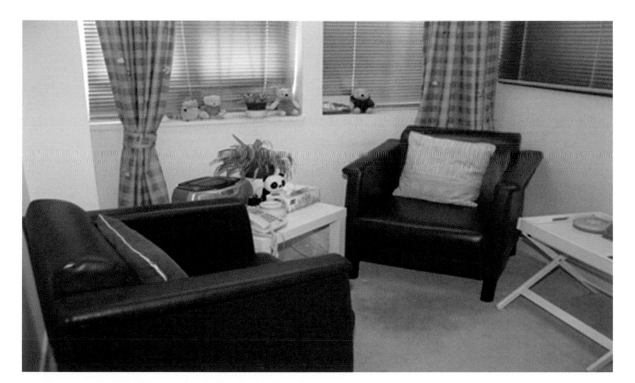

Figure 12.1 Interview room: comfortable chairs with some distance between them to allow victims to tell their ordeal to a trained crisis worker.

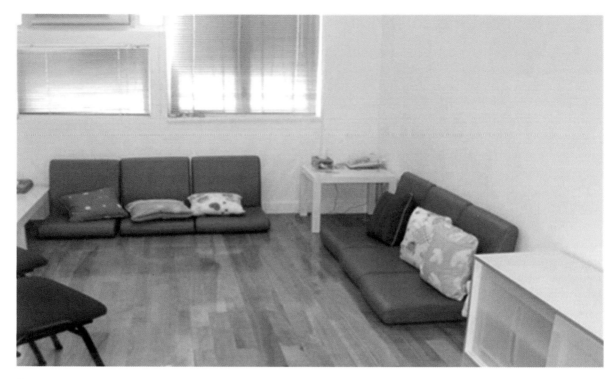

Figure 12.2 Counselling room: casual space for a more relaxed atmosphere and interaction. Useful for follow-up counselling sessions with survivors.

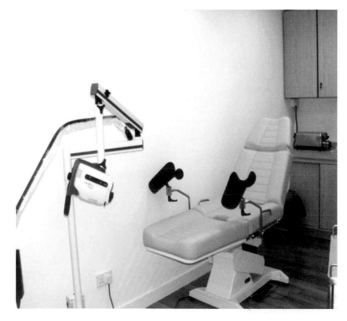

Figure 12.3 Medical examination room: shown here with a gynaecology examination couch, lighting, and a colposcope. Adequate storage cabinets are for forms, cotton swabs, containers, evidence bags, and labels. Ideally, surfaces are easy to clean to prevent cross-contamination between cases.

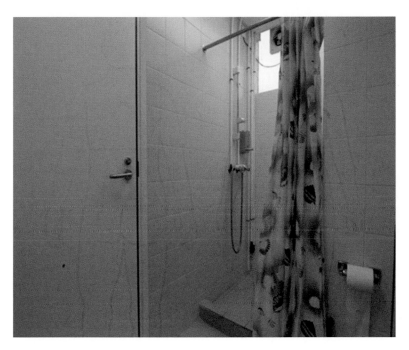

Figure 12.4 Shower facility to allow victims to wash after completion of the medical examination. A fresh set of clothing is also made available for victims to change into as it is likely that their clothing may be collected as evidence. Washing facilities are essential as they addresses a victim's need to 'cleanse' herself and also provides some time for the victim to settle her emotions before providing a long interview statement to the police.

facility as it serves an almost therapeutic role for many victims, who will frequently express a desperate need to wash and to cleanse themselves.

12.4 Attendance at scenes of sexual violence

It is uncommon for forensic doctors or nurses to be called to scenes of sexual assaults such as rape. Forensic scientists who do attend will have to decide what material will be needed and should be collected. It must be remembered that material collected may be important as a 'control' for establishing collaborating evidence of contact of the victim and/or offender with the scene. Material collected, commonly fibres from clothing, soil from clothing and shoes, head and body hair, blood and other body fluids, may also inform on the contact between the victim and the offender(s).

Fatal cases of sexual violence will always involve the pathologist, and similar care and attention should be in place to ensure that contact evidence that may be present on the body of the victim is not lost during the transfer of the body from the scene to the mortuary. It is common that forensic scientists or trained scene of crime officers will ensure good photographic recording of the body at the scene as well as collect body tapings to secure loose contact evidence such as hair, fibres, soil, etc., that may be on the body of the victim. Clothing should not be removed at the scene and should be examined and photographed as part of the process of autopsy photography. However, if a forensic DNA laboratory that is able to detect 'trace' or 'touch' DNA is involved, it may be preferable to securely collect the clothing at the scene to prevent possible further contamination.

The pathologist attending the scene of a sexual homicide or an auto-erotic death must be aware of some of the unique features present at a scene that may help understand what has happened. In auto-erotic deaths, evidence of previous occurrences such as 'worn-out' marks on suspension points, evidence of well-worn straps and restraints, and video recordings of previous activities may help give a sense of the background that may be associated with an auto-erotic death by helping to decipher if a death may be accidental due to inexperience or perhaps suicidal and intended. The examiner must, however, remain open minded and never forget that it is also possible for a sexual homicide to be 'staged'.

In sexual homicides, examination of the scene together with the autopsy findings of injuries associated with the death can help suggest a particular typology to the type of sexual homicide (Ressler et al. 1988). A sexual homicide associated with a violent struggle with extensive injuries on the victim as well as much blood splatter and damage of the scene suggests a 'disorganised' attacker. A 'clean' scene where there is evidence of post-attack activity and attempts at cleaning up or destroying evidence, on the other hand, suggests an 'organised' attacker. Most pathologists will not have enough experience of sexual homicides to develop such expertise, hence it is always important that in cases of sexual homicides the scene is well recorded in as much detail as possible. The development and use of extensive systematic scene photography and scene videography is invaluable under such circumstances. Such meticulous recording of details will allow others with such experience to review and comment in case the homicide becomes one of a serial killer's killing spree. Geberth (2003) offers a comprehensive crime-scene checklist for sex-related deaths.

12.5   Examination for injuries in sexual assault

It must be remembered that in the majority of victims of sexual offences there are no injuries. That said, the examination for injuries and their proper documentation is important and should be conducted in a systematic way. Many examination protocols and even rape examination kits have been developed around the world and some examples are provided by Crowley (1999). Protocols and examination kits do not make experts, and those charged with such duties or, preferably, those who have taken an informed interest in providing such services should ensure adequate training in such procedures before embarking on offering such services. There can be no dispute that victims prefer to be examined by a female doctor or a sexual assault nurse examiner (Chowdhury-Hawkins et al. 2008) despite dissent from male doctors (Templeton et al. 2010).

In the living victim of sexual violence, it is critical that the forensic examiner obtains informed consent directly from the victim. It must be made very clear to the victim that he/she only can agree to the examination, the extent of the examination, the recording of the examination (particularly if photography is needed), the collection and submission of samples, and the release of reports. It is often the practice that the victim is invited to stand on a 'ground sheet'. This 'ground sheet' is nothing more than a large piece of clean paper, plastic sheet or cloth. It must be clean and light in colour, preferably white. If the victim is still wearing the same clothing as was worn during the assault, he or she will then be invited to remove such clothing whilst standing on this 'ground sheet'. Debris that may drop off are hence collected. Clothing removed should be individually packed and labelled. The victim can then be offered an examination robe. The 'ground sheet' can then be collected, packaged and labelled for later examination.

The examination should be always systematic. It is quite common now in many jurisdictions that an examination proforma is used together with rape examination kits that are pre-packed with all the necessary swabs, evidence bags, containers, and labels. These are useful and helpful aids and if used as designed can serve to ensure a minimum quality in the examination. It must be remembered, however, that most such protocols are meant to be completely filled in to be effective. It is not uncommon to see the best designed protocol rendered useless because the examiner failed to use it appropriately.

A head-to-toe approach is simple and ideal and ensures that nothing is missed. It also ensures that examiners are not distracted by a specific area with injuries, only to then neglect others.

12.5.1 Head

Common injuries affecting the head in a case of sexual violence include:

a. *Hair pulling.* In extreme cases, chunks of hair may have been pulled out, leaving an obvious area of the scalp that is 'bare' with fresh evidence of bleeding. In less severe and obvious cases, victims are able to help the examiner by indicating regions of the head that are painful. Careful spreading of the hair may reveal an area of redness of the underlying scalp. Where possible, colour photography should be done. However, it is very difficult to demonstrate this easily and the examiner should describe the size of the area and its location adequately.

b. *Blunt impact to the head by or against a hard object.* Punches and kicks to the head are common and can result in bruising, abrasion, laceration or a combination of such injuries. These are usually irregular and are seen over the forehead, top, and back of the head. Where objects are used, the examiner should note the presence of patterns that may give some information about the object concern, e.g. hammer head imprints, etc. Such severe blunt traumas are rare in surviving victims of sexual assaults but can easily be present in fatal sexual assaults. Knife and gunshot wounds also may be found in fatal cases.

12.5.2 Face

The face is a common area where injuries and marks of violence can be found. Again, typically these are the result of blunt trauma usually as a result of blows by fists, kicking, and objects. Some common findings include the following:

a. Generalised facial congestion with petechial haemorrhages, found in fatal cases involving strangulation or smothering. This is also quite vividly seen in survivors where there was attempted strangulation or smothering.

b. Injuries to the eyes include direct trauma leading to bleeding and swelling of the eyelids and possible injury to the eyeball itself. In acute cases, victims may not be able to open their eyes and it may be painful for the victim to attempt to examine the eyelids properly. An ophthalmologist should be consulted for their assistance in such cases so as to repair and potentially save an eye and prevent permanent loss or damage to the eyesight.

c. Peri-orbital bruising and swelling may be a result of the gravitation of blood from trauma of the head (particularly injuries over the forehead). More sinisterly, subconjunctival haemorrhages may indicate the presence of intracranial injury and haemorrhage.

d. In cases of strangulation, petechial haemorrhages can be found in the conjunctivae along with petechial haemorrhages over the face.

e. Blows to the nose may also result in fractures of the nasal septum, resulting in swelling and bruising over the nose associated with nose bleeds.

f. Bruising and swelling over the cheekbones are also quite common following blunt impacts.

g. Where blows to or against the mouth have occurred, one may find broken tooth/teeth, lacerations to the mucosal surfaces of the lips, and swelling of the lip(s).

12.5.3   Neck

The neck may show the presence of discrete bruises that may be the result of grip marks in attempted manual strangulation or ligature marks from attempted ligature strangulation. There may also be abrasions associated with manual strangulation caused by the assailant or by the victim in an attempt to remove a strangulating ligature or hand(s).

It is not uncommon to see 'suction bruises', referred to as 'love bites' in some communities. The presence of such bruises should remind the examiner to swab the skin surfaces over them to collect possible saliva samples of the assailant for DNA analysis.

12.5.4   Trunk

All injuries present should be recorded. Bruises and swelling as a result of kicking or the body coming into contact with furniture, etc. may be found. The proper recording of such injuries and their measurement may sometimes be helpful and collaborative of accounts of the assault. Measuring the injury from the feet of the victim can help in case comparisons with the height of objects that might be involved in causing injury.

Common findings over the trunk, particularly in female victims, are bruises and bite marks of the breasts. Again, these injuries are a potential source of the offender's DNA. Bite marks should be properly photographed with scales to facilitate the possible need to create a life-size replica for comparison purposes. Injuries may also be found over the back of the trunk and buttocks where the body of the victim may be pressed down into protruding objects on the ground or floor. Abrasions may occur when a victim is dragged across a rough surface.

12.5.5   Limbs

Common injuries are likely to be bruises and abrasions. Fingertip bruises over the upper limbs are common in a struggle and efforts to restrain the movement of the victim by assailant(s). Occasionally ligature and handcuff marks may also be seen. Damage to the fingernail(s) may be found in victims with long and manicured nails. Breakage of one or more nails may be found in a struggle and broken parts of nails if recovered from a scene can provide good collaboration evidence. Victims may also have scratched an assailant and skin tissue and/or blood may be found underneath the finger-nails. Fingernail scrapings with a clean pointed piece of plastic or wooden object can help in the collection of such debris for forensic analysis.

In the lower limbs, bruises and abrasions may be found over the inner aspect of the thighs in forceful separation of a victim's lower limbs. Grip marks may also be found over the lower leg or ankles in attempts to grip and forcefully spread open the lower limbs of a victim.

Bruises and abrasions from bumps and falls in a struggle to escape are also quite common.

12.5.6 Ano-genital region

The examination of the ano-genital region should be approached in a sensitive manner. The examiner needs to explain clearly to the victim what will be done, how it will be done, and why it needs to be done. It is also important to reassure the victim that any part of the examination can be stopped if that is their wish.

Doctors or nurses performing such examination should familiarise themselves with the anatomy of the male and female genitalia and perineum. There are again many diagrams available and the uses of such charts is highly recommended (Crowley 1999).

In the examination of the ano-genital region, the lithotomy position with both legs raised, separated and supported on straps or pedestals is the recommended ideal position for visualisation and examination. Knee-chest position is embarrassing and should not be used in adults. In very young children, the knee chest position can be useful and appropriate.

A general examination of the perineum should be conducted and loose material such as hair and other debris collected. Obvious blood or fluid stains should be swabbed. Some examiners will also comb the pubic hair in an effort to collect fibres or loose hair that may be trapped.

Injuries such as bruises and abrasions to the vulva and perineum should be noted, measured, and recorded. Photography of the perineum is particularly sensitive and specific consent must be obtained. Injuries to the hymen, fourchette, and vaginal wall should be looked for and recorded when present. Proponents of colposcopy recommend their use and indeed if one is available, should be used as it allows for a better illumination and visualisation of the vaginal opening.

The presence of injuries is always associated with discomfort and there is rarely any difficulty identifying the presence of recent or fresh injuries. There may sometimes be bleeding and the assistance of a gynaecologist may be needed if bleeding is substantial as hidden vaginal wall injuries may need to be identified and treated.

Various devices have been used in the examination of the private parts such as the use of the vaginal speculum or the use of Glaister's globes to measure the size of the hymenal opening. It must be remembered that the introduction of such devices into a victim of a recent sexual assault is particularly traumatic and sensitive. Where injuries are present, they no doubt increase the discomfort, hence the use of such devices will need to be clearly established and justified.

The collection of appropriate vulval, vaginal, and cervical swabs can often be done without the need for such devices. The gradual increase in availability of paediatric flexible endoscopic instruments may allow their adaptation for use in such forensic settings in future.

The examination of the anal orifice and the collection of anal and rectal swabs must be guided by the history of the incident and the allegations made by the victim. It must be remembered that the examiner may need to gently ask specifically if anal or, for that matter, oral intercourse had occurred.

Table 12.2 List of exhibits from a victim of rape.

Item	Purpose	Packaging
Clothing	Examination for damage Examination for stains from body fluids Examination for contact trace evidence	Individual pieces of clothing packed in separate paper bags Clothing that is wet should ideally be dried before packing or delivered to the forensic laboratory immediately
Ground sheet	Collection of loose trace evidence	Folded and packed in evidence bags that are sealed
Hair combing	Loose hair and fibres	Sealed evidence bag
Cotton swab	Swabs of bitemarks, stains on skin, vulva, vagina, anal, rectum, mouth, etc., recovery of DNA	Swabs should be 'dried' and kept in a sealed plastic container or glass bottle in a fridge if there is delay in getting them to the forensic laboratory
Fingernail scrapings	Evidence of debris and skin and blood, trace contact as well as DNA	Kept in a sealed envelope or container
Fingernail cuttings	Comparison to broken fragment(s) of nail	Kept in sealed envelope or container
Loose debris, fibres, hair	Comparison with controls	Glass or plastic adhesive strips
Blood	DNA control, toxicology	Appropriate containers required by toxicology laboratory
Urine	Toxicology, pregnancy tests	Appropriate containers required by toxicology laboratory

At the end of the examination, the examiner should have a complete and detailed recording of the presence, type, size, and location of injuries over the body and a list of material collected and labelled for collection as exhibits. A list of common exhibits can be found in Table 12.2.

The collection of blood and/or urine for toxicological screening will have to be guided by the individual details of the assault, the time interval before the examination as well as the capabilities and capacities of the toxicology laboratory. It is important to remember that drug-facilitated sexual assault is increasing and victims may often not remember much of the assault to tell the examiner. Alcohol is still by far the most common drug involved but many other substances have also been reported (Table 12.3).

12.6   Interpretation of findings

It is critical that findings are interpreted fairly and in an unbiased manner. It must also be remembered that it is not the role of the forensic examiner to determine if rape has occurred; that is a question for the court to decide. The following myths must be avoided:

1. The absence of injuries generally negates the occurrence of rape – this is simply not true. Injuries occur when there is physical force used. Rape under threats, under the influence of drugs or when there are great discrepancies in physical size or even numbers of assailant can occur with no injuries to be found.

Table 12.3 Common drugs found in drug-facilitated rapes.

Substance	Form	Actions	Effects
Alcohol	Liquid	Central depression	Wide-range of effects from disinhibition to motor incoordination to coma and death
Rohypnol	Tablet	Tranquilliser/hypnotic	Memory impairment, drowsiness, muscle relaxation, confusion, unconsciousness
Benzodiazepiness	Tablet	Tranquilliser/hypnotic	Memory impairment, drowsiness, muscle relaxation, confusion, unconsciousness
Gamma-hydroxy-butyrate (GHB)	Clear, odourless liquid	Illegal drug (not approved for any clinical use)	Intense drowsiness, verbal incoherence, hampered mobility, antegrade amnesia
Ketamine	Liquid, powder	Anaesthetic agent	Drowsinees, confusion, psychogenic, loss of consciousness
Ecstasy	Pills, powder, liquid	Hallucinogenic and stimulant	Extreme relaxation and positivity towards others, hallucinations, hyperthermia, tremors, seizures, unconsciousness

2. The absence of genital injuries negates rape – this is again not true, particularly if the victim is sexually experienced and no foreign objects were used. Indeed, even victims who had no previous sexual experience may not have injuries after a rape (White and McLean 2006).

3. The presence of genital injuries must indicate that rape has occurred – it is again not true as many women have reported suffering genital injuries following consensual sexual intercourse (Sommers et al. 2006).

4. The presence of DNA from the alleged suspect indicates rape – this finding merely indicates that sexual intercourse was likely to have occurred; it does not help clarify the question of consent.

12.7 Examination of Fatal Sexual Assault

Fatal sexual assaults must always be at the back of the mind of any pathologist in a case involving the unexplained death of a female victim. It is a fallacy to only think of such a possibility when the victim is naked or semi-naked. Victims of sexual homicides may be 'dressed' up as part of a ritual, as part of the process of staging a crime scene or in an effort to move or transport the body from the primary scene for disposal or concealment purposes.

In dealing with a potential sexual homicide, the pathologist should remember to obtain anal and rectal swabs prior to the use of a rectal thermometer if there is a requirement for measuring postmortem body temperature. Photographs of the body in situ should be adequate to ensure that details of the presence of absence of clothing are clearly seen. It is again not uncommon for victims to be re-dressed, but improperly.

The collection of swabs for DNA is no different from those needed in a surviving victim of sexual assault. Several questions arise in cases of sexual homicides and attempts to document the any evidence of asphyxia or the manner (mode) of death can help answer questions that invariably arise during court trials.

12.7.1   Evidence of Asphyxia

A frequent and common scenario suggested by defendants in rape homicides involves the question of strangulation. Frequently, it is suggested that the individuals were engaged in consensual sexual activity and the victim enjoyed having some pressure applied to the neck to enhance the sexual experience. Hence, it is important for the pathologist to specifically look for and document the presence of generalised congestion of the face and upper neck, and petechial haemorrhages over the face, the conjunctivae, and the mucosal linings of the mouth. It is also important to document the presence or absence of any marks over the neck, or abrasions, bruises or even areas of 'blanching' that may be due to the application of a smooth soft ligature.

A careful layer-by-layer dissection of the neck should be carried out, looking carefully at the presence or absence of bruises of the soft tissues, injuries to the hyoid and thyroid cartilages, bruises around the carotid arteries, tear of the intimal lining of the carotid arteries. Such examination should allow a clear conclusion about the presence or absence of injuries over the neck that may or may not have caused death.

In some cases of sexual homicides there may be intentional disfigurement of the victim's face and removal of body parts. The psychology about such behaviour has been extensively written about by Geberth (2003). In some cases of necrophilia and dismemberments, sexual organs such as the breasts, penis, and female genitalia are cut out and removed. This may be a result of a 'warped attempt' to conceal the sexual identity of a body but may also be the result of a more complex psychopathy where the urge to humiliate the victim continues despite their death. It is not uncommon that serial sexual killers collect such 'trophies'. Sometimes, recovery of such artefacts may help in identifying the victims of the killer through DNA and/or anthropological analysis of bony artefacts.

12.7.2   Modes of death

In sexual homicide, it is not uncommon for a defendant to allege that the death was an 'accident' due to an unexpected result of a mutually consenting sexual act no matter how bizarre it may appear, as illustrated in the following case:

> Two males had just met but decided and agreed to engage in sexual acts involving bondage with chains and other paraphernalia. The activities occurred in the premises of one of the individuals and the activities were videotaped. Both individuals had taken some alcohol and some drugs, and it could be seen from the videos that as the evening wore on they were getting drowsy and tired. One of them was hog-tied with chains around his ankles as well as his neck, with a connecting length of chain between the neck and the ankles. He was also hand-cuffed with his hands behind his back. The individual was able to apply or loosen the pressure of the chain around his neck by flexing or extending his knees. The video recorded them falling asleep, only for the defendant to wake up to find the victim dead with a very congested face as a result of the pressure of the chain on the neck as the knees relaxed and pulled on the interconnecting chain. Death in this case was clearly a result of ligature strangulation and the defendant was convicted of manslaughter for engaging in a dangerous act that had caused the death.

Another common scenario raised by defendants is that of vaso-vagal death. Typically, it is suggested that both individuals were engaged in consensual sexual activity and one placed a hand or ligature over the neck of the deceased victim and the victim 'just collapsed'. Juries are more likely to give the benefit of the doubt in such cases if there is no evidence of any significant injury found. Clinically it is known that pressure over the carotid body can cause a transient loss of consciousness. Indeed this is refined into the so-called 'sleeper hold' that some law enforcement agencies adopt to train their officers on how to subdue violent or struggling individuals. When faced with such circumstantial accounts the pathologist must remain open-minded and accept that colleagues around the world have encountered similar cases of sudden deaths in the absence of obvious injuries (Saukko and Knight 2004).

Bizarre examples of sexual homicides are occasionally seen by forensic pathologists where an incredible assortment of objects may have been inserted into the vagina or rectum. In some instances death is a result of obvious perforating injuries resulting in blood loss. In others, it is less clear and the exact mode of death may just not be known. Pathologists should perhaps work with an open-mind and look for and exclude the presence of intentional injuries.

References

Burgess, A.W. and Holmstrom, L.L. (1973). The rape victim in the emergency room. *Am. J. Nurs.* 73: 1740–1745.

Chowdhury-Hawkins, R.A., Mclean, U., Winterholler, M., and Welch, J. (2008). Preferred choice of gender of staff providing care to victims of sexual assault in sexual assault referral centers (SARCS). *J. Forensic Legal Med.* 15: 363–367.

Crowley, S.R. (1999). *Sexual Assault – The Medical-Legal Examination*. Appleton & Lange.

Dunn, C. (2013). *Stolen Women in Medieval England: Rape, Abduction and Adultery*, 1100–1500. Cambridge University Press.

Geberth, V.J. (2003). *Sex-Related Homicide and Death Investigation – Practical and Clinical Perspectives*. CRC Press.

Heineman, E.D. (2013). *Sexual Violence in Conflict Zones – From the Ancient World to the Era of Human Rights*. University of Pennsylvania Press.

Ressler, R.K., Burgess, A.W., and Douglas, J.E. (1988). *Sexual Homicide: Patterns and Motives*. MA: D.C. Heath Lexington.

Saukko, P. and Knight, B. (2004). *Knight's Forensic Pathology*, 3e. Arnold.

Sommers, M.S., Zink, T., Baker, R.B. et al. (2006). The effects of age and ethnicity on physical injury from rape. *J. Obstet. Gynecol. Neonatal. Nurs.* 35: 199–207.

Templeton, D.J., Williams, A., Healey, L. et al. (2010). Male forensic physician have an important role in sexual assault care [correspondence]. *J. Forensic Legal Med.* 17: 50–52.

White, C. and McLean, I. (2006). Adolescent complaints of sexual assaults: injury patterns in virgin and non-virgin groups. *J. Clin. Forensic Med.* 13: 172–180.

World Health Organization (2003). *Guidelines for Medico-Legal Care of Victims of Sexual Violence*. World Health Organization.

Further reading

Gall, J. and Payne-James, J. (2011). *Current Practice in Forensic Medicine*. Wiley-Blackwell.

13
Paediatric Forensic Medicine

Philip Beh[1] and Peter Vanezis[2]
[1] Department of Pathology, University of Hong Kong, Hong Kong, PRC
[2] Queen Mary University of London, London, UK[3]

13.1 Introduction

This chapter will deal in the main with the subject of child abuse, although other areas of forensic interest in young infants and the newborn will also be discussed. Other categories of deaths in children will be dealt with elsewhere together with adult deaths.

13.2 Stillbirth/neonatal deaths

A stillbirth is defined in English law (Stillbirth (Definition) Act 1992) as a baby who, after 24 weeks of pregnancy and after being completely expelled from its mother, is not breathing or showing any other signs of life. Prior to this, the definition referred to stillbirths as those occurring after 28 weeks.

If a child is born dead in the circumstances set out in the Act, the doctor or midwife will issue a medical certificate of stillbirth that enables the stillbirth to be registered. This is entered on to the Stillbirth Register, which is separate from the standard Register of Births. The woman or couple is then issued with a Certificate of Stillbirth and the documentation for burial or cremation. There is no provision to allow the registration of stillbirths before the 24th week of pregnancy.

13.2.1 Child destruction

Child destruction is the intentional killing of an unborn child capable of being born alive before it has had an independent existence from its mother. The pregnancy must have been for a period of at least 28 weeks for there to be primâ facie proof that the child was capable of being born alive.

Essential Forensic Medicine, First Edition. Edited by Peter Vanezis.
© 2020 John Wiley & Sons Ltd. Published 2020 by John Wiley & Sons Ltd.

The situation arises where the mother is injured intentionally by someone for the purpose of killing the unborn child or by carrying out an illegal late abortion. Conviction of the felony carries a sentence of life imprisonment (Infant Life (Preservation) Act 1929). The Act, however, excludes situations where it is proven that the act that caused the death of the child was done in good faith for the purpose only of preserving the life of the mother.

13.2.2   Determination of Live Birth and Infanticide

The forensic pathologist's involvement is directed towards ascertaining whether or not the infant has had a separate existence from its mother and to determine whether the death might be infanticide or murder. (Legal definitions relating to deaths where the mother is responsible for the death of her newborn infant vary amongst different countries.)

Under the criminal law of England and Wales, the partial defence of infanticide provides a defence for both murder and manslaughter. The Infanticide Act 1938 describes infanticide as occurring in the following circumstances: 'Where a woman by any wilful act or omission, causes the death of her child, being a child under the age of 12 months, but at the time of her act or omission the balance of her mind was disturbed by reason of her not having fully recovered from the effect of giving birth to the child'.

In a case where infanticide is claimed for an offence that otherwise would have been framed as murder or manslaughter, the burden of proof is on the prosecution to disprove a claim of infanticide beyond a reasonable doubt. Although the maximum penalty for infanticide is life imprisonment, in practice a non-custodial sentence is usually the outcome, often subject to medical treatment or a hospital order.

The burden of proof is on the prosecution to demonstrate that an infant has had a separate existence when a woman is charged with infanticide. As most pathologists are aware, making such an assessment can be extremely difficult, particularly if some time has elapsed since delivery and the body has undergone significant post-mortem change. There needs to very strong evidence of a live birth and this would include lungs which are well expanded, the presence of food in the stomach, and signs of bruising around the umbilical stump or accompanying any other marks of possible injury which may have occurred after birth.

13.3   Sudden death in infancy syndrome

Sudden death in infancy syndrome (SIDS) can only be diagnosed by exclusion and only after thorough autopsy examination, examination of the scene, and investigation of the medical history of both the mother and infant. The term can only be correctly applied once all appropriate investigations have been carried out to look for all known identifiable conditions that may lead to sudden and unexpected death in an infant.

It has long been known that there are characteristic features commonly seen in such deaths. The deaths are rare in the first week or two after birth, rise to a peak incidence between the second and fourth months, and then decrease to become rare after six months of age (Fleming et al. 2000). There is an excess of cases in boys, who constitute around 60% of the deaths. In the 1970s and 1980s several studies showed an apparently increasing number of such deaths, and epidemiological studies in Europe and New Zealand showed an apparent association with the (relatively recently introduced) practice of putting infants down to sleep in a prone position. The dramatic reduction in the numbers of such deaths that followed attempts to dissuade parents from using the prone sleeping position for babies, in Avon County in England and in New Zealand, led to the widespread adoption of 'Back to Sleep' campaigns in many countries in the early 1990s. This resulted in a marked fall in the overall infant mortality rate and the post-neonatal mortality rate. Although there has been a major decrease in the incidence of SIDS cases, in most Western countries it is still the most common cause of infant mortality in the first 12 months of life. In this age group, unnatural deaths, including homicides, are infrequent and may be missed initially. It is essential therefore in all cases where the manner of death is not obvious to cultivate a high index of suspicion tempered with a sensitive approach to the bereaved family.

A number of environmental risk factors have been identified, including prone or side sleeping positions, exposure to tobacco smoke before or after birth, and sleeping in hazardous circumstances, particularly those in which the head might become covered or the baby might become covered with excess bedding, especially at the time of acute viral infections. There is clearly an association, the nature of which is controversial, between co-sleeping and the risk of SIDS. In the great majority of instances when infants die whilst co-sleeping (sharing a sleep surface) with an adult, there is no direct evidence that death has arisen by any identifiable mechanism such as overlying and thus such deaths may be appropriately categorised as SIDS even though some concern may have arisen as to the role of the adult in causing or contributing to the death. The 2014 National Institute for Health and Care Excellence (NICE) guidance on parents co-sleeping with infants recognised that co-sleeping may be intentional or unintentional, and concluded that whilst there is evidence of an association between co-sleeping and increased risk of SIDS the evidence was not sufficient to deduce a causal relationship. The guidance suggested that all parents should be made aware of this association, particularly for preterm or low birthweight infants and for parents who smoke or have been drinking alcohol or taking recreational drugs (NICE 2014). Unfortunately, this guidance did not distinguish between co-sleeping in a bed and co-sleeping on a sofa or armchair, which has been found to significantly increase the risk of SIDS compared with bed sharing (Fleming et al. 2015).

13.3.1 Scene examination

In all cases where there is the slightest suspicion, in addition to the post-mortem examination the scene needs to be carefully evaluated (Iyasu et al. 1994). Bass et al. (1986) conducted death scene investigations in 26 consecutive cases in which a presumptive diagnosis of SIDS was made. In six cases they found strong circumstantial evidence of accidental death. In 18 other cases they discovered various possible causes of death other than SIDS, including accidental asphyxiation by an object in the cot, smothering by overlaying whilst sharing a bed, hyperthermia, and shaken baby syndrome. Their study suggested that many sudden deaths of infants have a definable cause that can be revealed by careful investigation of the scene of death.

At the scene one should take into account the following:

- When and in what position, where and by whom was the child found dead?

- Was there any vomit at the nostrils or mouth?

- One should always examine the crib, cot or bed in which the child has been found dead, and take careful note of any wetness thereon due to secretions, vomitus, etc. present on it. Any soiled bedding or baby clothes should be retained if this is felt appropriate. There is still some uncertainty as to whether the mattress may be of importance in relation to the causation of the death (i.e. the presence of fungal growth on it), and this may have to be kept (Blair et al. 1995). If it is felt that there is a possibility that the design of the cot may have accounted for an accidental asphyxial death, this should also be retained and examined fully in the laboratory.

- One should take into account the general state of cleanliness of the house and other factors, which indicate lifestyle, socio-economic factors, and provision for adequate nourishment for the family.

- One should also take into account the finding of any noxious substances, medicines, and drugs of abuse.

In any investigation of a SIDS death the following matters should always be specifically addressed:

- findings at the actual time that the baby was discovered dead

- physical and socio-economic findings in the household within which the child has been living

- immediate past medical history of the child

- information about the parents and other siblings

- full history of the child's developmental progress since birth

- information about other current and previous members of the same household, including baby sitters and child minders.

13.4   Child abuse

Wherever one works in the world, it is very likely that the forensic practitioner will be asked to help diagnose and give expert opinions involving the detection of child abuse. It is fair to say that the concept of child abuse is a relatively new one with the establishment of organised child protection societies. History buffs would also note that societies and laws for the prevention of cruelty to animals were in place well before those for children. It is interesting to note that although the Declaration of the Rights of the Child was proclaimed by the General Assembly of the United Nations in 1959, the Convention on the Rights of the Child was adopted in 1989 and entered into force only in 1990 (United Nations Convention of the Rights of the Child 1989).

The UN Convention on the Rights of the Child defines a child as everyone under 18 unless, 'under the law applicable to the child, majority is attained earlier' (Office of the High Commissioner for Human Rights 1989). The UK has ratified this convention.

However, there are a number of different laws across the UK that specify age limits in different circumstances. These include child protection, age of consent, and age of criminal responsibility.

The broad definition of child abuse and neglect (child maltreatment) is referred to by the World Health Organization (WHO; WHO and the International Society for Prevention of Child Abuse and Neglect 2006) as encompassing all forms of physical and emotional ill-treatment, sexual abuse, neglect, and exploitation that result in actual or potential harm to the child's health, development or dignity. Within this broad definition, five subtypes can be distinguished: physical abuse, sexual abuse, neglect and negligent treatment, emotional abuse, and exploitation.

The WHO estimates that approximately 40 million children below the age of 15 are subject to child abuse and neglect each year and require health and social care (WHO 1999). In a 2005 study of 28 developing and transitional countries, it was found that a median of 83% of children in the African region experienced psychological abuse, 64% moderate physical abuse, and 43% severe physical abuse (Akmatov 2011).

Concerning homicides, there are an estimated 41 000 such deaths in children under 15 years of age (WHO 2014). This number underestimates the true extent of the problem, as a significant proportion of deaths due to child maltreatment are incorrectly attributed to falls, burns, drowning, and other causes.

In situations of armed conflict and refugee settings, girls are particularly vulnerable to sexual violence, exploitation, and abuse by combatants, security forces, members of their communities, aid workers, and others.

13.5   Types of child abuse

Differentiating the types of child abuse is done merely to facilitate an easier description of some of the features rather than suggesting that there are definitive delineations between the types of abuse. It is quite common that more than one type of abuse can be identified.

13.5.1   Physical abuse

This is by far the easiest type of abuse to diagnose and identify. Detection is usually triggered by the discovery of physical trauma on the body of a child which appears unusual in size, type or location. Suspicion is further aroused with the provision of an obviously inconsistent account of the causation of the injury. Attempts to obtain details are often met with denials and/or indignation.

13.5.1.1   Typical physical injuries
Cutaneous and other soft tissue injuries   Soft tissue injuries such as bruises, abrasions, and lacerations are common findings in an active normal growing child. The doctor should not jump to conclusions that the mere presence of such findings is suspicious and indicative of child abuse (Maguire 2010). However, when the cause of the injury is unclear and vague or improbable, greater care is required. Examples of soft tissue injuries which are associated with being caused in a non-accidental manner include laceration of superior frenulum of the lip, finger-tip bruises, bite marks, patterned bruises, and burns/scalds.

It is worthwhile remembering that babies that are unable to move about very much will not be able to fall and therefore hurt themselves. Bruises are common where there is underlying bony prominence; hence allowing the force of a fall or impact to break the underlying blood vessels. Bruises found over soft areas of the body, such as the cheeks, the abdominal wall, and inner aspects of the arms and thighs, will therefore require more detailed history taking and attention (Figure 13.1). The same also applies

Accidental bruising patterns   Abusive bruising patterns

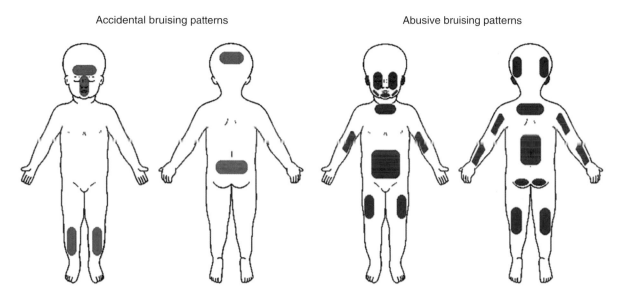

Figure 13.1   Accidental and non-accidental bruising patterns in infants. Source: Adapted from Maguire (2010).

to abrasions and lacerations. In addition, where lacerations occur it would be expected that medical attention would be sought promptly as there should be pain, bleeding, and concerns about infection. Delays in seeking attention for such injuries should be regarded as suspicious.

As a rule, injuries to the head, the eyes, and the mouth are worrying and should be carefully investigated. Injuries to the ears and the side of the head, injuries to the neck, and injuries to the mouth are uncommon injuries and should be looked at with extra care and concern.

Multiple soft tissue bruises with different colours suggest injuries over different periods of time. Clinicians should refrain from trying to age such injuries other than making a general categorisation of new, recent, and older injuries. They may, however, increase the suspicion of some degree of child abuse and/or neglect and warrant further investigation.

Bruise or other skin condition?   There are a number of congenital and acquired skin conditions that may resemble bruising. Mongolian spots, for example, which are congenital lesions, are often mistaken for bruises and reported as abuse. They appear as blue-grey areas of pigmentation (hence are sometimes called Mongolian blue spots) and commonly are found in the sacral area and the buttocks (Figure 13.2), but have also been seen on the back, legs, shoulders, upper arms, and scalp. They are predominately found in dark-skinned infants and tend to fade during childhood. They can be distinguished from bruises in that they do not fade or change colour as bruises do (Harris 2010).

Injuries that are infected and weeping denote a lack of care and attention to the well-being of the child and such children should be admitted even if it is for simply treating the wounds. Most carers would fuss over open wounds and an infected wound is worrisome of a lack of care or a poor quality of care, either of which requires attention and remedy.

Bite marks   Bite marks are sometimes identified and should be photographed with the presence of scales. The advice of a forensic odontologist would be particularly important if a serious attempt is to be made to identify the perpetrator. Bite marks are often difficult to identify because they are incomplete

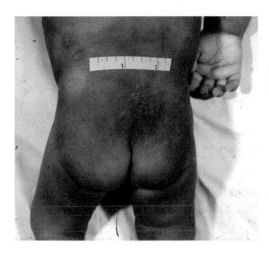
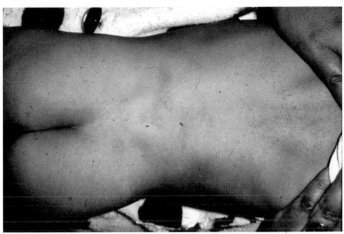

Figure 13.2 Mongolian spots in two children. The child on the left also has two healed cigarette burns in the left flank. The Mongolian spot of the child on the left is darker and situated in the sacral area and slightly beyond (the marks above the scale are bruises). The child on the right has fainter but more widespread marks over the buttocks and lower back which have a blue-grey appearance.

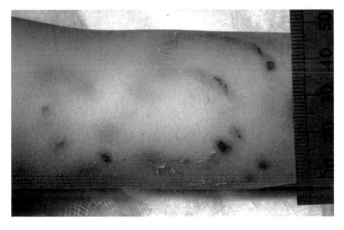

Figure 13.3 Four bite marks on a child's arm.

and may appear as bruises, abrasions, small lacerations, and a combination of these (Figure 13.3). It must also be remembered that bite marks may also be caused by other children and animals.

Scalds Scalds are quite commonly seen in accidents at home, usually due to an inquisitive toddler or young child running into another person holding a cup, bowl or pot of hot soup, etc. Children who are able to climb are often found to have pulled over a pot or kettle whilst exploring the kitchen. Such home accidents can and should be preventable and in some jurisdictions warrant questions about neglect. Most of these, however, are unfortunate and sometimes tragic accidents. The pattern of injuries is that of splashing, with a pattern of scalds with drip lines.

A more sinister pattern of scalding involves babies and young infants. Here, typically, a part of the body or occasionally the whole body is scalded by immersion into bathing water that was obviously too hot. The typical appearance of such scalds is a clear delineating line between the area of

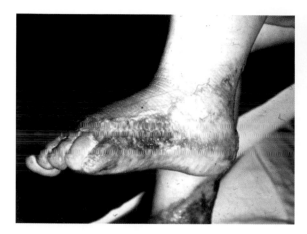
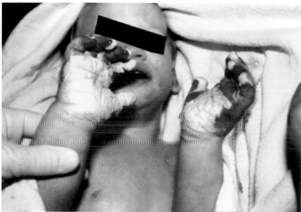

Figure 13.4   Demarcation lines in hands and feet seen in deliberate scalding.

scald and uninjured skin. The presence of such a line can help reconstruct the way the child was injured. It must also be remembered that a normal child would withdraw very quickly when they touch something that is so hot that it would scald, and such reflex withdrawal is very fast in order to prevent a more severe injury. The presence of such a line of demarcation in babies should make one suspicious that the carer had at the very least neglected to check the heat of the water before placing the whole baby into the bath. In older children, it suggests that the carer perhaps had been more deliberate as the limb or body must have been held in place for some time to become scalded (Figure 13.4).

Burns   Extensive burns are unusual and atypical, and are potentially related to home accidents where again questions of neglect may arise. The burns associated with child abuse are often much more deliberate and involve small discrete areas, although such burn injuries may be found all over the child's body. A common burn injury is that of burns caused by a lit cigarette end coming into contact with the skin, leaving a round or oval superficial burn injury (Figure 13.5). When fresh, this will often would blister or appear as an area of cratering with skin loss. As such wounds develop, they may scab and heal or they may become infected. Healing may or may not leave observable scars.

More than one form of burn wound involves the use of heated objects placed onto the skin; when these objects are 'patterned' they will leave marks that can be easily associated with the objects concerned, such as the heated parts of a cigarette lighter or the ends of a metal object (Figure 13.6). Occasionally the application of an open flame from a lit candle or cigarette lighter has been reported.

Skeletal injuries   The range of bony injuries can vary from fractures of the skull to multiple fractures of the rib cage and limb bones. In general, such extensive injuries are not difficult to identify and leave very little question as to the nature of the injury (Figure 13.7).

More subtle bony injuries such as metaphyseal fractures and spiral fractures of the upper limb bones are more difficult to detect and may require radiological examination and a paediatric radiologist's help to read the images. Such injuries typically arise from rough handling of a child leading to a twisting force causing a spiral fracture of the long bones and/or shearing of the metaphyseal growth plate/epiphysis that has not fused (Figures 13.8 and 13.9).

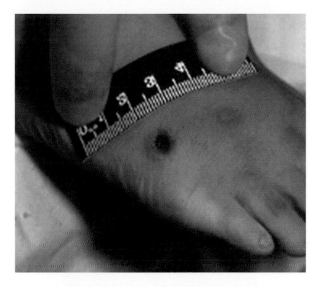

Figure 13.5 A typical recent cigarette burn is seen and medial to it a healed mark also caused by a cigarette.

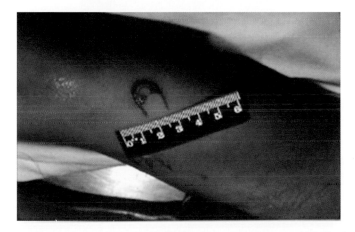

Figure 13.6 Burn mark made by the heated metal part of a disposable lighter.

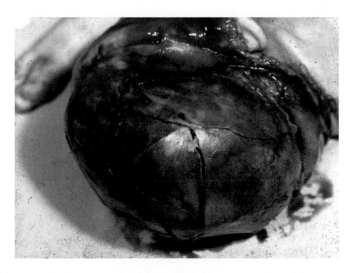

Figure 13.7 Angulated fracture of the right parietal bone caused by non-accidental impact against the edge of a table.

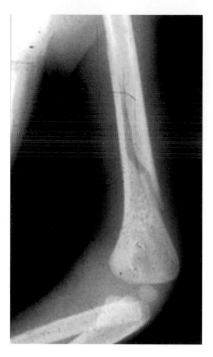

Figure 13.8   Spiral fracture of the left humerus.

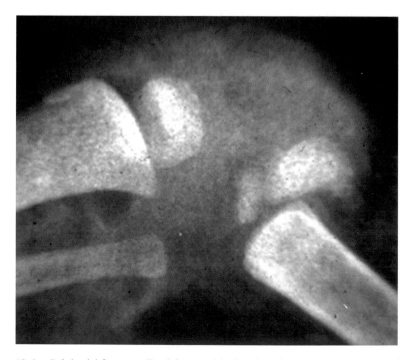

Figure 13.9   Epiphysial fracture distal femur with shearing of the metaphyseal growth plate.

Assessment of the age of fractures from radiological examination is commonly required in child abuse cases. However, this is an inexact science.

The healing process can be divided into the following stages:

- resolution of soft tissue injuries

- development of periosteal new bone

- loss of the fracture line's definition and the appearance of soft callus.

In the normal skeleton the rate of healing depends on a number of factors, including the site of injury. It is recognised that the ribs and upper limb bones heal at a greater rate than the lower limb bones, and that assessment of the age of a skull fracture is virtually impossible given that fracture line may take up to six to eight months to disappear.

Unusual healing patterns may be seen in systemic illness or some forms of metabolic bone disorders. Abundant callus is often found in Cushing's syndrome, those on steroids or those that are suffering from osteogenesis imperfecta. Poor callus formation is seen in patients with osteoporosis or osteomalacia.

It should be appreciated that the radiologic features of bone healing are a continuous process, with considerable overlap of the different stages and therefore estimates can only be based on a broad time frame in terms of weeks rather than days. However, recent fractures can be differentiated from old fractures and this evidence can be used to substantiate or refute accounts of multiple trauma at different times. A systematic review carried out by Prosser et al. (2005) concluded that periosteal reaction can be seen as early as four days and is present in at least 50% of cases by two weeks after the injury, with remodelling peaking eight weeks after injury (Figures 13.10 and 13.11).

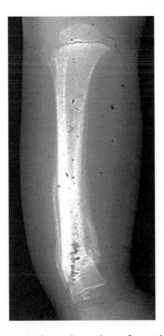

Figure 13.10 Periosteal new bone formation of tibia.

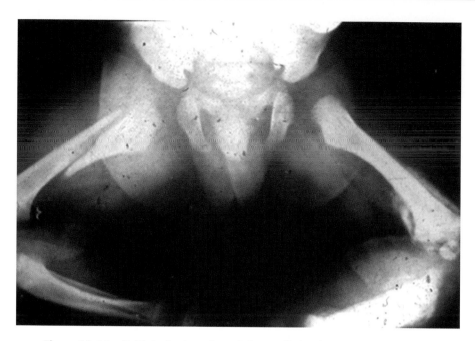

Figure 13.11   Multiple fractures in an infant suffering from congenital rickets.

Similarly, fresh and healing fractures provide a good indicator of the repetitive nature of the abusive episodes. The radiological evidence of callus formation and the different stages of healing can help in estimating the different timings of trauma events.

Visceral injuries   Injuries to the abdominal organs are occasionally seen and can include ruptures of the hollow structures such as the stomach or bowels. Lacerations of the liver and spleen with or without associated fractured ribs have been reported. Laceration of the pancreas where it is trapped against the spine by a force applied from the front of the abdomen has also been seen by the author.

Although such injuries may be caused by heavy punches to the abdomen of a child, they are more likely to occur when a child is lying on the floor and the attacker either steps or stamps forcefully on the abdomen or thorax. The use of the knee or elbow to deliver a blow can also lead to such visceral injuries. Visceral injuries are therefore more commonly seen in fatal cases of child abuse.

Unexplained loss of consciousness   Typically, a young child is rushed to an accident and emergency unit or to a doctor with an account that the child has suddenly became unresponsive. There may or may not be an associated episode of convulsion. The clinician must be aware that there can be many causes of unconsciousness in a child but whatever the cause, the child needs to be given adequate ventilator support. An urgent computerised tomography (CT) scan and magnetic resonance imaging (MRI) should be performed where available.

In the last 30 years, anyone dealing with children wil have become aware of shaken baby syndrome. The potential damage that may arise from the whiplash shaking of an infant was outlined by Caffey (1972) in his Abraham Jacobi Award Address. During this address he brought attention to the concept of whiplash injury resulting in bilateral subdural haemorrhage associated with bilateral retinal haemorrhage. Such injuries may be fatal but are more often associated with a resulting mental retardation. He further noted that skull fractures and scalp bruising are uncommon in such cases. He raised this as an attempt to discourage the practice of shaking of babies that was common practice then. He went further to ask for a careful study of child's play where the child's head may be subjected to this whiplash shaking to determine its safety for the child.

Currently there is a great deal of controversy regarding the very existence of shaking baby syndrome and the diagnostic triad on which it is based, i.e. subdural haemorrhage, retinal haemorrhages, and encephalopathy. Although it is accepted that in many cases of head trauma vigorous shaking has occurred, it is now accepted by many that there must also have been some impact to the head in most cases. In 2009 the American Academy of Paediatricians (Christian and Block 2009), followed by the UK Crown Prosecution Service (2011), stated that the term shaken baby syndrome should not be used because it did not exclusively explain the triad of findings, although confessions supported the role of shaking. The term non-accidental head injury or trauma (NAHI) has since been widely adopted (Squier 2011).

Despite the mechanism involved, it is vital that the child should be admitted to hospital and an urgent CT scan and/or MRI scan arranged, together with an ophthalmological examination. Issues about whether a carer should or should not be prosecuted should not be of concern to the clinician. Such matters can be properly discussed at the multidisciplinary committee meeting, where all relevant information can be considered. The challenge that is still unresolved is how much force is required and how we can differentiate between an intentional injury and routine, run-of-the-mill play.

As stated above, there have been changes in the labelling of injuries from shaken baby syndrome to shaken impact syndrome to abusive head injury or trauma. Regardless, the important issue is recognising that unexplained and unexpected incidences resulting in injuries to a young child should always be treated with some degree of suspicion and it is always important to bear in mind that the child's safety is paramount.

In the event that a child dies from such an injury, the death should be reported and a full and thorough autopsy made, including imaging and collection of samples for further investigation.

13.5.2 Emotional and psychological abuse

Detection of this in young babies is difficult; most cases are more readily detected in an older child where delays in developmental milestones can be documented and measured.

Children that are quiet and distant, avoiding eye contact, are of concern. Children that are destructive and/or abusive are similarly of concern. However, it is important to seek the advice of a child psychologist and child psychiatrist to exclude the increasing number of childhood disorders that are have been recognised in the last 10 years.

It is also not uncommon that emotional abuse is present together with other forms of abuse. In particular, the child is likely to have been neglected and would therefore suffer from poor nutrition and hygiene. Hence, such children appear sickly and are on the lower percentiles in terms of weight and height. Skin conditions are common, with infected rashes and wounds, and, in younger babies, infected nappy rashes. It must be remembered that neglected children can die from malnutrition and/or associated infection.

13.5.3   Child sexual abuse and exploitation

This is an extremely difficult area of paediatric forensic medicine and should be referred to individuals adequately trained and experienced in this area. Sexual exploitation of children can involve the taking of and sharing of naked pictures or videos of young children. It can, of course, involve the incitement and involvement of older children in sexual acts, including the actual sexual penetration of the child.

Physical penetration of the genitalia of a child can result in horrific tears and injuries to the perineum of a child or can result in no detectable physical findings. It is now commonplace to use video colposcopy (Figure 13.12) to examine the female genitalia in an attempt to identify the presence of healed injuries of the hymen in young children. Any clinician intending to take on such work would be well advised to familiarise themselves with the normal appearance and development of the paediatric hymen and the effects of different levels of oestrogen on them (Berenson et al. 1992; Heger and Emans 1992).

There should be no question that a proper assessment of the condition of the paediatric hymen can only be made with a careful colposcopic examination. It is highly recommended that good colour photographs be taken and if possible a video recording of the entire examination. Such material will allow for proper peer review (Heger 2011). Measurement of the size of the vaginal opening and other structures have been championed by some. There is, however, no consensus as the interpretation of such measurements is difficult. Similarly, the examination of the anus should be made in any cases involving penetration. Again, it is not uncommon that no injuries are observed even when anal penetration is certain. Clinicians must be cautious in their interpretation of the

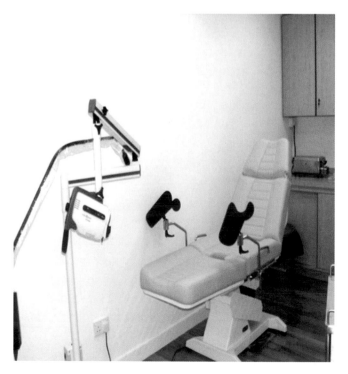

Figure 13.12   An obstetric examination couch with a digital colposcope.

findings, blind faith and interpretation, as in the use of the infamous reflex anal dilatation test. A positive reflex anal dilatation test is accepted by many to be a sign for suspicion, but it should be supported by other evidence.

13.5.4 Scene examination

Examination of the scene in cases of child abuse is necessary, particularly to ascertain whether injuries are compatible with being caused by various items or surfaces within that environment in the manner described by the custodians. Scene examinations in the vast majority of cases are retrospective, since most children are brought into hospital before the involvement of the police.

The investigators, including the pathologist, need to assess the credibility of any accounts given and may require an examination of the child's environment where the injuries were allegedly caused. In relation to the environment where the child may have been injured or was found dead, and in view of the fact that most injured children that are taken to hospital are either brought in dead or die at a later time, the scene is of necessity in the vast majority of cases examined retrospectively. In fact, scene examination and reconstruction of events, armed with a full knowledge of the extent of the injuries and possibly accounts by carers as to how injuries were caused, is much more preferable than examining the scene before the autopsy has been completed in the case of a deceased child. It has to be accepted, however, that because of the absence of a body from the scene in many cases, the scene examination is either neglected or not considered as thoroughly as is necessary (Wagner 1986).

Blunt head injury is the most common cause of death in physical child abuse cases, and perpetrators may give various explanations as to how the child was injured. Indeed, it is not uncommon for a suspect to attempt to explain a severe head injury by some accidental means. It is vital therefore to interpret such injuries in the light of explanations offered in conjunction with careful consideration of the scene. Head injuries should be evaluated, for example in respect to distance through which the child has reportedly fallen, to assess whether or not accounts given by accused are consistent with the injuries found. In this respect it is essential for the pathologist to take into account, for example, the height of the cot from the floor and evaluation of the height of furniture surfaces from the floor, such as a chair or a bed from which a child may have fallen, in conjunction with the type of floor covering. The height of furniture as well as window sills, balcony railings, etc. will also enable the examiner to assess whether or not it was feasible for the child to clamber up or over such structures.

Burns may have a characteristic pattern which can be matched, for example, with a radiator grill. Scalding by being held in a bath tub may occasionally be seen. The design of the bath or basin in which the child received scalds needs to be examined and measurements taken and related to the burns seen on the child.

In addition to the examination of specific items and surfaces, it is essential for the investigator to take note of the child's environment as a whole, i.e. the general appearance of the home, state of repair, degree of cleanliness, quality of clothing, food present, and state of basic amenities.

The boundaries of a scene or scenes in child abuse, because of the multiplicity and varying ages of injury in many cases, may be difficult or impossible to define. One should be guided by accounts available relating to circumstances surrounding the episode leading to death together with the post-mortem findings.

13.6   Management of child abuse

It is of paramount importance that the reader understands that the ideal setup for the management of victims of child abuse is through the co-ordinated, planned efforts of a multidisciplinary team of experts generally including representatives from social work, psychology, paediatrics, forensic doctors, and law enforcement. The co-opting of other experts can be arranged as the need arises. The second most important concept is that the team is there to serve the best interests of the child and to offer protection for the child. The identification of the perpetrator and the successful legal sanctions against such an individual should be left to those in the criminal justice system. Doctors and carers must be impartial at all times and not become child advocates, as such a role may result in a conflict of loyalties and interests.

Steps and protocols to be adopted should be agreed and established by the multidisciplinary team. Members of the team should all be properly trained and should have met regularly to ensure that the team works well together and any ambiguities are resolved.

A trigger event could be from teachers, child-minders, doctors, nurses, for example. Once the alarm is raised, such children should be admitted for observation and investigation in a paediatric unit in the local hospital. Paediatricians are ideal for obtaining a detailed history from the carer/parent to establish all that is needed for assessing the routines of care adopted by the carers of the child. Issues about previous illnesses, hospitalisations, immunisations, visits to doctors, etc. can also be documented and later checked if necessary. The approach is one of a clinician trying to establish what may be wrong with a patient. Such a process will allow the experienced paediatrician to decide on what types of investigation and tests may be needed.

The history taking should be followed by a thorough and methodological physical examination of the child. This can and should be done in the presence of the caregiver, and remarks and comments volunteered about injuries and marks should be noted in the clinical records.

Good colour photography with appropriate scale is of great help for future reviewers. Appropriate imaging should be ordered as indicated. In young children, a full skeletal survey is preferred as a very young child is unable to locate or describe pain and discomfort. In older children, radiological imaging of affected sites can be done and further comprehensive imaging guided by the findings.

It is essential that laboratory investigations should be carried out, including tests for bleeding disorders, particularly in cases where multiple bruises are found. In children with suspicion of skeletal and or joint injuries, screening for bone disorders and rare genetic conditions may be needed.

In children that are admitted unconscious, it is important that ophthalmological examination of the retina for haemorrhages is made and documented. CT and/or MRI scan of the brain should also be arranged as soon as possible to look for the presence of intracranial haemorrhages such as subdural haemorrhages and cerebral swelling.

A toxicological screen is recommended in communities where there is a high prevalence of drug abuse. In the unconscious child, a comprehensive toxicological screen may be critical if indeed the unconscious state is a result of drugs that could potentially be treated with an antidote.

The child should be kept in hospital for as long as is needed to establish if it is safe for the child to be returned to his/her carers. This should be achieved in as clinical a way as possible. Demands for the return of the child against the wishes of the clinician should be met with an approach to the police or the courts for a protection order. During the hospital stay, social workers should be able to visit and assess the family and the general situation at the home of the child. It is not infrequent that issues of parental immaturity, lack of a support network, poverty, and other factors are identified as affecting the child and the family.

Where more serious criminal acts may have taken place, the police should also be informed and investigations initiated. The taking of a formal statement from a child should be done only by well-trained individuals. In particular, the taking of a formal statement about child sexual abuse is a very delicate matter and should be left to professionals who are properly trained. Social workers, child psychologists, paediatricians, and specially trained police officers should receive training specifically on how to conduct such an interview. An ideal set-up is a purpose-built video-recording suite where the ambience is just like that of a comfortable child's room. Some toys will be available but too many will distract the child. The trained interviewer will put the child at ease and get the child comfortable. He/she will be on a one-way link to a command centre where other interested parties are present, possibly behind a one way mirror. In another situation, the relevant parties can watch the video and audio capture. Interviewers will ask generic questions and allow the child to use its' own vocabulary to describe the incident or incidents. The interviewer should avoid attempting to direct or suggest as it is very easy to contaminate such evidence. Some advocate the use of anatomically correct dolls to allow the child to demonstrate events that they may not be able to describe (Hlavka et al. 2010). A good example is the code of practice for pre-trial witness interviews promulgated by the UK Crown Prosecution Service (CPS 2008).

Many developed countries now have special legislation that allows the use of video-recorded interviews as evidence and the child is not required to repeat the account of incidents over and over again. Lessons learnt from survivors have highlighted that repeated requirements to give statements to different parties about an abusive incident has a long-term psychological impact on the individual and affects the recovery.

All cases should be discussed at a multidisciplinary meeting of all the various experts and a consensus reached and recorded on the recommendations on how to protect the best interest of the child. Such an approach allows for remedial societal support where appropriate and should limit criminal prosecution to cases that are clearly indicated and appropriate for the ultimate best interest of the child.

13.6.1 Safeguarding and protecting children

Child protection as defined by the Royal College of Paediatrics and Child Health is the process of protecting individual children identified as either suffering or likely to suffer significant harm as a result of abuse or neglect. It involves measures and structures designed to respond to abuse and neglect. Safeguarding and promoting the welfare of children is a broader term than child protection. It encompasses protecting children from maltreatment, preventing impairment of children's health or development, and ensures children grow up in safe circumstances.

13.6.2 The United Nations Convention on the Rights of the Child

In 1989, governments worldwide promised all children the same rights by adopting the UN Convention on the Rights of the Child, also known as the CRC or UNCRC. The Convention changed the way children are viewed and treated, in other words, as human beings with a distinct set of rights instead of as passive objects of care and charity (Office of the High Commissioner for Human Rights, United Nations 1989). These rights describe what a child needs to survive, to grow, and to live up to their potential in the world. They apply equally to every child, no matter who they are or where they come from. All children have rights, even those affected by conflict or emergencies.

The Children Act 1989 allows local authorities, courts, parents, and other agencies to ensure the safeguarding of children and the promotion of their welfare. Although the Act's central premise is that children are best cared for within their own families, provisions is made for instances when parents and families do not co-operate with statutory bodies. The Children Act 2004 amended the Children Act 1989, largely as a consequence of the Victoria Climbié inquiry (2003). This Act is now the basis for most official administration considered helpful to children, notably bringing all local government functions of children's welfare and education under the statutory authority of local directors of children's services. Each children's services authority in England must make arrangement to promote the following:

Co-operation to improve well-being.
S.10 The arrangements are to be made with a view to improving the well-being of children in the authority's area so far as relating to:

a.   Physical and mental health and emotional well-being;
b.   Protection from harm and neglect;
c.   Education, training and recreation;
d.   The contribution made by them to society;
e.   Social and economic well-being.

In making arrangements under this section, a children's services authority in England must have regard to the importance of parents and other persons in caring for children in improving the well-being of children.
S11 Arrangements to safeguard and promote welfare.
Each person and body to whom this section applies must make arrangements for ensuring that:

a.   their functions are discharged having regard to the need to safeguard and promote the welfare of children;
b.   any services provided by another person pursuant to arrangements made by the person or body in the discharge of their functions are provided having regard to that need.

13.6.3   Working together to safeguard children

In 2006 the government released *Working Together to Safeguard Children*, a document that sets out the ways in which organisations and individuals should work together to safeguard and promote the well-being of children to enable those children to have optimum life chances and to enter adulthood successfully. In 2010 this was superseded by *Working Together to Safeguard*

Table 13.1 Safeguarding risks.

Extrinsic to the child	Intrinsic to the child
Lone parents	Born at the wrong time (e.g. drug misuse distraction)
Income support (54%)	Result of forced, coercive or commercial sex
No wage earner (57%)	Premature, low birth weight, chronically ill and hospitalised
Domestic violence (27%)	Parental relationship breakdown
Family mental illness (13%)	Behaviour problems, temperamental or personality difficulties
Previously known to social services (65%)	Inconsolable crying and screaming
Previous investigation (45%)	Unwanted children, failure to meet parental expectations
Parents abused as children	'Wrong' gender
Drugs and alcohol misuse	Physical or learning disabilities
Parents with disabilities	Soiling and wetting past developmental age
Step parents	
Violence towards pets	
Adults who are a risk to children	
Multiple births	
Parental indifference or over-anxiousness	
Impoverished environment, poverty, social isolation	
Black and minority ethnic group parents	
Teenage parents	
Antisocial personality	

Children (2010 and 2018), which expanded the focus on interagency working. The document includes guidance on:

- protecting children from maltreatment

- preventing impairment of children's health or development

- ensuring that children are growing up in circumstances consistent with the provision of safe and effective care, and as adults are happy and making a positive contribution and achieving economic well-being.

13.6.4 Safeguarding risks to children

There are safeguarding risks to children which include parents, carers, and the environment in which they are living (extrinsic factors) as well as risk factors intrinsic to the child (Table 13.1).

References

Akmatov, M.K. (2011). Child abuse in 28 developing and transitional countries – results from the Multiple Indicator Cluster Surveys. *Int. J. Epidemiol.* 40: 219–227.

Bass, M., Kravath, R.E., and Class, I. (1986). Death scene investigation in sudden infant death. *N. Engl. J. Med.* 315: 100–105.

Berenson, A.B., Heger, A.H., Hayes, J.M. et al. (1992). The appearance of the hymen in prepubertal girls. *Pediatrics* 89: 387–394.

Blair, P., Fleming, P., Bensley, D. et al. (1995). Plastic mattresses and sudden infant death syndrome. *Lancet* 345: 720.

Caffey, J. (1972). On the theory and practice of shaking infants. Its potential residual effects of permanent brain damage and mental retardation. *Am. J. Dis. Child.* 124: 161–169.

Christian, C.W. and Block, R. (2009). Abusive head trauma in infants and children. *Pediatrics* 123: 1409–1411.

Crown Prosecution Service, Pre-trial witness interviews: Code of Practice http//www.cps.gov.uk/victims_witnesses/resources/interviews.html (February 2008).

Crown Prosecution Service (2011). Non Accidental Head Injury Cases (NAHI, formerly referred to as Shaken Baby Syndrome [SBS]) – Prosecution Approach – Legal Guidance, Domestic abuse, Violent crime. www.cps.gov.uk/legal-guidance/non-accidental-head-injury

Fleming, P.J., Blair, P.S., Bacon, C. et al. (2000). Sudden unexpected death in infancy. In: *The CESDI SUDI Studies 1993–1996*. London: The Stationery Office. ISBN: 0 11 322299 8.

Fleming, P.J., Pease, A., and Blair, P.S. (2015). Bedsharing and unexpected infant deaths. What is the relationship? *Paediatr. Respir. Rev.* 16: 62–67.

Harris, T.S. (2010). Bruises in children: normal or child abuse? *J. Pediatr. Health Care* 24: 216–221.

Heger, A.H. The Use of Video Colposcopy in Sexual Assault Examinations. http://www.obgyn.net/laparoscopy/use-video-colposcopy-sexual-assault-examinations (July 1 2011).

Heger, A.H. and Emans, S.J. (1992). *Evaluation of the Sexually Abused Child; Textbook and Atlas*. New York: Oxford University Press.

Hlavka, H.R., Olinger, S.D., and Lashley, J.L. (2010). The use of anatomical dolls as a demonstration aid in child abuse interviews: a study of forensic interviewer's perceptions. *J. Child Sex. Abus.* 19: 519–553.

HM Government (2018). Working together to safeguard children Infanticide Act, 1938 C.39, HMSO. www.legislation.gov.uk.

Infant Life (Preservation) Act, 1929 C.34, HMSO. www.legislation.gov.uk.

Iyasu, S., Hanslick, R., Rowley, D., and Wilinger, M. (1994). Proceedings of workshop on guidelines for scene investigation of sudden unexplained infant deaths. *J. Forensic Sci.* 39: 1126–1136.

Maguire, S. (2010). Which injuries may indicate child abuse? *Arch. Dis. Child. Educ. Pract. Ed.* 95: 170–177.

NICE Guidance (2014) Postnatal care. www.nice.org.uk.

Prosser, I., Maguire, S., Harrison, S.K. et al. (2005). How old is this fracture? Radiologic dating of fractures in children: a systematic review. *Am. J. Roentgenol.* 184: 1282–1286.

Squier, W. (2011). The 'shaken baby' syndrome: pathology and mechanisms. *Acta Neuropathol.* 122: 519–542.

Still-Birth (Definition) Act 1992 C.29, HMSO. www.legislation.gov.uk.

The Children Act 1984, HMSO. www.legislation.gov.uk.

The Victoria Climbié Inquiry. (2003). Report of an Inquiry by Lord Laming. CM5730.

UN Convention on the Rights of the Child (1989). Office of the High Commissioner for Human Rights, United Nations. www.unicef.org.uk.

United Nations (1959) Declaration of the rights of the child.

Wagner, G.N. (1986). Crime scene investigation in child-abuse cases. *Am. J. Forensic Med. Pathol.* 7: 94–99.

WHO (1999). Report of the Consultation on Child Abuse Prevention. Consultation on Child Abuse Prevention. World Health Organization, Geneva.

WHO (2006). *Violence and Injury Prevention Team Global Forum for Health Research Issue*. Geneva: World Health Organization.

WHO. (2014) Child maltreatment. Fact sheet N°150.

WHO and the International Society for Prevention of Child Abuse and Neglect (2006). Preventing child maltreatment: a guide to taking action and generating evidence.

14
Sudden Natural Death

Peter Vanezis

Queen Mary University of London, London, UK

14.1   Introduction

This chapter will briefly review deaths which are sudden, unexpected and thought to be due to natural causes which nevertheless may have medico-legal significance. It is outside the scope of the text to give a detailed account of each type of death, but more germane to familiarise the reader with the types of cases that are encountered, including those where establishing the cause of death may be challenging because of the paucity of findings at autopsy.

The World Health Organization defines sudden death due to natural causes or otherwise unexplained as occurring within 24 hours of onset of symptoms (WHO ISCD 2015), although the term is sometimes used to cover a wider margin of time.

In forensic pathology practice, potentially any death from natural causes that is sudden and/or unexpected may be the subject of a medico-legal autopsy (case referred to the coroner or procurator fiscal) for various reasons as discussed elsewhere.

By the very fact that many such deaths are unexpected, they need to be fully assessed to see whether they are of forensic significance. The vast majority of cases are straightforward natural deaths and the coroner or procurator fiscal is satisfied that no further investigation is required. This is discussed in detail in Chapter 2.

Sudden natural deaths may occur in a previously apparently fit and healthy individual with no significant medical history or could also occur in someone with a known illness who dies suddenly. The deceased person may or may not have suffered a complication of an existing condition. This is a common occurrence in the elderly, who may have a number of significant co-morbidities but who may die suddenly or unexpectedly with no obvious explanation for their death. Establishing the

Essential Forensic Medicine, First Edition. Edited by Peter Vanezis.
© 2020 John Wiley & Sons Ltd. Published 2020 by John Wiley & Sons Ltd.

cause of death in such cases may on occasions be problematic, bearing in mind the need to assess the contribution to death of various conditions present, if there is no obvious catastrophic event, for example a cerebral haemorrhage, ruptured aortic aneurysm or pulmonary thromboembolism.

Certain types of natural death may well have important forensic significance bearing in mind the circumstances in which they occur. A good example is the situation where a bus driver may die suddenly as a result of a cardiac arrhythmia from ischaemic heart and crash his vehicle, causing injury to passengers and pedestrians. The same person dying at home from the same condition would obviously have no forensic implications.

Some deaths usually classified as natural in most circumstances may be classified as unnatural if there is an external factor or factors related to the cause of death. An example of this is the effect of external stress causing a myocardial infarction following some physical activity such as running away from an assailant or being placed in fear of one's life by an intruder.

One of the important issues in relating natural deaths to an external incident is identifying a chain of causation. This may cause problems for the coroner in deciding what category to place the death into, whether it be clearly natural or otherwise. This problem is explored by Roberts and his collaborators (2000), who state that there are no guidelines to help doctors in dealing with such cases and death certification is often arbitrary and inconsistent.

For a number of reasons, it is an essential part of forensic practice to determine the cause of death in cases where the cause of death is unknown but thought to be natural and has occurred suddenly or unexpectedly:

- to provide information in the interest of public health by identifying public health risks and monitoring disease trends

- to identify epidemiological data about diseases and their changing patterns, to assist in their control and treatment

- to allow relatives to seek medical advice where there is a significant hereditary factor in the cause of death

- to provide information to relatives, particularly where death was sudden and unexpected, so as to assist them in their bereavement.

14.2 Sudden/Unexpected deaths where findings at autopsy are non-specific

There are a number of recognised syndromes which refer to different situations or conditions in which sudden death occurs with few or non-specific morphological changes at autopsy and which require further investigation.

14.2.1 Sudden infant death syndrome

The term sudden infant death syndrome (SIDS) (see also Chapter 13) was defined in 1965 under code 795 of the International Classification of Diseases (ICD-8) for infant deaths as the sudden unexpected death of an infant with no apparent cause. SIDS is a category of exclusion for designating the death of an infant where a post-mortem examination (and often a death scene investigation) fails to determine a specific cause (Willinger et al. 1991).

14.2.2 Sudden unexplained death in infancy

When a death does not fulfil the criteria for SIDS it is referred to by many pathologists as unexplained or unascertained, usually referred to as Sudden unexplained death in infancy (SUDI), and there is still doubt about its cause. However, there is evidence to suggest that these terms are used interchangeably by coroners (Limerick and Bacon 2004) and research has shown that the characteristics of babies dying of these two causes are very similar (Corbin 2005).

14.2.3 Sudden adult death syndrome

Sudden adult death syndrome (SADS) is associated with a plethora of others, essentially referring to sudden death in adolescents or adults where the cause is unknown, including sudden unexpected death syndrome, sudden unexpected nocturnal death syndrome (SUNDS), sudden arrhythmic cardiac death syndrome (SADS), sudden unknown death syndrome, and bed death, many of which occur during sleep (de la Grandmaison 2006). Undoubtedly, on a few occasions pathologists will be unable, despite a thorough post-mortem examination, including examination of the cardiac conduction system, to ascertain the cause of death. Genetic testing in such circumstances is essential since a number of these conditions are inherited (see also Chapter 5).

Cardiac channelopathies/arrhythmia syndromes are a group of relatively rare diseases that affect the electrical functioning of the heart without affecting the heart's structure and are often the cause of a SADS death. There are several different types of ion channelopathies, including:

- long QT syndrome

- Brugada syndrome

- catecholaminergic polymorphic ventricular tachycardia (CPVT)

- progressive cardiac conduction defect (PCCD)

- short QT syndrome

- early repolarisation syndrome

- sodium channel disease.

Less frequently, SADS can be caused by other cardiac abnormalities, such as extra electrical pathways or even subtle heart muscle disease (cardiomyopathies).

14.2.4 Sudden unexpected death in epilepsy

People with epilepsy have a higher risk of mortality compared to healthy individuals. A subgroup of patients with epilepsy are classified as sudden unexpected death in epilepsy (SUDEP) when they die suddenly, in otherwise apparently good health, from an unknown cause of death.

SUDEP is reported to occur in up to 18% of all deaths in people with epilepsy, the most frequent epilepsy-related cause of death.

A number of risk factors for SUDEP have been proposed, including:

- young age

- presence of generalised tonic–clonic seizures

- poor anti-epileptic drug (AED) compliance

- use of multiple AEDs

- duration of seizure disorder ranging from 15 to 20 years

- early onset of epilepsy.

The exact mechanisms underlying SUDEP remain unknown. Seizure-related abnormalities of respiratory and cardiac function have both been implicated as possible contributors, and the most commonly suggested terminal event is a cardiac arrhythmia during and between seizures (Tu et al. 2011).

14.2.5   Dead in bed syndrome

Dead in bed syndrome (DIBS) is a rare but devastating condition that is generally thought to affect only people with type 1 diabetes (Hsieh and Twigg 2014). Several large-scale population studies reporting sudden unexpected deaths that in combination have helped to formalise the DIBS definition and criteria, which include:

- previously generally well individuals with type 1 diabetes mellitus

- no obvious cardiovascular complications

- unwitnessed sudden unexpected death in an undisturbed bed

- no clear anatomical cause for death at the time of autopsy.

While the exact cause(s) and mechanism(s) leading to DIBS are unknown, there is growing evidence implicating both autonomic neuropathy and nocturnal hypoglycaemia. Autonomic neuropathy in diabetes can cause impaired parasympathetic activity, resulting in some cases in sympathetic predominance, which can cause abnormal cardiac repolarization and prolong the QTc interval. Hypoglycaemia can act in a similar way on the heart.

In addition, at this point it is appropriate to state that diabetes mellitus (Type 1 and 2) is one of the group of metabolic diseases commonly encountered by the pathologist in day to day practice. Usually the long term complications of diabetes contribute to the cause of death mainly through the cardiovascular system and the kidneys, but occasionally when poorly controlled it may directly be responsible for leading to death, through either the acute effects of hypoglycaemia or from hyperglycaemia, including hyperosmolar hypergylcaemic state or diabetic ketoacidosis.

14.2.6 Sudden Unexpected Death in Alcohol Misuse

Sudden unexpected death in alcohol misuse (SUDAM) refers to deaths related to chronic alcohol abuse where there is no morphological cause of death but frequently just the presence of a fatty liver with little or no alcohol detected in the body fluids. Most deaths in this category are due to ketoacidosis (Thomsen et al. 1995). Alcoholic ketoacidosis (AKA) occurs in patients with prolonged alcohol intake or after an episode of binge drinking. Typically, there may be a brief period of starvation induced by alcoholic gastritis. β-hydroxybutyrate is characteristically elevated in AKA. In a very small number of such deaths, the cause remains undetermined and may be due to cardiac arrhythmia or a number of other as yet unknown causes.

14.3 Deaths involving different body systems

14.3.1 Cardiovascular deaths

The most common conditions causing sudden natural deaths seen in coroners' cases are within the cardiovascular system.

14.3.1.1 Ischaemic heart disease This is the most common cause of sudden and/or unexpected death in cases which are reported to the coroner. Thomas et al. (1988) examined 322 autopsied cases of sudden deaths in one coroner's jurisdiction and found that ischaemic heart disease accounted for 189 deaths (59%). In a study by Rutty et al. (2001) assessing 568 deaths, there were 207 from ischaemic heart disease (36%), 46 cases (8%) were combined hypertensive and ischaemic heart disease, and there were 39 deaths (7%) from myocardial infarction.

14.3.1.2 Hypertensive heart disease As shown above, hypertensive heart disease is commonly associated with ischaemic heart disease caused by coronary atherosclerosis. Hypertension causes hypertrophy of cardiac muscle, giving rise to cardiomegaly, and causes relative ischaemia of the myocardium. In 2013 hypertensive heart disease resulted in 1.07 million deaths as compared with 630 000 deaths in 1990 (GBD 2015). However, since high blood pressure is a risk factor for atherosclerosis and ischemic heart disease (Grossman and Messerli 1996), death rates from hypertensive heart disease provide an incomplete measure of the burden of disease due to high blood pressure.

14.3.1.3 Valvular heart disease Valvular stenosis or incompetence, particularly calcific aortic stenosis in the elderly, is not uncommon. Bacterial endocarditis may also occasionally be seen, with the tricuspid valve being particularly involved in intravenous drug users.

14.3.1.4 Cardiomyopathies Cardiomyopathies are a heterogenous group of diseases that have caused a great deal of confusion in relation to definition and nomenclature, reflected in the large number of classifications over the last 30 years (Sheppard 2011). They comprise a number of complex conditions, which makes classification very difficult. A classification from the American Heart Association (AHA) (Maron et al. 2006) divides cardiomyopathies into primary cardiomyopathies, which affect the heart alone, and secondary cardiomyopathies, which are the result of a systemic illness affecting many other parts of the body. These categories are then further broken down into subgroups incorporating new genetic and molecular insights.

14.3.1.5 Other cardiac conditions

Other conditions, including congenital heart disease and myocarditis, are occasionally encountered in routine coroners' autopsies.

14.3.1.6 Pulmonary thromboembolism

Pulmonary embolism is one of the most underdiagnosed causes of death where no autopsy is performed; it has been estimated that less than half of fatal pulmonary emboli are recognised clinically.

In relation to trauma, a non-lethal injury may be followed by death from pulmonary embolism following venous thrombosis, in which case a simple accident or common assault may be converted into homicide.

There are a number of reasons why a victim of trauma may be at risk from developing pulmonary embolism:

- Blood coagulability is increased for several weeks after injury, the peak being between one and two weeks.

- Injury to the tissues, especially the legs or pelvic region, may give rise to local venous thrombosis in the contused muscles or around fractured bones.

- The injury may confine the victim to bed, thus decreasing mobility, particularly in the elderly. This would increase the pressure on the calves and reduced venous return and stasis due to lessened muscular massage of the leg veins.

The various aspects of pulmonary embolism have been investigated in several retrospective autopsy surveys. Knight and Zaini made a survey of 38 406 post-mortem investigations of the Institute of Pathology at the Welsh National School of Medicine between the years 1908 and 1977. In 1176 subjects the cause of death was recorded as being due to pulmonary embolism. In trauma cases the peak incidence was at about two weeks after injury, whereas in a series by Lau the peak time of death following trauma and/or immobilisation was one week.

A study carried out by Menaker et al. (2007) on patients with pulmonary embolism demonstrated that the condition occurred as early as the first day of the trauma. They found that in days 1–4 after trauma there were 35 patients (37%) with pulmonary embolism. On day 5–7 the condition was seen in 17 patients (18%), on day 8–14 in 22 patients (23%), and after 14 days in 20 patients (21%).

In Knight's survey, more than three-quarters of the victims had predisposing factors such as injury, surgical operation or immobility in bed, but the remaining 20% were ambulant and apparently healthy. This has important medico-legal implications because if fatal pulmonary embolism can strike an appreciable proportion of the population who have not suffered one of the recognised predisposing factors, then the cause–effect relationship after trauma is weakened. If the standard of proof in criminal trials must be 'beyond reasonable doubt', then the fact that up to 20% of pulmonary embolism deaths have not followed trauma or immobility must surely remove the cause–effect relationship from near-certainty to mere probability, which is sufficient for a civil decision, but not for a criminal conviction. This is a legal matter for the judge, however, who may or may not let the matter go to the jury, and if it does, it is for the jury to decide. There is marked variation in these decisions from case to case.

In almost all cases the source of the embolus will be found in the vessels draining into the femoral veins, though rarely pelvic vessels are involved (usually in relation to pregnancy or abortion). Here pelvic veins may be thrombosed, with extensions into the iliac system and exceptionally into the inferior vena cava. An even rarer source is from jugular thrombosis, sometimes seen as extensions of intracranial venous sinus thrombosis. Axillary and subclavian vein thrombosis is equally unusual, the legs accounting for the vast majority of emboli.

14.3.1.7 Dating of pulmonary emboli and deep vein thrombi As discussed above, it can be a matter of considerable medico-legal importance to know if a pulmonary embolus arose prior to or subsequent to some traumatic event. A major difficulty is that the embolus may be the most recent addition to an extending venous thrombosis that is considerably older.

It is also difficult to use histological criteria to date the free embolus from the lungs, as it is the thrombo-endothelial junction that provides the most information. The best method, therefore, is to examine the residual thrombus, almost always in the leg veins, to see if the oldest part could have formed as far back in time as the suspected traumatic event.

Chronological evaluation is an important factor, especially to determine whether the causation coincides with the date of a specific accident/operation or instead there is an earlier onset of pulmonary thromboembolism.

14.3.1.8 Intracranial vascular conditions There are two main intracranial vascular conditions:

- Subarachnoid haemorrhage: rupture of an aneurysm of the arteries at the base of the brain (circle of Willis) (this may also occur as a result of a vascular malformation).
- Cerebrovascular accident (CVA, stroke): intracerebral haemorrhage or infarction.

14.3.1.9 Aneurysms Aortic aneurysms and dissections frequently present as sudden and unexpected deaths. Most frequent are abdominal aortic aneurysms that present as an unexpected finding at autopsy with extensive haemorrhage into one or other side of the retroperitoneal space. Occasionally dissection of the thoracic aorta is seen, presenting as a haemopericardium, and may be associated with collagen disease, in particular cystic medionecrosis, which is seen in Marfan's syndrome in older adults as a consequence of atherosclerosis with rupture of an atherosclerotic plaque.

14.3.2 Other intracranial causes

14.3.2.1 Epilepsy SUDEP (see above) is thought to be associated with a fit and may occur during sleep. There is an increased risk of SUDEP when there is poor control of seizures. There are frequently no specific anatomical findings seen at autopsy (Leestma et al. 1985). Occasionally, therefore, particularly if death has occurred in a young person and when it is not expected, it may be treated initially as suspicious. The deceased may, for example, die in bed with asphyxial changes because the face may have been pressed into a pillow. Schwender and Troncoso (1986) found that 23 of 29 cases had been found dead in their bed or elsewhere in the bedroom. There may be injuries from fits or the deceased may have fallen into a bath and drowned. Investigation of the scene can therefore be crucial in eliminating any suspicion of foul play as well as differentiating from unnatural causes. The scene, particularly if there are injuries present, should be examined to assess where the deceased could have received such injuries in relation to the position of the body. Distribution of any blood and other body fluids and materials should also be noted; epileptics may bite their tongue and lose blood and saliva from the mouth, lose bladder control, and occasionally may also defecate. The house should also be searched for any medication.

14.3.2.2 Other conditions Meningitis, occasionally tumours, and on a very few occasions hydrocephalus are seen from time in autopsies.

Meningitis is not an uncommon finding presenting as sudden death. Invariably, acute bacterial meningitis is secondary to a bacteraemia in adulthood, and is most commonly caused by pneumococci and meningococci. At necropsy, the brain may be greatly swollen and the sulci filled by a cloudy, pale yellow/green exudate, which, in meningococcal meningitis, may be so slight as to be difficult to identify. Acute bacterial meningitis is frequently associated with social and economic deprivation and alcohol abuse, and is classically associated with pneumonia, a compromised immune system, and an absence of the spleen. It is usually possible to culture pneumococcus from samples taken after death, but this is uncommon in the case of meningococcal meningitis, although the diagnosis may be suspected if there is other evidence of meningococcal disease, such as petechial haemorrhages and purpura of the mucous membranes and skin, and haemorrhagic necrosis of the adrenal glands. This diagnosis can be confirmed by the detection of specific meningococcal capsular polysaccharides in the blood.

14.4 Sudden death in Schizophrenia

Schizophrenia is associated with premature mortality and a high rate of sudden unexpected death. Although a significant number of deaths remain unexplained, post-mortem data indicate that the most common cause of sudden natural death in schizophrenia is coronary artery disease. Furthermore, the rate of sudden cardiac death is 0.8% in a psychiatric hospital, well above the rate in the general population (Ifteni et al. 2014).

14.5 Respiratory causes

14.5.1 Bronchial asthma

Sudden death from bronchial asthma is still a significant cause of sudden and unexpected death both in children and adults of all ages despite improvements in treatment. The mortality risk factors in asthma include poor disease management and adverse psychosocial circumstances. Bronchial asthma causes characteristic histological changes in the mucosa of the airways which are present even before the clinical diagnosis of asthma can be made. These include fibrous thickening of the lamina reticularis of the epithelial basement membrane, smooth muscle hypertrophy and hyperplasia, increased mucosal vascularity, and an eosinophil-rich inflammatory cell infiltrate. In addition, mucoid plugging of the airway lumen is frequently associated with fatal asthma. The recognition of these changes can allow the diagnosis of asthma to be made for the first time at autopsy in those cases where asthma goes undiagnosed in life. Acute severe asthma may be accompanied by pneumothorax and surgical emphysema of the mediastinum (Sidebotham and Roche 2003). Disorders which may mimic asthma include pulmonary embolism, chronic obstructive pulmonary disease (COPD), and anaphylaxis, but careful post-mortem examination and appropriate investigations should reveal the true cause of death.

14.5.2 Chronic obstructive pulmonary disease

The primary cause of COPD is exposure to tobacco smoke (either active smoking or second-hand smoke). Other risk factors include exposure to indoor and outdoor air pollution and occupational dusts and fumes. Globally, it is estimated that about three million deaths were caused by the disease in 2015 (5% of all deaths globally in that year). More than 90% of COPD deaths occur in low- and middle-income countries (World Health Organization 2016).

COPD may either be the main cause of death by exacerbation of symptoms interacting with respiratory failure or be associated with or complicated by a chest infection, most frequently bronchopneumonia.

Less commonly other conditions which have led to sudden death are seen, including haemoptysis associated with pulmonary malignancy where there has been erosion of a major blood vessel by the tumour.

14.5.3 Aspiration of gastric contents

Aspiration of gastric contents is frequently found at autopsy and its significance should be carefully considered. Many instances of aspiration found at post-mortem examination occur during the process of dying as a result of another cause or occur after death in association with resuscitation. From time to time inhaled stomach contents may be found in the lungs of small infants, notably in relation to deaths categorised as SIDS, and one should be very careful in assessing the significance of such findings and reinforcing guilt felt amongst the parents. Knight (1975), from a series of 100 consecutive routine autopsies, found 25 cases with macroscopical gastric contents in the air passages. In no case did the clinical history suggest regurgitation of stomach contents and this was not related to the primary cause of death. However, one must not lose sight of the fact that aspiration in many cases, particularly where the person has been suffering from other conditions, and especially in the very young or the elderly, may indeed be the primary cause of death.

14.5.4 Tuberculosis

Mycobacterium tuberculosis may be encountered in routine coroners' autopsies, occasionally as a previously undiagnosed infection causing death or as a co-morbidity in cases reported to the coroner. Persons suffering from diseases in which the body is immunocompromised, alcoholics, persons living 'rough' or others who may be at risk, particularly if they have returned from countries where the disease is endemic.

Chapman and Claydon (1992) examined 4600 cases from Ealing and Charing Cross hospitals (both in West London) over a three-year period and found 13 cases of tuberculosis (an incidence of 0.28%).

Six were from the Indian subcontinent, six were indigenous Caucasians, and one was Afro-Caribbean. Of the six Caucasians five were known to drink heavily, and three of them led a semi-vagrant life.

Flavin et al. (2007) found unsuspected tuberculosis cases in 10 out of 15 (67%) from a total of 4930 cases (incidence of 0.3%) Their patients tended to be middle aged and male with complex clinical histories; two were HIV positive. Two patients were brought in dead to hospital, with no clinical indication of tuberculosis. They concluded that the risk of unexpectedly encountering the disease at autopsy continues even in a low-risk European setting.

Mortuary technical staff and pathologists and others working in a mortuary environment face an ever-present risk of contracting tuberculosis when exposed to cases. The transfer and handling of a corpse expels air from the lungs of the diseased and this aerosolizes the bacilli. It is for this reason that personal protective equipment and work space precautions such as ultraviolet germicidal irradiation are necessary.

14.6   Gastrointestinal causes

There are a number of gastrointestinal conditions which may commonly present as sudden death. One of the most common presentations is that of acute abdomen (Ng et al. 2007). The authors examined 2121 autopsy cases from 1997 to 2000 of patients aged 70 or above, and they gave 'acute abdomen' as a primary cause of death in 111 cases. Peptic ulcer disease was the most common underlying cause of death. Twenty-nine (26.1%) cases were due to its complications, namely gastrointestinal haemorrhage and perforation. Armstrong and Whitelaw (1988), in a 10-year study of all 9653 autopsies performed in the Plymouth Health District, UK from 1977 to 1986, found 154 patients who died from undiagnosed peptic ulcer complications. In all, 118 of these patients died suddenly at home and 36 died in hospital. Most patients were elderly, although 47 were under 70 years and 2 were under 50 years of age. Anti-inflammatory drugs were being used by 81 of these patients, an incidence of 60% where full drug histories were available. Women who died were much more likely to be using these drugs than men.

Haematemesis is the vomiting of blood (not to be confused with haemoptysis, which is the coughing up of blood). It is seen in peptic ulceration, erosive gastritis, and occasionally from oesophageal varices in persons with chronic alcoholic liver disease.

Acute intestinal obstruction can be seen from various causes, including previous adhesions from surgical intervention, volvulus with or without infarction, incarcerated hernia, faecal impaction, and obstruction by a tumour.

Peritonitis, particularly from perforated peptic ulcer, diverticular disease, appendix or tumour (Hayashi et al. 2013), is occasionally reported to the coroner. These fatalities are mainly related to spontaneous perforation of parts of the gastrointestinal tract.

Acute pancreatitis can present as sudden death, although the condition may represent a spectrum of morbidity from mild to the rapidly progressing haemorrhagic type producing extensive necrosis. A retrospective study of 883 cases of acute pancreatitis by Appelros and Borgström (1999) revealed that from 31 fatalities, only 15 were diagnosed before death. They confirmed that biliary disease (usually related to gall stones) was the main aetiological factor in first attacks whereas alcohol was the predominant factor when relapses were included. In 27 cases of acute pancreatitis presented as sudden unexpected death Tsokos and Braun (2007) found that alcohol was the predominant causative mechanism in medico-legal autopsies rather than gall stones.

References

Armstrong, C.P. and Whitelaw, S. (1988). Death from undiagnosed peptic ulcer complications: a continuing challenge. *Br. J. Surg.* 75: 1112–1114.

Chapman, R.C. and Claydon, S.M. (1992). *Mycobacterium tuberculosis*: a continuing cause of sudden and unexpected death in West London. *J. Clin. Pathol.* 45: 713–715.

Corbin, T. (2005). Investigation into sudden infant deaths and unascertained infant deaths in England and Wales, 1995–2003. *Health Stat. Q.* Autumn (27): 17–23.

Flavin, R.J., Gibbons, N., and O'Briain, D.S. (2007). *Mycobacterium tuberculosis* at autopsy – exposure and protection: an old adversary revisited. *J. Clin. Pathol.* 60: 487–491.

GBD 2013 Mortality and Causes of Death Collaborators (2015). Global, regional, and national age-sex specific all-cause and cause-specific mortality for 240 causes of death, 1990–2013: a systematic analysis for the Global Burden of Disease Study 2013. *Lancet* 385: 117–171.

Grossman, E. and Messerli, F.H. (1996). Diabetic and hypertensive heart disease. *Ann. Inter. Med.* 125: 304–310.

Hayashi, T., Ingold, B., Schönfeld, C., and Tsokos, M. (2013). Sudden unexpected death due to perforation of an unclassified small intestinal tumor. *Forensic Sci. Med. Pathol.* 9: 581–584.

Hsieh, A. and Twigg, S.M. (2014). The enigma of the dead-in-bed syndrome: challenges in predicting and preventing this devastating complication of type 1 diabetes. *J. Diabet. Complicat.* 28: 585–587.

Ifteni, P., Correll, C.U., Burtea, V. et al. (2014). Sudden unexpected death in schizophrenia: autopsy findings in psychiatric inpatients. *Schizophr. Res.* 155: 72–76.

International Statistical Classification of Diseases and Related Health Problems 10th Revision (ICD-10)-2015-WHO Version for 2015. Chapter XVIII. Symptoms, signs and abnormal clinical and laboratory findings, not elsewhere classified. (R00-R99).

Knight, B.H. (1975). The significance of the post-mortem discovery of gastric contents in the air passages. *Forensic Sci.* 6: 229–234.

de la Grandmaison, G.L. (2006). Is there progress in the autopsy diagnosis of sudden unexpected death in adults? *Forensic Sci. Int.* 156: 138–144.

Leestma, J.E., Hughes, J.R., Teas, S.S., and Kalelkar, M.B. (1985). Sudden epilepsy deaths and the forensic pathologist. *Am. J. Forensic Med. Pathol.* 6: 215–218.

Limerick, S.R. and Bacon, C.J. (2004). Terminology used by pathologists in reporting on sudden infant deaths. *J. Clin. Pathol.* 57: 309–311.

Maron, B.J., Towbin, J.A., Thiene, G. et al. (2006). Contemporary definitions and classification of the cardiomyopathies: an American Heart Association Scientific Statement from the Council on Clinical Cardiology, Heart Failure and Transplantation Committee; Quality of Care and Outcomes Research and Functional Genomics and Translational Biology Interdisciplinary Working Groups; and Council on Epidemiology and prevention. *Circulation* 113: 1807–1816.

Menaker, J., Stein, D.M., and Scalea, T.M. (2007). Incidence of early pulmonary embolism after injury. *J. Trauma* 63: 620–624.

Ng, C.Y., Squires, T.J., and Busuttil, A. (2007). Acute abdomen as a cause of death in sudden, unexpected deaths in the elderly. *Scott. Med. J.* 52: 20–23.

Roberts, I.S.D., Gorodkin, L.M., and Benbow, E.W. (2000). What is a natural cause of death? A survey of how coroners in England and Wales approach borderline cases. *J. Clin. Pathol.* 53: 367–373.

Rutty, G.N., Duerden, R.M., Carter, N., and Clark, J.C. (2001). Are coroners' necropsies necessary? A prospective study examining whether a "view and grant" system of death certification could be introduced into England and Wales. *J. Clin. Pathol.* 54: 279–284.

Appelros, S. and Borgström, A. (1999). Incidence, aetiology and mortality rate of acute pancreatitis over 10 years in a defined urban population in Sweden. *Br. J. Surg.* 86: 465–470.

Schwender, L.A. and Troncoso, J.C. (1986). Evaluation of sudden death in epilepsy. *Am. J. Forensic Med. Pathol.* 7: 283–287.

Sheppard, M.N. (2011). *Practical Cardiovascular Pathology*, 133–192. Hodder Arnold Chapter 5.

Sidebotham, H.J. and Roche, W.R. (2003). Asthma deaths: persistent and preventable mortality. *Histopathology* 43: 105–117.

Thomas, A.C., Knapman, P.A., Krikler, D.M., and Davies, M.J. (1988). Community study of the causes of 'natural' sudden death. *BMJ* 297: 1453–1456.

Thomsen, J.L., Felby, S., Theilade, P., and Nielsen, E. (1995). Alcoholic ketoacidosis as a cause of death in forensic cases. *Forensic Sci. Int.* 75: 163–171.

Tsokos, M. and Braun, C. (2007). Acute pancreatitis presenting as sudden, unexpected death: an autopsy-based study of 27 cases. *Am. J. Forensic Med. Pathol.* 28: 267–270.

Tu, E., Bagnall, R.D., Duflou, J., and Semsarian, C. (2011). Post-mortem review and genetic analysis of sudden unexpected death in epilepsy (SUDEP) cases. *Brain Pathol.* 21: 201–208.

Willinger, M., James, L.S., and Catz, C. (1991). Defining the sudden infant death syndrome (SIDS): deliberations of an expert panel convened by the National Institute of Child Health and Human Development. *Pediatr. Pathol.* 11: 677–684.

World Health Organization. Chronic obstructive pulmonary disease (COPD). Fact sheet, November 2016. http://www.who.int/mediacentre/factsheets/fs315/en.

15

Heat, Cold, and Electricity

Peter Vanezis
Queen Mary University of London, London, UK

15.1 Deaths from the effects of heat

15.1.1 Fires

15.1.1.1 Introduction The vast majority of deaths in relation to heat in temperate climates result from the effects of fire.

Fire-related fatalities have also been on a downward trend for many years from a peak of 485 fatalities in 1999/2000 down to a low of 261 in 2016/2017 (National Statistics 2017) (Figure 15.1) The period included in this report does not cover the tragic fire at Grenfell Tower in June 2017, a 24-storey high-rise block of flats in west London in which 72 people lost their lives. It is undoubtedly the worst residential fire disaster in the UK since the Second World War. The fire apparently started from a malfunctioning fridge-freezer on the fourth floor and its rapid spread has been blamed on building materials, especially the building's external cladding. Further information is available at Grenfell Tower.Gov.UK (2017).

The majority of fire-related fatalities occur in dwellings, around 80% in 2016/2017 (213 fire-related fatalities), with very low numbers of fire-related fatalities occurring in other locations. Of the fire-related fatalities which occurred in dwellings the majority, 86% in 2016/2017 (183 fatalities), occurred in accidental fires (Bryant and Preston 2017) (Figure 15.2).

The most common cause of death in fires was inhalation of noxious substances in smoke. Death from burns alone or a combination of burns and smoke is less common.

The vast majority of fires in dwellings are accidental. The main cause is usually careless handling of fire or hot substances (e.g. careless disposal of cigarettes).

Essential Forensic Medicine, First Edition. Edited by Peter Vanezis.
© 2020 John Wiley & Sons Ltd. Published 2020 by John Wiley & Sons Ltd.

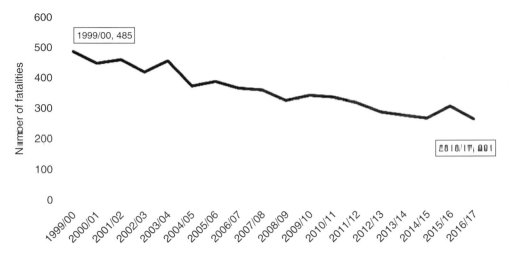

Figure 15.1   Number of fire-related fatalities in England, 1999/2000 to 2016/2017 (National Statistics 2017).

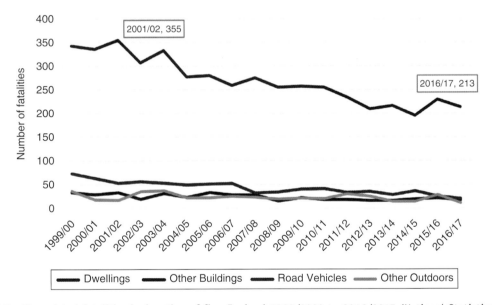

Figure 15.2   Fire-related fatalities by location of fire, England 1999/2000 to 2016/2017 (National Statistics 2017). As stated previously, please be aware that this report covers the period up to the end of March 2017, and therefore the Grenfell Tower fire is not included in these figures.

In England around 10% of fires in which fatalities occur are started deliberately and it is important that every fatal fire be treated as a suspicious death until the cause of the fire has been established (National Statistics 2017). It goes without saying that a multidisciplinary approach to fire investigation is essential. In situations where a fire has been started deliberately, the issues are whether the person of persons found were alive or dead at the time it was started.

15.1.1.2   The scene   The very first consideration at any fire scene should be for the safety of those persons who will be responsible for recovering the body and investigating the cause of the fire. Before entering the premises, an assessment of structure safety should be made and appropriate caution taken by the persons entering the scene. The pathologist's role at this stage, if the body is still present at the scene and has not been recovered prior to his/her arrival, may be limited to a general view of the position of the body and its surroundings because of the severity of the conflagration and debris. Investigation of the cause of the fire will take priority. Examination of the body or bodies is best carried out in the mortuary. Establishing the cause of the fire, whether accidental or deliberate, will be the role of the fire investigators. In relation to fires involving multiple fatalities these are dealt with in chapter 17.

The concept of so-called 'spontaneous' human combustion is a myth. The combustion is not spontaneous. A source of heat is required near the body. It commonly involves the elderly who may also be alcoholic, according to Levi-Faict and Quatrehomme (2011). In some fires the body of the victim may display exceptionally severe localised damage while materials in the immediate vicinity appear to be unaffected. Often the victim's torso is partly or completely consumed and large bones reduced to a crumbly grey ash.

15.1.1.3 Findings in fire deaths As noted above, a person who is in a fire may die from the inhalation of fire fumes, or from burns alone or in combination with the inhalation of toxic fire fumes. Occasionally death may result from falling masonry.

It is also essential to assess whether the victim was dead or alive when the fire started and if dead, if there is evidence of foul play. Disposal of a homicide victim by burning them is not an uncommon method of concealing such a death and misleading investigators (Figure 15.3). Hence, in all fire deaths the investigating team must be careful to assess the true nature of the death and include radiographic imaging prior to commencement of the autopsy.

In the vast majority of cases, where the person was alive at the time of the start of a fire within a building, there is evidence of inhalation of toxic gases and it is very likely that the person died prior to the body becoming significantly burnt. In such instances the findings can range from very little or no evidence of burns and just evidence of toxic gas inhalation, to bodies which are severely burnt with extensive charring of soft and bony tissues.

Amongst the usual findings seen in such deaths are skin defects from skin splitting and blistering. In addition, there may be a heat-induced fractured skull and heat haematomas, especially in an extradural position. It is important that such artefacts are differentiated from injuries occurring during life. Heat contractures to muscle groups, particularly to the arms, may give rise to the so-called 'pugilistic attitude' (Figure 15.4).

Internally one may see thermal injuries to the upper airway (to subglottic level) from the inhalation of hot gases, as well as soot deposition (Figure 15.5). The latter is an extremely important and regular finding in those who have inhaled smoke and on examination of the blood nearly all will have significantly raised carboxyhaemoglobin (further information about carbon monoxide can be found in Chapter 10). The resulting hypoxia is frequently contributed to by cyanide poisoning. There may also be lower respiratory tract irritation from other noxious chemicals.

Overall, without the assistance of the presence of carboxyhaemoglobin and soot deposits in the lower airways, it may be difficult for the pathologist to assess whether the victim was dead or alive when the fire started and clearly such cases will raise suspicions. This is compounded by the fact that it may be difficult, if not impossible, to distinguish between ante-mortem and post-mortem injury when the body has been severely carbonised, as seen in many house and vehicle fires.

(a)

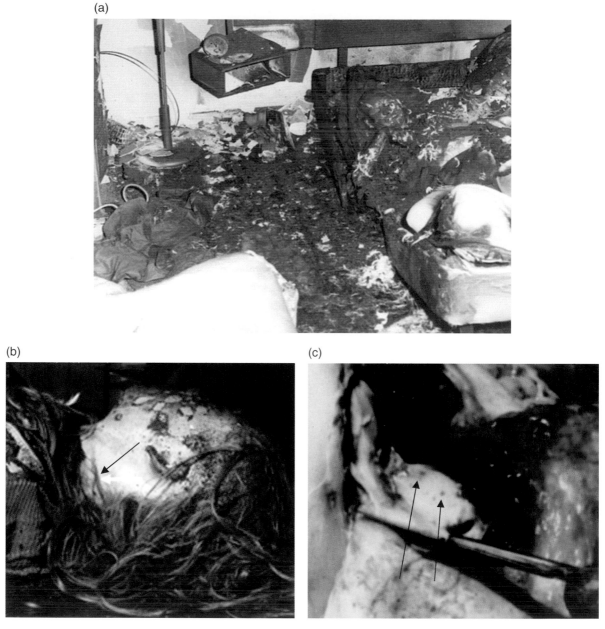

(b)

(c)

Figure 15.3   (a) Woman found dead in a fire in her bedroom. The seat of the fire was by her right side, where she was thought to have dropped a lit cigarette. (b) Examination of the neck showed a narrow ligature mark (arrowed) and her eyes (c) revealed scleral petechial haemorrhages (arrowed). She had been strangled and the room set on fire to conceal the homicide.

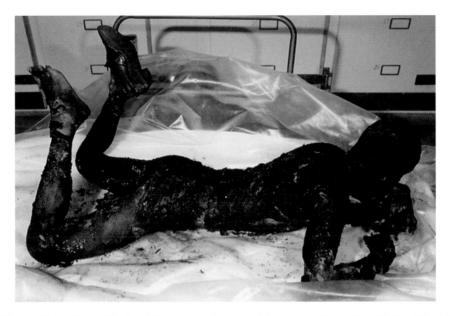

Figure 15.4 Charred body with contracted arms and legs resembling a 'pugilistic attitude'.

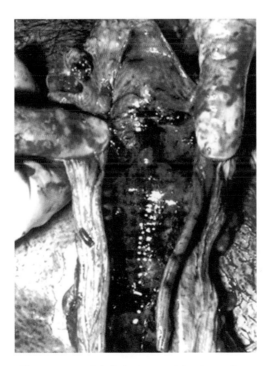

Figure 15.5 Inhaled soot particles in trachea.

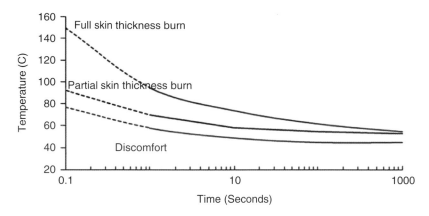

Figure 15.6   Time taken to cause thermal injury against temperature (adapted from various sources).

15.1.1.4   Burns   The production of burns depends on the temperature to which the skin is exposed and the length of exposure. Temperatures above 65 °C will result in instantaneous burns. Lower temperatures (40–55 °C) can still result in burns but after many seconds (Figure 15.6). The aged and children are more susceptible the effects of heat.

The classification of burns is related to the depth and extent of changes in the skin.

–   First-degree burns are the mildest form of burn, causing reddening of the skin, which is transitory.
–   Second-degree or partial thickness burns extend to some of the dermal layers with blistering but there is return to normal, with healing within 10–14 days. Such burns retain the ability for potential regeneration.
–   Third-degree burns or full thickness burns, extend to all layers of the skin. Irreversible damage is caused to all layers of the skin and will require grafting.
–   There may be further extensive damage to deeper tissues, sometimes called fourth-degree burns.
–   Massive damage of tissue may occur such that the burnt areas dry out if exposed to air and produce dessicated eschars (scar tissue).
–   Carbonisation occurs if the temperature reaches about 300 °C.

'The rule of nines' (Figure 15.7) is used for calculating the area of damage on the body surface caused by heat. It allows the clinician to estimate the extent of the spread of the burns on the skin. A total affected body surface area of 30–50% has a generally poor prognosis, although with intensive treatment in a specialised burns unit survival with much greater body coverage may be possible.

15.1.1.5   Scalds   Scalding results from heated fluids such as boiling water or steam (moist heat). Most are considered as first- or second-degree burns, although occasionally third-degree burns can result if there is prolonged contact. Accidental water scalds are commonly seen in the home and in most instances resemble burns from dry heat. Scalds tend to have a well-defined edge and this can be helpful, especially when dealing with burns in children, in deciding whether the configuration of the burn is likely to have been produced in an accidental or deliberate manner (see the section on child abuse in Chapter 13).

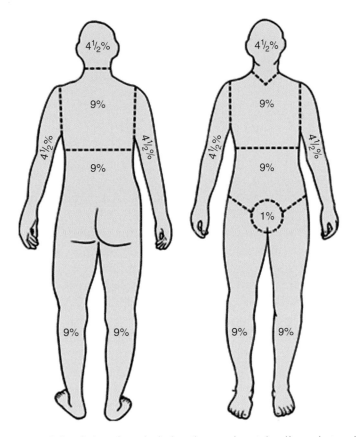

Figure 15.7 Rule of nines for calculating the area burnt (applies only to adults).

15.1.2 Heatstroke and Hyperthermia

Hyperthermia occurs when a body absorbs more heat than it can dissipate and thus cannot regulate its temperature. In humans, hyperthermia is defined as a temperature greater than 37.5–38.3 °C (99.5–100.9 °F), depending on the reference used, that occurs without a change in the body's temperature set point, which characteristically occurs in concert with an increased hypothalamic set point, from severe infection or central nervous system haemorrhage. Hyperthermia is diagnosed clinically by a core body temperature more than 40 °C and occurs when the body's thermoregulatory mechanisms are no longer capable of effectively dissipating heat.

The most common causes of hyperthermia include heatstroke and adverse reactions to drugs. The National Association of Medical Examiners Ad Hoc Committee on the Definition of Heat-Related Fatalities (Donoghue et al. 1997) recommends the following definition of heat-related death: 'a death in which exposure to high ambient temperature either caused the death or significantly contributed to it and excluding other causes of hyperthermia'.

Heatstroke is caused by exposure to excessive heat or a combination of heat and humidity that overpowers the heat-regulating mechanisms. Increased physical activity will also elevate the body temperature and is particularly a problem when the ambient temperature is high at the same time. It is particularly a problem in the very young, the elderly, and chronic alcoholics, who are less likely to have efficient central thermoregulation.

Various classes of legal and illicit drugs, including anticholinergics, antihistamines, antidepressants (monoamine oxidase inhibitors, tricyclics), antiparkinsonian, antipsychotics (butyrophenones, phenothiazines, thioxanthenes), alcohol, amphetamines, phencyclidine hydrochloride, cocaine, and lysergic acid diethylamide, can raise the metabolic rate and cause hypohidrosis, resulting in increased heat production. Diuretics, used often by the elderly, give rise to hypovolemia. Drug-induced hyperthermia (DIH) syndromes are a rare and often overlooked cause of body temperature elevation and can be fatal if not recognised promptly and managed appropriately. There are five major DIH syndromes: neuroleptic malignant syndrome, serotonin syndrome, anticholinergic poisoning, sympathomimetic poisoning, and malignant hyperthermia. The differential diagnosis of DIH syndromes can be challenging because symptoms are generally non-specific, ranging from blood pressure changes and excessive sweating to altered mental status, muscle rigidity, convulsions, and metabolic acidosis.

Social and environmental factors, such as bed confinement, living on the top floor of an apartment building, lack of access to air conditioning, and social isolation with the inability for self-care, all predispose to preventable, yet often deadly, hyperthermia.

Lack of heat acclimatisation is frequently associated with exercise and work-related hyperthermia in hot conditions. Acclimatisation, incremental tolerance to a warmer environment, requires one to two weeks. Without proper dissipation of heat, the increased heat production can result in body temperature increase at a rate of $1.1\,°C\,h^{-1}$. Unacclimatised individuals undergoing strenuous activity generate and retain heat energy up to $1000\,kcal\,kg^{-1}\,h^{-1}$, which may result in severe heat illnesses or death. Initially, exposure to excessive heat raises the body temperature because inadequate sweat production or anhidrosis yields inadequate evaporative heat loss to keep the body normothermic. During small periods of 'protected' exposure, core temperatures adjust and the individual can gradually tolerate the heat longer.

In classical heatstroke the elderly or chronically ill are passively affected in heatwave situations and in addition to hyperthermia, experience anhydrosis and mental status changes. Exertional heatstroke, which occurs in unacclimatised young people involved in vigorous physical activity in hot weather, is the second most common cause of death in high school athletes. They develop tachycardia, tachypnea, hypotension, and mental status alterations with persistent sweating in 50% of victims and elevated muscle and liver enzymes and creatinine secondary to rhabdomyolysis, with hepatic and renal injury.

In cases where the measured ante-mortem body temperature at the time of collapse was $>40.6\,°C$ ($>105\,°F$), the cause of death should be certified as heatstroke or hyperthermia. Deaths may also be certified as heatstroke or hyperthermia with lower body temperatures when cooling has been attempted prior to arrival at hospital and/or when there is a clinical history of mental status changes and elevated liver and muscle enzymes.

A significant number of these deaths will occur in persons having some pre-existing conditions known to be exacerbated by heat stress, such as hyperthyroidism, obesity, and burns, which complicate the usual liberation of heat because of the increased metabolism, decreased activity, increased subcutaneous fat or inability to sweat properly.

Hyperthermia deaths in children younger than four years are often seen in association with vehicular entrapment. They have either gained access to an unlocked car or intentionally or accidentally been left in cars by an adult. The ambient temperature within a parked car on a temperate, sunny day can reach dangerous temperatures within minutes, resulting in heatstroke and death.

The diagnosis of heat-related death is based principally on investigative information; autopsy findings are non-specific. In cases of heat-related death occurring during a heatwave, toxicological analyses will usually not affect the determination of the cause of death but may help identify risk factors and contributory conditions.

If survival is prolonged, measured in hours before death, laboratory, macroscopic, and histopathologic findings vary greatly and may consist of acute renal failure with rhabdomyolysis, acute tubular necrosis, and disseminated intravascular coagulation, hepatic failure with centrilobular necrosis, acute pancreatitis, pulmonary oedema with diffuse alveolar damage, and cerebral oedema with diffuse neuronal injury.

15.2 Deaths from the effects of cold

15.2.1 Hypothermia

Hypothermia is characterised by an unintentional drop in core body temperature to less than 35 °C. It is noteworthy that deaths related to environmental conditions occur equally as frequently indoors as outdoors and are also recorded in temperate climates. A debilitated elderly person may become hypothermic at home in temperatures as high as 22–24 °C.

Unlike secondary hypothermia, which results from diseases disrupting hypothalamic thermoregulation, hypothermia from exposure to cold (primary accidental hypothermia) supervenes when heat retention by the protective body mass and excess heat production produced by shivering are insufficient to maintain a normal body temperature.

The risk for hypothermia is particularly great during prolonged exposure to sub-zero ambient temperatures. Furthermore, the wind chill index, calculated by factoring ambient temperature, wind velocity, and thermal radiation, is an accepted, reliable measure of conditions contributing to cold stress. At above-freezing temperatures, an overriding wind chill factor can hasten hypothermia. For example, individuals have experienced hypothermia clinically in hurricane conditions at 4.4 °C in wind and rain, and at 15.6 °C.

The elderly and the very young are especially susceptible to fatal cold exposure. There are multiple mechanisms of action which put the aged at risk of hypothermia, including:

- reduced heat production because of loss of physiological reserves in chronic disease
- increased heat loss from malnutrition and diminished subcutaneous muscle and fat
- impaired thermoregulation primarily from primary or secondary pathologies of the central nervous system
- inactivity related to senility.

In infants, increased body surface area–body mass index coexists with underdeveloped thermoregulatory mechanisms.

A variety of commonly prescribed drugs, including antidepressants, barbiturates, opioids, benzodiazepines, phenothiazines, and reserpine, adversely affect the body's ability to sense cold. In addition, ethyl alcohol promotes rapid cooling by effecting continuous peripheral vasodilation and inhibiting heat production by shivering. Alcohol, whose intoxicating effects cloud appropriate decision making in cold environments, is the chemical most commonly detected in the blood of victims succumbing to primary hypothermia.

15.2.1.1 Thermoregulation and features of hypothermia Heat loss occurs at two levels: intrinsic from the core to the skin or respiratory tract and extrinsic from the skin to the environment. The intrinsic pathway is predominantly derived from circulating blood and maintained by subcutaneous tissues. The extrinsic pathway of heat dissipation occurs from four environmentally mediated heat transferring mechanisms: conduction, convection, radiation, and evaporation.

Once the internal thermoregulatory controls are compromised by excesses in environmental temperatures, signs and symptoms of hypothermia or hyperthermia ensue. As skin and core temperatures fall to a critical degree in severe exposures, hypothalamic control of body temperature fails and the warm-blooded individual converts functionally to a poikilotherm.

The ensuing peripheral vasodilation results in a sudden rush of warmer blood to the extremities. This exaggerated heat sensation, as perceived by the mentally confused, severely hypothermic individual, leads to the rare volitional act of undressing prior to coma and death and is known as *paradoxical undressing*. Some investigators postulate that the first stage of hypothermia causes paralysis of the vasomotor centre, producing the aberrant sensation of a higher body temperature. A variant of this phenomenon, termed the *hide-and-die syndrome*, arises when the strange location of the body at the scene suggests to investigators that the deceased attempted concealment.

Only in rare cases are there reports of survival without profound brain injury following extreme hypothermia, most commonly seen in children submerged in freezing water for as long as 30 minutes. Indeed, if the victim is rewarmed promptly, death may not result.

In fatal cases, the skin of the extremities may exhibit patches of poorly circumscribed pink to red-brown discoloration in association with bright red hypostasis (frost erythema), which may be confused with carbon monoxide or cyanide intoxication. The red colour of the skin and soft tissues is attributed to the increased percentage of oxyhaemoglobin in the blood engorging the vasculature. Cutaneous blistering may accompany hyperaemia and oedema. Abrasions on the palms of the hands and flexor surfaces of the arms and legs often are associated with stumbling. Other non-specific findings at autopsy may include multifocal haemorrhages of the gastric and duodenal mucosa (termed *Wischnewski spots*) (Figure 15.8), haemorrhagic pancreatitis (Figure 15.9), and haemorrhage of the iliopsoas muscle. However, in the majority of cases the gross and microscopic findings are non-diagnostic: only pulmonary oedema may be present.

The problematic issue of non-specific diagnostic findings in hypothermia has been discussed by Palmiere C et al (2014) as well as the possibility of employing biochemical parameters for clarifying the diagnosis.

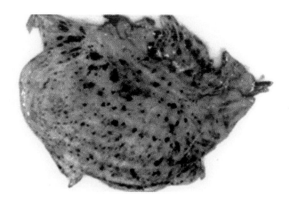

Figure 15.8 Wischnewski spots.

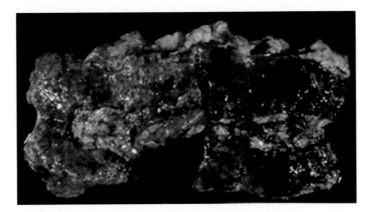

Figure 15.9 Haemorrhagic pancreatitis.

In presumptive hypothermic deaths, the investigator should conduct a scene investigation as early as possible. Determination of the rectal temperature by a non-standard thermometer specially calibrated from 28.9 to 43.2 °C at this stage may assist in the diagnosis. It goes without saying that evaluation of hypothermia goes hand in hand with knowledge of the environmental conditions prevalent during the relevant window of time when death could have occurred.

15.3 Deaths from electricity

15.3.1 Epidemiology

It is estimated that approximately 1000 people die of exposure to electricity annually in the USA (Skoog 1970; Cawley and Homce 2003). The age distribution of deaths shows two peaks, in young children under six years of age and in young adults. With children, the electrocution occurs within the domestic environment whereas most adult deaths are related to their occupation. This is particularly the case with construction workers and miners, with rates of 1.8–2.0 deaths per 100000 workers (John et al. 2003).

15.3.2 Electrocution

Deaths involving electrocution are most frequently accidental. It is an infrequent mode of suicide (Fernando and Liyanage 1990) and an exceedingly rare mode of homicide (Al-Alousi 1990). Wright and Davis (1980) state that proper investigation of injury and death from electrocution requires a high level of suspicion, as examination of the victim will often prove negative. There must be careful photographic documentation of the scene in every case. In low-voltage cases, the equipment that may have been involved should be photographed, X-rayed, and examined electrically. Autopsy examination of the victim in cases of electrocution due to high-voltage alternating or direct current usually reveals burns and occasionally non-specific findings of asphyxia. Victims of low-voltage alternating current often have no electrical burns and this absence is characteristic of ventricular fibrillation. Low-voltage direct current rarely produces death.

The effect of electricity on a person depends on many factors, including the nature of the current with respect to its frequency, voltage, amperage, and duration as well as whether the body is effectively earthed and the path of current through body.

15.3.2.1 Mechanism of injury High-voltage electric shocks (1000V or more) are expected to result in more severe injury per time of exposure. Typical household electricity is 110–230V and high-tension power lines have voltages of more than 100000V. Lightning strikes can produce 10 million volts or more.

There are four effects of electrocution:

- direct effect of current on body tissues, leading to asystole, ventricular fibrillation or apnoea
- blunt mechanical injury from lightning strikes, resulting in muscle contraction or falling
- conversion of electrical energy to thermal energy, resulting in burns
- electroporation, defined as the creation of pores in cell membranes by means of electrical current. Unlike thermal burns, which cause tissue damage by protein denaturation and coagulation, electroporation disrupts cell membranes and leads to cell death without clinically significant heating. This form of injury occurs when high electrical field strengths (defined as volts per metre) are applied.

Direct current causes a single muscle contraction, often throwing the person receiving the electrical shock away from the source of electricity. Alternating current is considered more dangerous than direct current because it can lead to repetitive, tetanic muscle contraction. In the case of contact between the palm and an electrical source, alternating current can cause a hand to grip the source of electricity (because of a stronger flexor than extensor tone) and lead to longer electrical exposure. The amount of alternating current needed to cause injury varies with the frequency of the current. Skeletal muscles become tetanic at lower frequencies, ranging from 15 to 150Hz. Household electricity (60Hz) is particularly arrhythmogenic and may lead to fatal ventricular arrhythmias. Alternating current is the most frequent cause of electrocution.

The outcome of electrical contact, which depends on amperage, varies with the resistance of the body tissues. Tissues that have a higher resistance to electricity, such as skin, bone and fat, tend to increase in temperature and coagulate. Nerves and blood vessels that have low resistance to electricity conduct electricity readily. The skin has a wide range of resistance to electricity and plays the crucial role of gatekeeper when the body is exposed to electricity. Dry skin, which has a higher resistance to electricity than moist skin, may have extensive superficial tissue damage but may limit conduction of potentially harmful current to deeper structures. Moist skin receives less superficial thermal injury but allows more current to pass to deeper structures, resulting in more extensive injury to internal organs. Rubber gloves and rubber or leather soles provide adequate protection.

Death in electrocution usually results from ventricular fibrillation or suppression of activity of respiratory centres in the brain stem.

15.3.2.2 Injuries

Skin Burn injuries are categorised into four groups: electrothermal burns (Figures 15.10 and 15.11), arc burns, flame burns, and lightning injuries. The electrothermal burn is the classic injury pattern and creates a skin entrance and exit wound. Regardless of the mechanism involved, wounds due to exposure to electricity can be classified as partial thickness, full-thickness or skin burns involving deeper subcutaneous tissue. High-voltage injuries commonly produce greater damage to deeper tissues, largely sparing the skin surface.

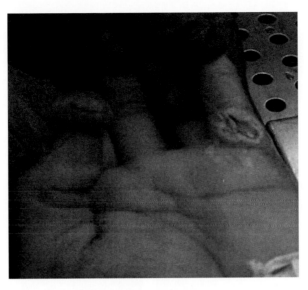

Figure 15.10 Electric burn of left hand caused by contact with a live electric cable. Note on the palm opposite the fifth finger there is an area of pale contact burn where the cable was gripped in the hand between the two surfaces.

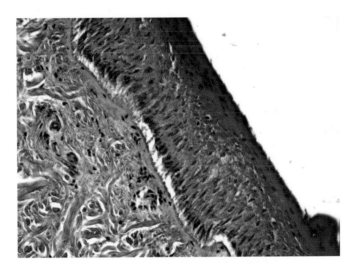

Figure 15.11 Area of skin burn on the hand. Note the presence of palisade-like nuclei in the stratum spinosum of the epidermis, lysis in the stratum granulosum. and incomplete detachment from the underlying dermis (Haematoxylin & Eosin, 10×) (Bellini et al. 2016).

Respiratory Respiratory arrest immediately following electrical shock may result from inhibition of the central nervous system respiratory drive, prolonged paralysis of respiratory muscles, tetanic contraction of respiratory muscles or a combined cardiorespiratory arrest secondary to ventricular fibrillation or asystole. In the last case, respiratory arrest may persist after restoration of spontaneous circulation.

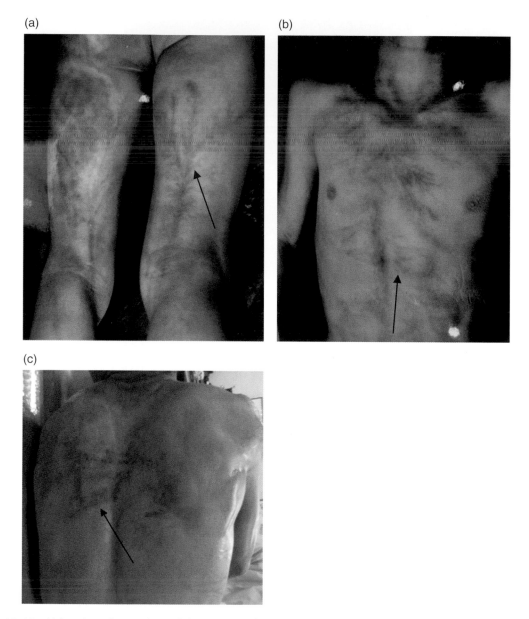

Figure 15.12 Lichtenberg figures (arrows) in two case of lightning strike: Case 1 (a) legs and (b) front of chest; Case 2 (c) back. (Courtesy of Dr Alex Lee Jiun Yih.)

Cardiovascular Cardiac effects of electrical shock can be divided into arrhythmias, conduction abnormalities, and myocardial damage. The last category can be further separated into injury due to direct electricity exposure and secondary myocardial injury due to induced ischemia. These effects are not mutually exclusive. Sudden cardiac death due to ventricular fibrillation is more common with low-voltage alternating current, whereas asystole is more frequent with electric shocks from direct current or high-voltage alternating current.

Musculoskeletal Bone has the highest electrical resistance and experiences the most severe electrothermal injuries, including periosteal burns, destruction of bone matrix, and osteonecrosis. Forceful tetanic contractions or falls can cause fractures and large-joint dislocation. Electrothermal injury of the musculature may manifest as oedema formation and tissue necrosis, and may lead to compartment syndrome and rhabdomyolysis. The extent of muscle tissue damage can be assessed with serum measurements of creatine kinase.

Neurological Electrical shock can damage the central and peripheral nervous system. Loss of consciousness, generalised weakness, autonomic dysfunction, respiratory depression, and memory problems are frequent manifestations. *Keraunoparalysis* is a specific form of reversible, transient paralysis that is associated with sensory disturbances and peripheral vasoconstriction and is seen in some patients following lightning injury. Central nervous system complications also include hypoxic encephalopathy, intracerebral haemorrhage, and cerebral infarction.

15.4 Lightning

Lightning strike is unique because it causes cardiac and respiratory arrest, resulting in a 25–30% mortality rate. Lightning delivers a large amount of direct-current electricity (up to hundreds of millions of volts during a very short period (milliseconds)). Thus, according to Joule's law, the actual amount of energy delivered may be less than with other high-voltage electrical injuries because of the short exposure time. Those struck by lightning rarely sustain extensive tissue destruction or large cutaneous burns. The mode of cardiac arrest in patients struck by lighting is asystole, with frequent spontaneous restoration of an organised cardiac rhythm. However, concomitant respiratory arrest is often prolonged, and without ventilator support apnoea results in hypoxia-induced ventricular fibrillation. Thus, the duration of apnoea, rather than the duration of initial asystole, has been considered the critical factor in the survival of patients who have been struck by lightning. Although rarely seen, Lichtenberg figures (tree branch pattern) are pathognomonic skin manifestations in persons struck by lightning (Resnik and Wetli 1996) (Figure 15.12).

References

Al-Alousi, L.M. (1990). Homicide by electrocution. *Med. Sci. Law* 30: 239–246.

Bellini, E., Gambassi, G., Nucci, G. et al. (2016). Death by electrocution: histological technique for copper detection on the electric mark. *Forensic Sci. Int.* 264: 24–27.

Bryant, S. and Preston, I. (2017). *Focus on Trends in Fires and Fire Related Fatalities*. Home Office.

Cawley, J.C. and Homce, G.T. (2003). Occupational electrical injuries in the United States, 1992–1998, and recommendations for safety research. *J. Safety Res.* 34: 241–248.

Donoghue, E.R., Graham, M.A., Jentzen, J.M. et al. (1997). Criteria for the diagnosis of heat-related deaths: National Association of Medical Examiners – position paper. *Am. J. Forensic Med. Pathol.* 18: 11–14.

Fernando, R. and Liyanage, S. (1990). Suicide by electrocution. *Med. Sci. Law* 30: 219–220.

Grenfell Tower: Information relating to the fire at Grenfell Tower. Published 22 June 2017. Last updated 12 June 2018. http://www.gov.uk/government/collections/grenfell-tower.

John, B.A., Bena, J.F., Stayner, L.T. et al. (2003). External cause specific summaries of occupational fatal injuries. Part I: an analysis of rates. *Am. J. Ind. Med.* 43: 237–250.

Levi-Faict, T.W. and Quatrehomme, G.J. (2011). So-called spontaneous human combustion. *Forensic Sci.* 56: 1334–133952.

National Statistics. Detailed analysis of fires attended by fire and rescue services, England, April 2016 to March 2017. Focus on trends in fires and fire-related fatalities.GOV.UK http://www.gov.uk/government/statistics/detailed-analysis-of-fires-attended-by-fire-and-rescue-services-england-april-2016-to-march-2017.

Resnik, B.I. and Wetli, C.V. (1996). Lichtenberg figures. *Am. J. Forensic Med. Pathol.* 17: 99–102.

Skoog, T. (1970). Electrical injuries. *J. Trauma* 10: 816–830.

Wright, R.K. and Davis, J.H. (1980). The investigation of electrical deaths: a report of 220 fatalities. *J. Forensic Sci.* 25: 514–521.

Palmiere, C., Teresiński, G., and Hejna, P. (2014). Postmortem diagnosis of hypothermia. *Int J Legal Med.* 120, 607 611.

16
Diagnosing Death and Changes after Death

Peter Vanezis
Queen Mary University of London, London, UK

16.1   Introduction

Historically the recognition of death has been defined through cultural and religious practices and various other taboos and over time has evolved through the development of medical science (Figure 16.1).

The definition of death has changed over the years to take into account advances made in medicine and in reality, from the medical point of view, is inextricably linked to procedures relating to organ donation for transplantation.

Pallis' definition is 'Human death is a state in which there is irreversible loss of the capacity for consciousness combined with irreversible loss of the capacity to breathe (and hence to maintain a heartbeat) – alone neither would be sufficient' (Pallis 1983). In most deaths, whether at home or on general hospital wards, once the heart stops beating that is the point at which a person is accepted as being dead. In another group of patients, those who have sustained head injuries, massive strokes or cerebral anoxia for whatever reason and are in ICU and kept 'animated' by life support systems, the story is very different. It is in such cases, particularly where the possibility of the donation of organs exists for transplantation, that the criteria for ensuring that the person is, without question, irretrievably dead have been extensively studied and debated.

Nowadays, the concept of brain stem death is virtually universally accepted as the point from which there is no return (Mohandas and Chou 1971). Charlton summarises the position as follows: 'The diagnosis of death is made by excluding all possible signs of life. Thus, to avoid apparent death

Essential Forensic Medicine, First Edition. Edited by Peter Vanezis.
© 2020 John Wiley & Sons Ltd. Published 2020 by John Wiley & Sons Ltd.

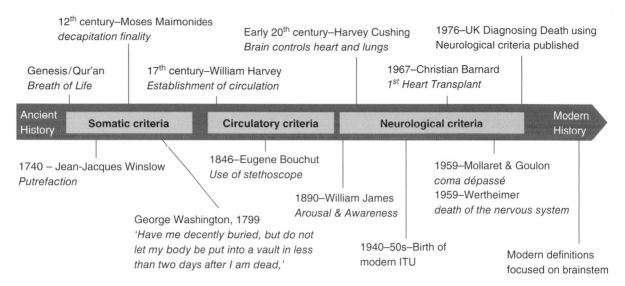

Figure 16.1   History of diagnosing death timeline. (Source: Courtesy of Dr Andrew Vanezis, personal communication.)

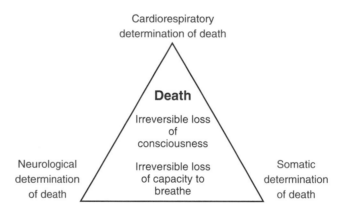

Figure 16.2   Relationship between criteria for the diagnosis and confirmation of death. (After Oram and Murphy 2011.)

being mistaken for actual death and to ensure that opportunities for resuscitation are not missed, corners should never be cut in making this ultimate diagnosis.' (Charlton 1996).

The World Health Organization (WHO, 2014) defined death as '… the permanent loss of capacity for **consciousness and all brainstem function**. This may result from permanent cessation of *circulation* or catastrophic *brain injury*. In the context of death determination, [the term] **permanent** refers to loss of function that cannot resume spontaneously and will not be restored through intervention.'

The inter-relationship between the various criteria used to diagnose and confirm death is shown in Figure 16.2.

16.2   Is the person really dead?

In the nineteenth century, fear of premature internment resulting from the person not being dead was very common (Figure 16.3).

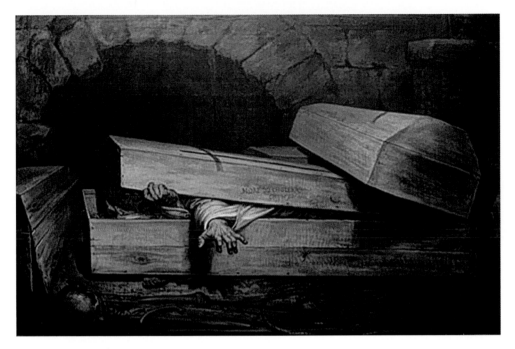

Figure 16.3 Wiertz's painting of a man buried alive – L'Inhumation précipitée, 1854, depicts a cholera victim awakening after being placed in a coffin (Antoine Joseph Wiertz 1806–1865).

Much of this fear stemmed from the population not having much faith in the medical profession of the time. Indeed, the Victorians took a number of precautions to prevent live internment. For example, the deceased were left lying in their caskets for days or weeks on end before being deemed sufficiently dead to bury. When the Duke of Wellington died in 1858, he was not buried until two months after his death!

A simpler method of allaying premature-burial anxiety was to place crowbars and shovels in the deceased's caskets; if they revived, they could dig their way out. Also used was a pipe that went through the ground and into the casket, to be used for emergency communications (Figure 16.4). Such 'safety coffins' were fitted with a mechanism to prevent premature burial or allow the occupant to signal that they have been buried alive. A large number of designs for safety coffins were patented during the eighteenth and nineteenth centuries and variations on the idea are still available today.

There are a number of conditions which may be mistaken for death:

- Hypothermia: The elderly in particular are at risk from hypothermia for a number of reasons. Any condition which causes coma can impair temperature regulation and lead to hypothermia.

- Drug overdose: Tricyclic antidepressants and barbiturates are known to mimic brain death, as well as alcohol, and anaesthetic agents.

- Metabolic states: Myxoedema, coma, uraemia, hypoglycaemia, hyperosmolar coma, and hepatic encephalopathy.

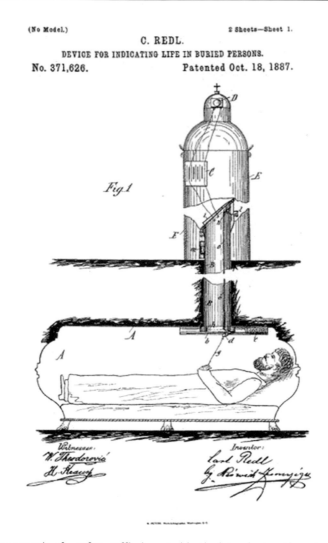

Figure 16.4   An example of a safety coffin invented in the late nineteenth century (C. Redl, 1887).

16.3   Types of death

16.3.1   Somatic death

Initially there is overall loss of all bodily functions, including:

- irreversible loss of sensory feeling

- inability to communicate with or be aware of their environment

- inability to initiate any voluntary movement

- loss of vital signs.

There may be continuation of reflex activity (nervous, circulatory, respiratory), spontaneous or with artificial support.

For approximately six minutes after somatic death – a period referred to as clinical death – a person whose vital organs have not been damaged may be revived. For example, there may be sudden cessation of vital functions in a number of conditions and be amenable to successful resuscitation in, e.g. in drowning, airway obstruction and electric shock or lightning strike.

16.3.2 Cellular death

The death of tissues and constituent cells results from ischaemia and anoxia following somatic death. Different cells die at different rates after cessation of the circulation. The cerebral cortex develops anoxia after only a few minutes of cessation of the circulation. On the other hand, other tissue such as connective tissue and muscle will remain viable for a number of hours.

Somatic death is followed by a number of irreversible changes that are of legal importance. These are discussed below and are especially significant in estimating the time of death. They include rigor mortis, hypostasis, cooling of the body, autolysis, and putrefaction.

The following personnel with appropriate training are authorised to pronounce/diagnose death in the UK:

- A doctor of any grade.

- First level registered nurse (band 6–8) with specific training in relation to the death of adult patients in cases when the patient's death is expected within the context of a medical facility.

- Paramedics in hospital or out-of-hospital deaths.

- Emergency services technicians with appropriate training (minimum 12 months) for out-of-hospital deaths.

Usually in the context of out-of-hospital deaths there are established criteria for the purpose of recognition of life extinct (ROLE) by paramedics:

- massive cranial and cerebral destruction

- hemicorporectomy

- massive truncal injury incompatible with life, including decapitation

- decomposition/putrefaction

- incineration (full thickness burns + charring of 95% of the body surface)

- hypostasis

- rigor mortis.

16.4   Diagnosis of circulatory death

Death after cardiorespiratory arrest is identified by the simultaneous and irreversible onset of apnoea, unconsciousness, and absence of the circulation. There are no standardised criteria for the confirmation of death following irreversible cessation of cardiorespiratory function as exists with confirmation of brainstem death. UK best practice (in the absence of somatic identifiers such as rigor mortis/hypostasis) includes:

- absence of a central pulse on palpation (five minutes)

- absence of heart sounds on auscultation (five minutes)

- absence of respiratory effort and breath sounds on auscultation (five minutes)

- absence of pupillary responses to light, corneal reflexes, and motor response to supra-orbital pressure (greater than five minutes after continued cardiorespiratory arrest).

In hospital, the above can be augmented with:

- asystole on a continuous electrocardiograph (ECG) display

- absence of pulsatile flow using direct intra-arterial pressure monitoring

- absence of contractile activity using echocardiography.

Other considerations:

- Full/extensive attempts at reversal of any contributing cause to the cardiorespiratory arrest have been made.

- One of the following is fulfilled:
  - the individual meets the criteria for not attempting CPR
  - attempts at CPR have failed
  - treatment aimed at sustaining life has been withdrawn because it has been decided to be:
    - of no further benefit to the patient
    - and not in his/her best interest to continue
    - and/or is in respect of the patient's wishes via an advance decision to refuse treatment.

Any spontaneous return of cardiac or respiratory activity during the five minute period of observation should prompt a further five minutes of observation from the next point of cardiorespiratory arrest.

The time of death is recorded as the time at which these criteria are fulfilled.

16.5 Diagnosis of brain death

Brain death is used in the scenario of a comatosed patient (Glasgow Coma Scale 3), usually in the setting on an ITU on ventilator support. Hospital staff are aware of the need to make decisions that are in patient's best interest. In the UK, Canada, and India, the focus is on the brainstem whereas in other countries, such as the USA and Australia, brain death includes assessing higher cortical functions as well as the brain stem.

Diagnosis is made after the cause and depth of the coma have been determined and an attempt has been made to maintain life and restore function (respecting any valid advance decision to refuse treatment) and based on criteria proposed by the Academy of Royal Colleges (2008]), with subsequent revisions. Courts in England and Northern Ireland have adopted these criteria for the diagnosis of death.

The patient's situation before performing brain death testing should be such that:

1. there is no doubt that the patient's condition is due to irreversible brain damage of known aetiology or

2. a final diagnosis is never fully established despite extensive investigation and includes:
   a. presumed hypoxic brain injury
   b. cerebral air or fat embolism
   c. drug overdose
   d. encephalitis.

The patient who is in apnoeic coma, i.e. unresponsive and on a ventilator, is only subjected to brain death testing if, after continuing observation/investigation, there is no possibility of finding a reversible/treatable underlying cause.

Reversible causes of coma which need to be excluded include:

• coma due to depressant medications

• primary hypothermia

• potentially reversible circulatory, metabolic, and endocrine disturbances causing coma (cause and effect sometimes difficult to establish, e.g. ↓Na^+).

Reversible causes of apnoea which need to be excluded:

• neuromuscular blocking agents/other drugs

• cervical spine injury following trauma. In such cases apnoeic brainstem tests are invalid. Only other brain stem reflexes should be used. Furthermore, ancillary tests should be considered. The latter are used less in the UK than in North America and include the use of EEG, transcranial dopplers, four vessel angiography and CT and MR angiography.

Other prerequisites are necessary before performing brain death testing. There must be two doctors to carry out the tests who have been registered for over five years and are competent in the procedure. One of the doctors should be a consultant. They must undertake the tests together and perform them successfully and completely on two occasions. The doctors must not have or be perceived to have any clinical conflict of interest and must not be members of the transplant team. It is also good practice to have the family present during the testing.

16.6   Diagnostic tests for brain stem death

There will an absence of brain stem reflexes:

* no pupillary responses to light

* no corneal reflex

* no vestibulo-ocular reflex

* no cranial nerve motor responses

* no gag or reflex responses to tracheal suction

* no oculocephalic reflex 'dolling' (important to test although not in UK code of practice).

Testing for apnoea should also be done:

* preoxygenate with 100% oxygen for 10 minutes

* reduce ventilation rate or administer 5% carbon dioxide.

It is important to note the difference between brain stem death and persistent vegetative state. Persistent vegetative state is irreversible destruction to the cortex, but the brain stem is not damaged. The patient may develop permanent unconsciousness, but cardio-respiratory functions continue unassisted. This is may occur from a period of hypoxia, trauma or toxic insult.

16.7   Organ donation

In the UK approximately 8000 patients are actively waiting for an organ transplant and over 1000 patients die each year before a suitable organ becomes available.

In relation to consent for organ donation the General Medical Council in their Good Medical Practice guidelines state the following:

* 'If a patient is close to death and their views cannot be determined, you should be prepared to explore with those close to them whether they had expressed any views about organ or tissue donation, if donation is likely to be a possibility.'

• 'The doctor should follow any national procedures for identifying potential organ donors and, in appropriate cases, for notifying the local transplant coordinator. He/she must take account of the requirements in relevant legislation and in any supporting codes of practice in any discussions that they have with the patient or those close to them. The doctor should make it clear that any decision about whether the patient would be a suitable candidate for donation would be made by the transplant coordinator or team, and not by the doctor and the team providing treatment.'

The National Health Service organ donation taskforce produced guidelines recommending the minimum conditions for referral for donation. It included patients where the intention is to confirm death:

• by neurological criteria for donation after brain-stem death (DBD)

• after a clinical decision to withdraw active treatment had been made for donation after circulatory death (DCD).

16.7.1 Management of the brain dead person

Initiating mechanical ventilation in those patients thought to have irremediable brain damage, who stop breathing *before* brain stem death testing can occur, is both justified and legal. On the other hand, elective ventilation, i.e. initiating mechanical ventilation in those patients *already declared brainstem dead* to preserve organ function, was a practice started in Exeter but deemed illegal in the UK in 1994 and classed as battery (the 'dead donor' rule) (Mental Capacity Act 2005). No test case has yet been through the courts.

16.7.2 Donation after circulatory death

There is an increasing proportion of donors in this category. They can be classed as controlled or uncontrolled. *Controlled* organ retrieval occurs after death which follows the planned withdrawal of life-sustaining treatments that have been considered to be of no overall benefit to a critically ill patient on ICU or in the emergency department. *Uncontrolled* organ retrieval occurs after a cardiac arrest that is unexpected and from which the patient cannot/should not be resuscitated. A surgical retrieval team must be immediately available in a nearby theatre before death (by implication before cardio-respiratory support withdrawal) (see also the Maastricht Classification of Donation after Circulatory Death 2013) (Thuong et al. 2016).

16.7.3 Organ donation (opt in/out) policy in the UK

England, Scotland, and Northern Ireland have an *opt-in* policy (for England in the Human Tissue Act 2004, for Scotland in the Human Tissue [Scotland] Act 2006, and for Northern Ireland in common law). Since December 2015 Wales has an *opt-out* policy (Human Transplantation [Wales] Act 2013).

16.7.4 Family's role in organ donation

There is no provision in any of the Acts for family members to be able to overturn an individual's intentions. Scottish legislation, however, allows families to complete a written waiver should they seek to obstruct a loved one's decision to be a donor. If the wishes of the individual are not known/cannot be determined, then the authority for decision making passes to:

- a nominated/appointed representative (England and Northern Ireland)

- a person in a qualifying relationship (England, Scotland, and Northern Ireland)

- In Wales, deemed consent would normally be applicable. Only if it is not (e.g. in the case of a child) would those in a qualifying relationship be approached for consent.

16.7.5   Position of the coroner

In some circumstances it is necessary for the coroner to determine if an objection to organ donation will be raised. The specialist nurse ensures all relevant information is relayed to the coroner so that they may make a decision in relation to raising an objection to organ donation.

16.8   Early Indications of Death

16.8.1   Within a few minutes of death

One of the very first signs noticeable after death is pallor of the body and loss of elasticity of skin. All reflexes are lost and there will be no reaction to painful stimuli. Although all muscle tone is lost, it still physically capable of contraction for many hours. Due to the loss of muscle tone and skin elasticity, contact flattening in areas in contact over surfaces will be noticeable and is usually seen over the shoulder blades, buttocks, and calves.

The eyes also show characteristic early changes, including:

- reflex loss from insensitive corneas and fixed unreactive pupils
- fall in intra-ocular tension
- the corneas appear cloudy
- dessication of exposed sclerae nown as 'tache noir' (Figure 16.5)
- 'trucking' in retinal vessels (loss of blood pressure causes blood to break up into segments).

16.8.2   Early changes after death up to 12 hours

Once somatic death has occurred, cellular death proceeds and is manifest by various post-mortem changes. Those of forensic importance which appear from within a few minutes up to the first 12 hours are:

- ocular and other signs (described above)
- cooling of the body
- hypostasis
- rigor mortis.

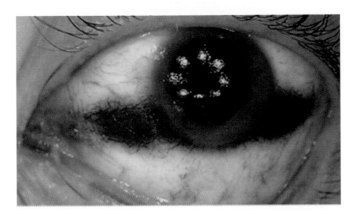

Figure 16.5 Dessication of the scleral after death causing 'tach noir'.

16.8.2.1 Cooling of the body The skin surface begins to cool and a gradient is set up and followed by cooling of the centre or core of the body. Initially there will be a plateau on measurement of the rectal temperature until the steep curve of the gradient forms, taking the form of an exponential curve.

As the difference between the core body temperature and the ambient temperature approaches zero, the curve flattens (Figure 16.6).

Although one would expect to use the straight steep gradient of the curve to assess the post-mortem interval, assuming the core body temperature at the point of death was 37 °C, there are too many variable factors affecting heat loss so that an accurate assessment in case work is not possible.

The factors which can affect the use of cooling for time of death estimation include:

- an initial higher temperature, which may be caused as a result of emotional stress and increased physical activity, febrile disease states or from an increased metabolic rate caused, for example, by hyperthyroidism
- a lower initial temperature, which may be found in persons with exposure to a severe cold environment or suffering from peripheral circulatory disorders or from metabolic disorders such as hypothyroidism
- other factors, for example children have higher rectal and oral temperatures (37.5–38 °C) and there may thermoregulatory system problems in some conditions which prevent heat loss or heat production.

In addition to the above, consideration should be given to the way the body losses heat. This can be by radiation, vaporisation, convection, and conduction. It is important to be aware of the interaction of these variables as well as the difference between the core temperature and temperature of the surroundings. Investigation of the body and its surroundings should therefore note the following:

- coverings on the torso
- air movements
- air humidity
- posture of the body

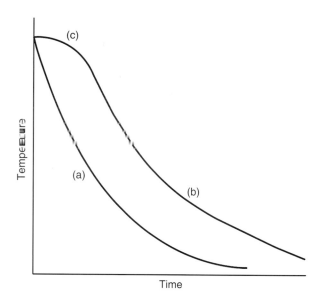

Figure 16.6   Cooling curves: the Newtonian single exponential curve (a) does not occur in practice, except on the surface of the body. Because of the variable plateau (c), the true curve for deep core temperature (b) assumes a double exponential shape. The sigmoidal shape of the cooling curve is best described by Marshall and Hoare's two-exponential term (Marshall and Hoare 1962).

- medium in which the body is found
- body dimensions.

16.8.2.2   Use of a nomogram for estimating the time of death   The nomogram published by Henssge (1988) (Figure 16.7) is based on accumulated research data and conventional calculations. Adjustments are built in for body weight, ambient temperature, dry or wet clothing, still or moving air, and still or flowing water. The result is provided with different error ranges different ranges with a 95% probability of the true time of death falling within these ranges. The ranges vary from ±2.8 hours at best, down to 7 hours at worst.

16.8.2.3   Rigor mortis   Rigor mortis is the stiffening of both voluntary and involuntary muscles after death which follows the primary flaccidity. Rigor mortis is associated with slight shortening of muscles.

Biochemical changes associated with rigor mortis   In life there is a dynamic balance between utilisation and synthesis of ATP. This balance is disturbed after death. After molecular death, the following occur:

- ATP synthesis ceases

- no energy for calcium ions transport

- calcium ions continue to combine troponin – continuous activation of contraction

- troponin/tropomycin is not formed and there is no inhibitory effect on contraction

- no relaxation of muscle.

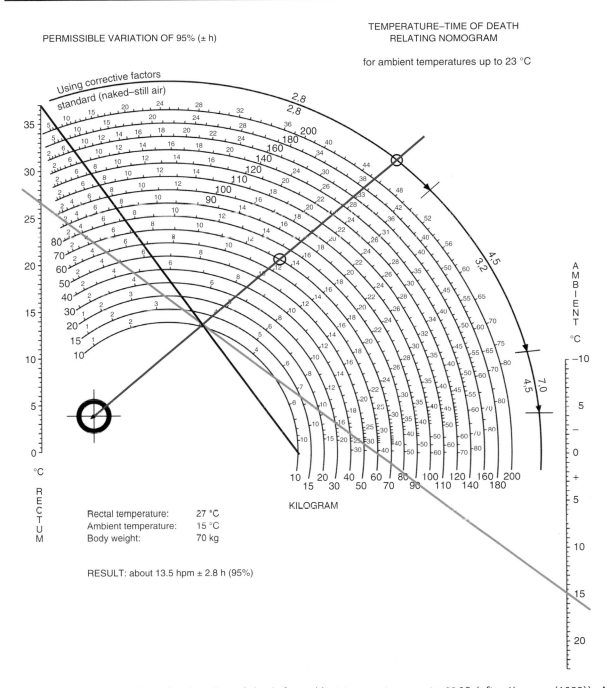

PERMISSIBLE VARIATION OF 95% (± h)

TEMPERATURE–TIME OF DEATH
RELATING NOMOGRAM

for ambient temperatures up to 23 °C

Rectal temperature: 27 °C
Ambient temperature: 15 °C
Body weight: 70 kg

RESULT: about 13.5 hpm ± 2.8 h (95%)

KILOGRAM

Figure 16.7 Nomogram for estimating time of death for ambient temperatures up to 23 °C (after Henssge (1988)). A rectal temperature of 27 °C at an ambient temperature of 15 °C is measured. First, the points of the measured rectal temperature and ambient temperature are joined by a straight line (green) that crosses the diagonal of the nomogram at a specific point. A second straight line is then drawn passing through the centre of the circle (below left of the nomogram) and the intersection of the first line and the diagonal (red line). The second line crosses the semicircles for different body weights. The time since death (in this case, for a 70-kg body weight) can be read at the intersection of the semicircle of the given body weight. The intersection gives the mean time since death and the intersection with the outer circle gives the 95% limit of confidence, which may be higher if corrective factors must be used (Madea 2016).

PERMISSIBLE VARIATION OF 95%

TEMPERATURE–TIME OF DEATH
RELATING NOMOGRAM

for ambient temperatures above 23 °C

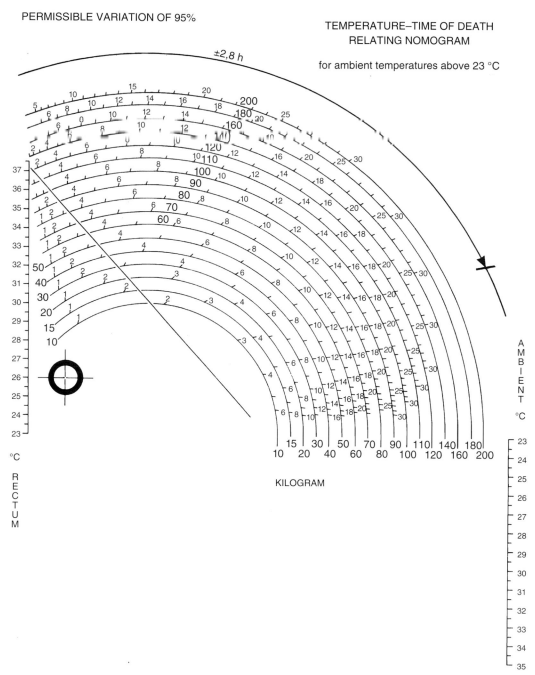

The nomogram expresses the death-time (t) by:

$$\frac{T_{rectum} - T_{ambient}}{37.2 - T_{ambient}} = 1.11 \exp(B\,t) - 011 \exp(10\,B\,t); \quad B = -1.2815\,(kg^{-.625}) + .0284$$

Figure 16.7 (Continued)

The detection of and degree of rigor mortis of the muscles or its absence may, along with other post-mortem changes such as body cooling, be of some use in forensic pathology practice in allowing the pathologist to give a rough estimate as to when death occurred. It should be appreciated that it appears and fades at variable post-mortem intervals depending on numerous factors. It is therefore by itself a poor determinant of the time since death. As a general rule, in a temperate climate, rigor mortis usually appears 3–6 hours from death. It is apparent in the smaller muscle groups because smaller joints are more easily immobilised although it begins in all groups. Rigor becomes complete in 6–12 hours and may remain full from 18 to 36 hours, thereafter fading in approximately the same order in muscle groups as it appeared.

As stated above there are a number of factors affecting the timing of rigor mortis, including the following:

- Temperature of the environment: rigor develops more slowly in a colder environment and takes longer to wear off. In bodies found in cold conditions rigor should not be confused with cold stiffness. The opposite is the case if the temperature is warm.

- Increased physical activity: rigor develops faster with increased physical activity shortly before death, for example the deceased being involved in a fight.

- Deaths associated with a temperature rise: these include various infections, malignant hyperthermia, and conditions involving agitation, such as excited delirium from the effects principally of cocaine.

- Some toxicological deaths will also lead to a rapid onset of rigor, such as poisoning from organophosphates, fluorine, and strychnine.

- Electrocution may also increase the speed of onset of rigor mortis.

A number of other conditions may be seen which involve muscle contraction, including the following:

- Cadaveric spasm, which is an instantaneous form of rigor that develops at the moment of death without primary flaccidity. It is rare, its cause is unknown, and it usually affects one group of muscles. Cadaveric spasm is seen in fatalities associated with intense emotion and muscular exertion.

- Heat stiffening involves contraction of muscles and ligaments as a result of the action of heat on the body as in a fire. Many fire victims are found with extensive burns, although the vast majority of fires in enclosed spaces result in death by the inhalation of fire fumes, including carbon monoxide. The contraction of the arms in particular results in flexion so that they appear to be in a pugilistic attitude (as if boxing).

- Cold stiffening occurs when the body is found in a very cold environment and should not be considered as a delayed form of rigor in a cold environment.

16.8.2.4 Hypostasis (syn. Livor mortis)   Hypostasis is the post-mortem discolouration of the skin (usually bluish red) and internal organs caused by gravitation of the blood to the dependent parts of the body (Figure 16.8).

Onset and Progression   Hypostasis occurs once the circulation has ceased, usually within half an hour after death but it may be delayed for many hours. Its development is complete usually within 6–12 hours post-mortem. Its appearance can be confluent or patchy, and may on occasions resemble bruising. It generally fixes with the onset of putrefaction. Its use in estimating the post-mortem interval in the past has been of subjective and limited value, although more recent studies show potential value as an objective measure of time since death (Vanezis and Trujillo 1996; Usumoto et al. 2010; Romanelli et al. 2015).

Distribution   Hypostasis may show a pattern where an object or material has produced pressure on the skin (Figure 16.9). Its distribution may indicate a previous position of the body, prior to

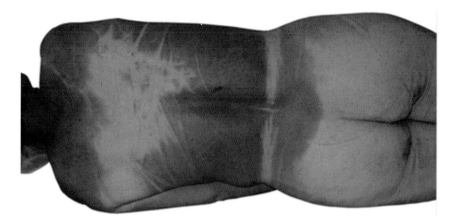

Figure 16.8   Hypostasis distributed on the back. The blanched areas are where there has been contact with a surface.

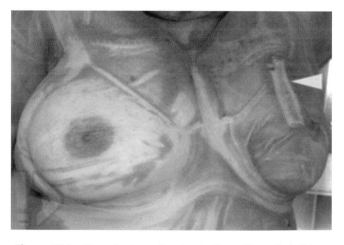

Figure 16.9   Hypostasis conforming to the pattern of clothing.

moving. If a body is moved from its primary position at death, hypostasis will move partially or completely to the newly dependent zones. This is true for a considerable time after death, depending on putrefaction. The rate of movement and reallocation of hypostasis is faster in the early hours after death and slows down as the post-mortem interval progresses. In drowning, its appearance on the body may be indistinct and may vary according to the movement of the water.

Colouration   The usual colour of hypostasis is bluish-red, but this may vary depending on the state of oxygenation at death (reduced haemoglobin is deeper in colour). The cause of death may be associated with the colouration where combinations of haemoglobin other than oxyhaemoglobin are present, e.g. carboxyhaemoglobin in carbon monoxide poisoning gives a cherry pink appearance, as does cyanmethaemoglobin in HCN poisoning. A brownish or chocolate red colour is associated with methaemoglobin, e.g. in poisoning by potassium chlorate, aniline or ethylene glycol (antifreeze). Hypostasis can also appear cherry pink in a low environmental temperature both before and after death.

As the post-mortem interval advances and the body becomes putrified, a green-black colour is seen due to the formation of sulfmethaemoglobin.

On occasions, however, hypostasis may appear faint or absent where there has been a large amount of blood loss or the deceased suffered from severe anaemia.

Differential diagnosis   Bruising may sometimes be mistaken for hypostasis and vice versa. While it is developing hypostasis may have a patchy appearance and resemble bruising. It may also be the case that there may be bruising within an area of hypostasis which masks it and thus the bruising could easily be missed. In the fresh cadaver, once the skin has been incised in the area in question it is relatively easy to differentiate between hypostasis and bruising. However, in the putrefied body this is much more difficult and frequently not resolved by incising the skin or by histological examination which, in such circumstances of decomposition, is problematical or of no use.

Purpuric haemorrhages are frequently seen in very congested areas of hypostasis, as in postural asphyxia deaths. These are produced after death and appear to become more prominent as the post-mortem interval increases.

In terms of the appearance in internal organs, to an inexperienced pathologist hypostasis may give the appearance of some form of morbidity such as:

- intestinal infarction

- pulmonary congestion

- posterior haemorrhagic myocardial infarction

- post-pharyngeal haemorrhage

- meningeal haemorrhage.

16.8.3   Intermediate changes after death

The early changes after death overlap to some extent with later changes. Changes due to decomposition are continuous and dependent on many factors, principally environmental, in particular the prevailing climatic conditions and access to predation. Essentially, we are moving from the appearance of the fresh body to its gradual destruction until full skeletonisation. As can be appreciated the timescale of these changes varies greatly, even on the same corpse.

Following the early stages, the breakdown of the body tissues is referred to as putrefaction. This process develops more quickly in some cells and organs than in others and is affected by the presence and type of bacteria as well as conditions prior to death involving infective processes, such as septicaemia.

Post mortem changes as the body decomposes may include the following, which may be seen in combination at different stages:

- putrefaction

- adipocere formation

- mummification

- post-mortem damage by predators

- late changes – skeletonisation.

16.8.3.1 Putrefaction   Putrefaction is the process by which the tissues of the body are finally broken down and disintegrated. The rate of its progression is variable, depends on many factors, and can only be used as a rough guide for estimating the post-mortem interval.

Autolysis   This is the softening and liquefaction of tissues in sterile conditions. It is caused by the action of enzymes released by the cells after death. Autolysis can be prevented by freezing the tissues.

Stages of putrefaction

- In temperate climates, in spring and autumn putrefactive changes are usually visible from two days after death and general disruption of the body after four weeks.

- Putrefaction in submerged bodies where the water is cool takes approximately twice as long to develop.

Putrefactive changes and their approximate order of occurrence

- Progressive greenish discolouration to a blackened and bloated appearance with marbling of veins, blistering, and sloughing of skin occurs from about two, up to 28 days. Despite the discoloured nature of the skin, it is still possible to see scars, tattoos, and other blemishes.

- Fungal growth, which may prevent visual identification of the face (e.g. Figure 16.10).

- Purging of body fluids from orifices (Figure 16.11).

- Bloating results from bacterial action and a feature of gaseous production is the distention seen in the intestine (Figure 16.12).

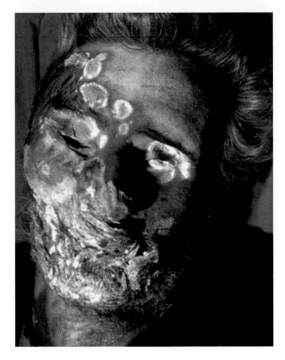

Figure 16.10   Fungus growing on the face.

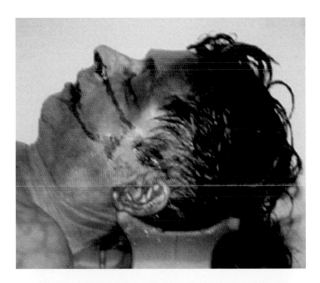

Figure 16.11   Blood-stained fluid purged from mouth and nose.

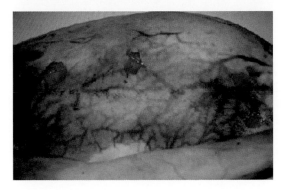

Figure 16.12   Bloated abdomen with marbling of the veins and blistering of the skin.

- Bloating progresses until about the third week when body cavities may burst.

- Organs with the largest blood supply putrefy first.

- The prostate and uterus may survive for months after death.

Factors involved in the progression of putrefaction   There are a number of factors which influence the progression of putrefaction:

- Bacteria may act externally or internally. *Clostridium welchii* and its production of the enzyme lecithinase plays a particularly important part.

- Insect larvae produce lytic enzymes.

- Animal intervention may cause post-mortem changes on land and in water.

16.8.3.2   Adipocere

- Putrefaction is modified or arrested with adipocere formation and can occur in different parts of the same body, resulting in partial preservation of body (Figure 16.13). The process involves the hydrolysis or saponification of body fat and requires damp conditions for its formation. Acidity is also important factor.

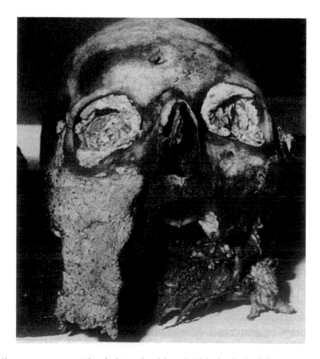

Figure 16.13   Adipocere on a partly skeletonised head. This body had been recovered from the sea.

- Adipocere is firm, initially yellowish brown then becomes white and friable.

- It is more prominent in women and well-nourished children.

16.8.3.3 Mummification Dry conditions are required for mummification and usually higher temperatures. The tissues become hardened, dry out, become contracted, and appear dark brown in colour.

16.8.3.4 Post-mortem action by predators Insects and larger animals are commonly involved in predation (Figure 16.14). In particular insect predation may allow estimation of the minimum post-mortem interval.

The insects which have been most studied are blowflies (Diptera: Calliphoridae), in particular their larvae or maggots. This is because they are found in greater numbers than most other insect groups, colonise the body most rapidly after death (Figure 16.15), and usually provide the most accurate information regarding time of death.

Blowfly larvae featured in the first successful use of entomological evidence in the UK, in the Buck Ruxton case, a Lancaster doctor who killed his common law wife and maid, and dumped their decomposing and dismembered remains in a stream running into the river Annan, 2 miles north of Moffat in Scotland, in September 1935. The maggots were aged at Sir Sidney Smith's forensic pathology laboratory at the University of Edinburgh, and provided a vital clue as to when the bodies were dumped. Dr Ruxton was subsequently found guilty of the murders and was hanged in 1936 (Glaister and Brash 1937).

Adult blowflies are attracted in large numbers within a few hours after death by the decaying odour of corpses, finding them with precision even in hidden locations such as through air vents in the walls of buildings and in suitcases (Bhadra et al. 2014).

After the ability to identify entomological specimens from forensic cases, the most fundamental need is to age them, to provide the minimum estimate of the post-mortem period. It will not be the time of death that is determined, rather the time that the flies laid eggs or larvae on the body.

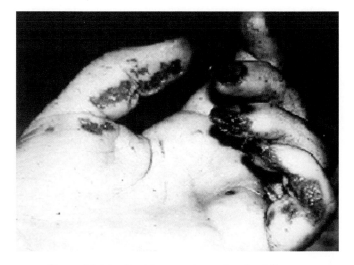

Figure 16.14 Rat bites on tips and pads of fingers.

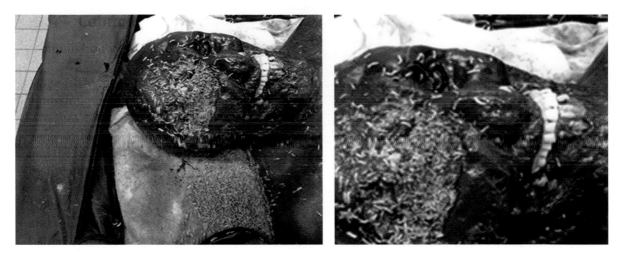

Figure 16.15   Maggots from blowflies on male's decomposing face with close up showing holes bored into skin.

It should be appreciated that there may have been a significant delay in placing the body in a location which would allow insects to have access (Reibe and Madea 2010; Anderson 2011) or the body may have been covered so that insect access was prevented.

Determining the age of eggs, larvae or other stages requires a detailed knowledge of the flies' lifecycle and development processes. Blowflies and flesh flies have four life stages, i.e. egg, larva, pupa, and adult (Figure 16.16). The larval stage is divided into three instars and between each instar the larva sheds its skin (cuticle) to allow for growth in the next instar. The pupa is a transition stage between larva and adult. It is found inside the barrel-shaped puparium, which is actually the hardened and darkened skin of the final, third instar larva. As an example of the timing of the lifecycle, averaged data for the common bluebottle fly, *Calliphora vicina*, one of the most commonly encountered species in forensic investigations in the UK, reared at 26.7 °C (see Kamal, 1958 in Smith 1986) are egg duration after oviposition (laying) 24 hours, first instar larva 24 hours, second instar larva 20 hours, third instar larva (feeding) 48 hours, third instar larva (post-feeding, prepupa) 128 hours, pupa 11 days, total immature (egg to adult) 18 days.

Toxic substances in or on a dead body can be accumulated by feeding larvae (Pounder 1991). An area of increasing importance is the effects of such toxins on the rate of larval development. For example, cocaine and heroin significantly increase the rate of development of larvae, thereby affecting the accuracy of post-mortem intervals if not taken into account (Goff et al. 1989, 1991; de Carvalho 2010). In contrast, clothes permeated with lubricants, paints or combustibles may double the time to insect colonisation of a corpse and significantly retard its decomposition (Greenberg 1991).

16.8.3.5 Late changes   Soft tissue loss resulting in skeletonisation can vary enormously depending on many factors relating to the environment. Where bodies are preserved, either accidentally or by design, skeletonisation may not occur, for example the Ice man (Otzi), Tollund man, and many other examples.

It important when human remains are discovered to assess whether they are of forensic interest, i.e. within living memory. The context in which the remains are discovered is important, together with the use of radiocarbon dating.

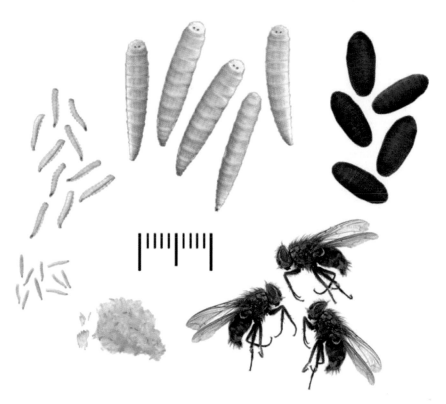

Figure 16.16 Lifecycle of a typical bluebottle blowfly, *Calliphora vicina* (Diptera: Calliphoridae). Clockwise from bottom left: eggs, first instar, second instar, third instar larvae, puparia containing pupae, adults. (Source: Courtesy Hall MJ, Natural History Museum.)

References

Academy of Medical Royal Colleges (2008). A code of practice for the diagnosis and confirmation of death.

Anderson, G.A. (2011). Comparison of decomposition rates and faunal colonization of carrion in indoor and outdoor environments. *J. Forensic Sci.* 56: 136–142.

Bhadra, P., Hart, A.J., and Hall, M.J. (2014). Factors affecting accessibility to blowflies of bodies disposed in suitcases. *Forensic Sci. Int.* 239: 62–72.

de Carvalho, L.M.L. (2010). Toxicology and forensic entomology (Chap. 9). In: *Current Concepts in Forensic Entomology* (ed. J. Amendt, C.P. Campobasso, L.M. Goff and M. Grassberger), 163–178. Springer.

Charlton R. Editorial (1996). Diagnosing death. *BMJ* 313: 956–957.

Glaister, J. and Brash, J.C. (1937). *Medico-Legal Aspects of the Ruxton Case.* Edinburgh: Livingstone.

Goff, M.L., Omori, A.I., and Goodbrod, J.R. (1989). Effect of cocaine in tissues on the development rate of *Boettcherisca peregrina* (Diptera: Sarcophagidae). *J. Med. Entomol.* 26: 91–93.

Goff, M.L., Brown, W.A., Hewadikaram, K.A., and Omori, A.I. (1991). Effect of heroin in decomposing tissues on the development rate of Boettcherisca peregrina (Diptera: Sarcophagidae) and implications of this effect on estimation of postmortem intervals using arthropod development patterns. *J. Forensic Sci.* 36: 537–542.

Greenberg, B. (1991). Flies as forensic indicators. *J. Med. Entomol.* 28: 565–577.

Henssge, C. (1988). Death time estimation in case work I. The rectal temperature time of death nomogram. *Forensic Sci. Int.* 8: 209–236.

Madea, B. (2016). Methods for determining time of death. *Forensic Sci. Med. Pathol.* 12: 451–485.

Marshall, T.K. and Hoare, F.E. (1962). Estimating the time of death: the rectal cooling after death and its mathematical expression. *J. Forensic Sci.* 7: 56–81.

Mohandas, A. and Chou, S.N. (1971). Brain death: a clinical and pathological study. *J. Neurosurg.* 35: 211–218.

Oram, J. and Murphy, P. (2011). Diagnosis of death. *Contin. Educ. Anaesth. Crit. Care Pain* 11: 77–81.

Pallis, C. (1983). ABC of brain stem death: the arguments about the EEG. *BMJ* 286: 284.

Pounder, D.J. (1991). Forensic entomo-toxicology. *J. Forensic Sci. Soc.* 31: 469–472.

Reibe, S. and Madea, B. (2010). How promptly do blowflies colonise fresh carcasses? A study comparing indoor with outdoor locations. *Forensic Sci. Int.* 195: 52–57.

Romanelli, M.C., Marrone, M., Veneziani, A. et al. (2015). Hypostasis and time since death: state of the art in Italy and a novel approach for an operative instrumental protocol. *Am. J. Forensic Med. Pathol.* 36: 99–103.

Smith, K.G.V. (1986). *A Manual of Forensic Entomology*. British Museum (Natural History), London & Cornell University Press [Ithaca] 205 pp.

Thuong, M., Ruiz, A., Evrard, P. et al. (2016). New classification of donation after circulatory death donors definitions and terminology. *Transpl. Int.* 29: 749–759.

Usumoto, Y., Hikiji, W., Sameshima, N. et al. (2010). Estimation of postmortem interval based on the spectrophotometric analysis of postmortem lividity. *Leg. Med. (Tokyo)* 12: 19–22.

Vanezis, P. and Trujillo, O. (1996). Evaluation of hypostasis using a colorimeter measuring system and its application to assessment of the post-mortem interval (time of death). *Forensic Sci. Int.* 78: 19–28.

World Health Organisation (2014). *International guidelines for the determination of death*. Montreal Forum Report 2012–2014, endorsed by WHO.

17

Identification: General Principles, including Anthropology, Fingerprints, and the Investigation of Mass Deaths

Peter Vanezis

Queen Mary University of London, London, UK

17.1   Introduction

Establishing the identity of a person, living or dead, is an essential part of a forensic investigation. It is carried out in a number of different circumstances and for a number of reasons.

In the living, identification is a universal requirement to confirm who the individual claims to be, for a myriad of reasons. Where the identity of an individual is at issue, verification is required from known individual parameters and assessment of biological questions such as paternity, age, stature, ancestry, and occasionally gender.

In the deceased, both individual and biological identification is carried out. There is also the added problem of assessing how post-mortem change has affected the ability to correctly identify the individual. The issue becomes more complex with fragmented and, in some cases, co-mingled remains, as in mass catastrophes or exhumation from mass graves.

In every forensic investigation involving an individual, identification is essential, whether it is treated as a straightforward formality or is a more complex undertaking. There are some circumstances, however, where a forensic investigation is not relevant or is not the primary consideration, as in the identification of persons exhumed from graveyards for reburial in another location, e.g. for redevelopment or for reburial of war dead.

Essential Forensic Medicine, First Edition. Edited by Peter Vanezis.

© 2020 John Wiley & Sons Ltd. Published 2020 by John Wiley & Sons Ltd.

17.2   Reasons for identification

As stated above, there are many reasons for ascertaining the true identity of a living or deceased person. Some of the reasons apply to both categories whilst others are only applicable to one or other of the two groups.

17.3   Reasons for identification in deceased individuals

- To satisfy the basic human rights of an individual to be properly identified before legal disposal.

- Humanitarian and ethical: to ensure that the needs of surviving relatives, to find out whether their loved one is dead, are satisfied and to allow them to properly inter the body according to their religious or cultural practices.

- To satisfy the requirements of coroners, fiscals, examining magistrates, and other legal authorities and to facilitate medico-legal enquiries such as inquests, fatal accident inquiries, and other hearings.

- To assist a police investigation where one is dealing with a death in suspicious circumstances or one which is clearly a homicide.

- To establish the fact that a person has died for administrative, statistical, and legal purposes.

- To allow discharge of legal claims, property, estate, life insurance, survivor's pensions, debts etc.

17.4   Reasons for identification in living persons

- To establish the perpetrator of a crime.

- To assess fraudulent claims in relation to immigration.

- To assess the age of an individual in offences related to the age of an individual.

- To establish who the individual claims to be or in cases of amnesia or dementia where the individual is not sure of who they are.

- To establish kinship.

17.5   Approach

Identification can be a fairly straightforward process or it may be complex. The aim must be to prove identity and this may be achieved by one reliable means such as odontology, DNA or fingerprints, although these so-called primary methods of identification have some limitations and are dependent on their interpretation and presentation in the circumstances of each case. It is always preferable, however, wherever possible to corroborate identity by more than one method, including consideration of secondary and accessory means of confirming identity. The approach to any identification of an individual will depend on the prevailing circumstances and in particular, in relation to the deceased, on the condition or state of preservation of the individual, i.e. whether fresh, decomposing or skeletonised and whether partial or complete and/or co-mingled with other remains.

17.6   Biological (general) identification (what type of individual are we trying to identify?)

All general identification characteristics corroborate to a variable degree personal identification. The more personal features, such as scars or tattoos, may be sufficient individually to constitute positive identification in their own right, or corroborate other methods of identification. The main biological characteristics which are assessed include the stature, age, gender and ancestry of an individual, bearing in mind that in many instances we may be dealing with decomposing and skeletonised, fragmented, and/or mutilated remains rather than a complete recently dead cadaver and therefore could be presented with a challenging task.

17.6.1   Stature

Assessment of stature is not as straightforward as one would imagine, even in a non-decomposed complete cadaver. Indeed, measuring the height of a deceased person may be inaccurate for a number of reasons, including rigor mortis resulting in muscle flexion, which may shorten the individual. Contracted muscles from being in a fire give rise to a contracted posture and thus apparent shortening. When rigor mortis has worn off and the body is flaccid, such loss of tone may cause apparent lengthening of the body.

Destruction of extremities in a fire, or dismembered or skeletonised limbs requires the use of formulae that have been constructed by anthropologists for different ethnic groups, assessing one or more long bones (Trotter and Gleser 1958; Krogman and Iscan 1986).

17.6.2   Age

There is a wide margin of error when assessing age. There are many unreliable indicators or changes that occur with age, many of which are related to nurture as well as nature. For example, hair colour and distribution with age show great variation and are unreliable as indicators of age.

There are a number of ageing changes to the skin which are most obvious in the elderly and include loss of skin elasticity, thinness, and hyperkeratosis and red Campbell de Morgan spots, although they cannot accurately assist with the age of the deceased.

Joints may show increasing osteoarthritic changes with age but assessment of age can only be assessed with a broad margin of error.

Degenerative cardiovascular changes, due to the effect of atherosclerotic changes in arteries with increasing age, may assist to some extent, although the speed of such changes is also affected by the presence of other conditions such as diabetes mellitus and hypertension. Eyes may show evidence of arcus senilis, which is unusual below 60 years. Cataracts are most commonly due to ageing but may be found in other conditions.

Teeth are an especially useful indicator up to the age of about 20–25 years (see Chapter 19).

Examination of the bones provides a number of established parameters for ageing, including the appearance of ossification centres and epiphyseal fusion.

17.6.3 Ancestry

Recognition of ancestry in the non-decomposed body is relatively straightforward bearing in mind that with ethnic interbreeding there is a wide range of biological variability.

Occasionally the clothing or ornaments may be of assistance. Physical artefacts such as body piercing or types of tattoos may also be helpful. Facial appearance and skin pigmentation may be characteristic.

17.6.4 Gender

Determining gender is usually obvious in the non-decomposed cadaver but may be problematic in dismembered, mutilated or severely decomposed individuals.

One should also take care to assign the correct gender in transgender individuals who have had surgical realignment, and exercise care and sensitivity in communicating findings to family members and friends. Furthermore, in determining gender it is essential to examine the internal organs and not rely on just the external appearance.

17.7 Personal identification

17.7.1 Recognition

Recognition relies on remembering in particular, the face of the person.

17.7.1.1 Recognition in the deceased   This is by far the most common way in which a dead body is identified before putrefaction renders gross distortion and discoloration of the facial features. It is generally carried out by someone who is well acquainted with the deceased, particularly near the time of their death. Occasionally, the next of kin or other close relatives may not have seen the deceased for some time and may therefore not be best placed to carry out the identification. Such a visual method, although quick and in most cases uneventful, carries the risk of misidentification for the following reasons:

- Effect of psychological stress on the ability to identify. Relatives may be in denial or the person carrying out the identification, usually a close relative, is very distressed and can easily make a mistake.

- The appearance of a corpse, frequently in a supine position, has an appreciably dissimilar appearance to the person during life because of pallor, loss of muscle tone, distribution of hypostasis etc.

- Facial injuries or other disfiguring factors, such as bruises, associated swelling or lacerations, can have a profound effect on the appearance of the deceased's face.

- The inanimate face, particularly under different lighting conditions, may have an entirely different appearance. In some instances where the image of the deceased's face is relayed to relatives via closed circuit television, the potential for error increases because not only does one have the problems described above, but additionally one is looking at an inferior two-dimensional image and not the person in the flesh. The same difficulty applies if identification is attempted from photographs of the deceased.

- Publication of a facial image in order to try and establish a putative identity must always be followed by confirmatory means from comparison with ante-mortem information.

17.7.1.2 Recognition in the living   In the living, recognition may be of a familiar person or of someone who is unfamiliar and may have only been seen for a short period of time, for example whilst carrying out an assault. In both circumstances the person familiar with the individual or the person who has witnessed the offence will rely on their recall facilities for identification. Situations in which recognition is used include the use of CCTV cameras for viewing an individual carrying out an armed robbery in a bank, for example, or another situation where an offence is being committed and captured on camera. Images from such equipment as well as images from other sources may be used to assist with recognition or by someone who is not familiar with a subject in the questioned image to assess whether there are similarities between the images in question and other images of the known individual in order to make a positive identification. Along with the introduction of CCTV cameras in private premises and public places there has been some renewed interest in anthropometry as a means of identification, which has its origins in the work of Alphonse Bertillon (Bertillon 1893). He was a French physical anthropologist who devised a formula for identification based on a series of 11 measurements which remained unchanged after full maturity, various body marks, and personality characteristics. The formula was accepted until the early 1900s, when it was supplanted by fingerprints. Its credibility was questioned in a number of cases, including the case of Will and William West (National Law Enforcement Newsletter 2011) (Figure 17.1). In 1903, a man named Will West (Figure 17.1b) was committed to the penitentiary at Leavenworth, Kansas, where he was photographed and measured using the Bertillon system. Will West's measurements were found to be almost identical to a criminal at the same penitentiary named William West (Figure 17.1a), who was committed for murder in 1901 and was serving a life sentence. Furthermore, their photographs showed that the two men bore a close physical resemblance to one another, although it was not clear that they were even related. In the ensuing confusion surrounding the true identities of the two men, their fingerprints conclusively identified them and demonstrated clearly that the adoption of a fingerprint identification system was more reliable than the older Bertillon system.

Recognition is employed in identification line-ups, publication of an artist's sketch working with the assistance of an eye witness, and making use of photographs, for example, in fraudulent passport imagery. In addition to recognition of the appearance of the individual in question, it may also be possible to recall behaviour characteristics such as gait or their voice if they had spoken and perhaps other features of the demeanour of an individual.

FEDERAL BUREAU OF INVESTIGATION
UNITED STATES DEPARTMENT OF JUSTICE
J. Edgar Hoover, Director

History of the
"West Brothers" Identification..

Bertillon Measurements are not always a Reliable Means of Identification

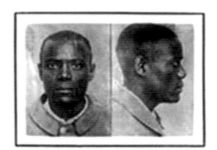 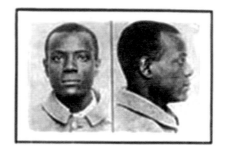

Figure 17.1   Misidentification of William West and Will West (FBI National Archives Catalogue). They were apparently not related in any way, as suggested in the figure.

17.7.1.3   Comparative methods using ante-mortem information

In the case of a deceased person, ante-mortem information is collected in order to compare what is found on the unidentified deceased person with an individual thought to be the deceased (there may be more than one putative identity and therefore there is the need for exclusion of other individuals in such cases, particularly when dealing with multiple deaths).

Comparative methods of identification involve reliable (usually stand-alone) techniques of identification or corroborative (secondary/accessory) methods. The three primary methods of identification are *DNA*, *odontology* and *fingerprints*. These three techniques are described in detail in this and the following two chapters (fingerprints in Section 17.11, DNA in Chapter 18, and odontology in Chapter 19).

There are many other findings on a deceased which are considered secondary or accessory to achieving identification. These include the type of clothing, documentation, scars, tattoos, adornments etc. Such information may assist or corroborate a much more reliable means or may, by a combination of corroborative and circumstantial factors, be in a position to provide a positive identification. Very occasionally there may be individual findings on a body which are regarded as unique to that person and may therefore be acceptable as stand-alone for positive identification.

An internal post-mortem examination is also helpful in assisting identification. It may be possible to confirm disease which was present during life and confirmed by medical records. In addition, degenerative conditions may assist with age estimation. Furthermore, lifestyle choices may be corroborated, such as cirrhosis of the liver in an alcohol-dependent individual.

Confirmation of personal identification may be acceptable with the discovery of surgical implants with unique identifying marks (e.g. cardiac pacemaker) or anomalies which are considered likely to be individual, such as fracture sites and comparison of mastoid and frontal sinus patterns, where ante-mortem information for comparison is available.

In living persons, comparative techniques involve in particular the identification of perpetrators of crimes, or the verification of claimed identity, including age assessment of an individual (the reader is recommended for further reading to Black et al. 2010).

17.7.1.4 Identification of skeletal remains Assuming that the skeletal remains have been identified as human, there are a further two stages necessary to achieve personal identification. The first is to establish the biological or anthropological characteristics of the remains and the second to establish the personal identity of the individual.

As stated above, prior to carrying out the anthropological assessment, in certain instances, particularly when dealing with partial remains or fragmented bones, the question may arise as to whether the remains are true bones, e.g. plastic student's skeleton, and whether they are human or animal. It is relatively easy with large and complete bones which are not markedly fragmented to categorise them on gross anatomical inspection. The assistance of a veterinary anatomist is useful in difficult cases. However, with smaller samples serological investigation is essential to examine for species-specific proteins where the post-mortem interval does not exceed 5–10 years.

Biological identification Before one can proceed to a personal identification it is necessary to assess various biological parameters which allow the individual to be placed into a particular anthropological grouping. The four basic parameters are age, ethnicity, sex, and stature (see Section 17.6.1).

Age assessment based on skeletal remains is more likely to be accurate with those from immature or young adults. In any assessment of maturation, one has to take into account nutrition, state of health, and genetic factors amongst others. Parts of the skeleton useful in age estimation include:

- the skull and teeth

- the post-cranial skeleton:

    o appearance of ossification centres

    o epiphysial union

    o pubic symphysis

    o sternal rib

- degenerative changes.

The accuracy of sex determination varies with the age of the subject and the degree of fragmentation of the remains. The most useful for bones for sex determination are:

- skull

- pelvis

- sacrum

- long bones.

Stature estimation is discussed in detail Section 17.6.1.

Determination of ethnicity may be extremely difficult because of ethnic mixing. For further information the reader is referred to Krogman and Yscan (1986).

Personal identification   In virtually all instances personal identification involves comparing the skeletal remains in question with ante-mortem data. The only exception is facial reconstruction, attempted in the first instance in order to achieve recognition as a first step to identification where no ante-mortem data are available.

Skull

The skull (apart from the use of dental information as described in Chapter 19) contains the frontal and paranasal sinuses and mastoid air cells, which have proven useful for identification where ante-mortem radiographs or other related medical information is available (Quatrehomme et al. 1996; Rhine and Sperry 1991; Fernandes 2018). Cranial suture patterns have also occasionally been used (Rogers and Allard 2004).

Cranio-facial identification using the whole or fragmented skull to relate it to a face for possible identification has been widely used. There are two principle ways in which this is carried out: *superimposition* and *reconstruction* (*approximation*). Superimposition techniques compare ante-mortem photographs with the skull. With reconstruction, the aim is to produce a face which corresponds as far as possible with the general shape and anthropological characteristics of the skull in order to assist with the recognition of a particular individual. Iscan and Helmer (1993) provide a comprehensive review of the methodologies employed. The manual method of reconstruction has been in use for forensic purposes since the early twentieth century and is still currently employed and used alongside three-dimensional computer-generated images (Gatliff and Snow 1979; Vanezis et al. 1989; Vanezis and Vanezis 2000).

Post-cranial Skeleton

There may be fractures or deformities to the skeleton which prove useful for personal identification where ante-mortem records exist, such as radiographs, CT scans, or medical notes. Sometimes the general configuration of the bones, where ante-mortem radiographs are compared with post-mortem radiographs, may be remarkably similar, for example osteoarthritic lipping in vertebral bodies (Brogdon 1998; Scott et al. 2010).

17.8   Victim identification and management in disasters (mass fatality incidents)

A mass fatality incident is defined as 'any incident where the number of fatalities is greater than normal local arrangements can manage'. There are many types of disasters, both natural and man-made, classified into 'open' or 'closed' or a combination of the two. An example of an open disaster would be deaths in a town following an earthquake where there are many tourists coming and going. A closed disaster would be an incident where there is manifest of passengers, such as on an aircraft.

Types of mass fatality incidents include:

- natural causes, e.g. flooding, earthquakes

- major transportation accidents, including road, rail, sea, and air

- hostile acts, including terrorism and criminality

- crowd-related incidents, often involving disorder and overcrowding

- contamination and/or pollution incidents

- structural failures

- industrial incidents (e.g. mining disasters)

- health-related incidents

- chemical, biological, radiological or nuclear incidents.

Any plan for dealing with fatalities needs to be integrated with all aspects of the response to and recovery from such situations and incidents. Organisations need to work in collaboration with others on key activities and ensure their own plans are robust. Any response to a mass fatality incident will require special arrangements to be implemented at a local, regional or national level, depending on the capabilities at each level and the scale and complexity of the emergency.

There are two main functions to any investigation of a mass disaster incident: the investigation of the cause of the disaster and identification of the victims. As stated above, there are obvious reasons why identification of the victims is of primary consideration. Interpol Resolution AGN/Res/13 (1996) recognises that for legal, religious, cultural, and other reasons human beings have the right not to lose their identity after death, and that the identification of victims is of importance for police investigations. There is a protocol that exists between 181 member countries to agree a standard of disaster victim identification (DVI) in the event that they suffer fatalities within their country.

The investigation of all mass disasters, whatever their nature and magnitude, requires the same degree of careful and meticulous preparation and degree of preparedness, and involves all the disciplines that are expected to play a part. The overall legal responsibility for the deceased in England, Wales and Northern Ireland falls to the coroner. In Scotland it is the procurator fiscal, and it is different again in other jurisdictions. The primary responsibility, however, falls on the police on behalf of the coroner for control of the remains of the deceased.

The UK Government has an agreed policy for the management of a mass disaster and has produced guidance and legislation on dealing with fatalities in emergencies (Civil Contingencies Act 2004; Home Office Communications Directorate 2004; Emergency Response and Recovery 2013; Dealing with Disasters 2017). It has been put in place to facilitate the co-ordination of the various relevant agencies to work together to manage all aspects of a disaster, including the identity of the victims, and at the same time ensure that all activities are closely controlled and regularly reviewed, at national as well as local level.

The police in the event of a disaster will normally co-ordinate all the activities of the responding agencies at and around the scene of a land-based emergency. Co-ordination of the various aspects of dealing with fatalities in emergencies will require close working with coroners, local authorities, and others as necessary. It is usual for the police to regard the scene as a crime scene unless, or until, a decision is made to the contrary. Where fatalities are involved this will often be the case. The police will appoint a senior investigating officer (SIO) to lead the investigation, though it must be remembered that other responsible authorities such as the Health and Safety Executive may also carry out an investigation.

A senior identification manager (SIM) will be appointed to lead police arrangements regarding the identification of victims. Specific areas of responsibility for this role include:

- recovery of victims and human remains from the scene, with the consent and agreement of the coroner

- establishing police mortuary teams

- setting up a police casualty bureau

- establishing police family liaison teams

- establishing and co-ordinating meetings of the Identification Commission under the chairmanship of the coroner

- collation of ante-mortem and post-mortem data for presentation to the Identification Commission.

The officers undertaking the critical roles of SIO and SIM should be trained and experienced investigators appointed by the police strategic (Gold) commander. Clearly these arrangements require effective co-ordination between commanders, their teams, the response arrangements, and other agencies and key roles. The SIM will be a key member of the Identification Commission. In some cases the SIO may also be a member of the same group.

Post-mortem and ante-mortem teams will be set up to co-ordinate their findings, in particular with respect to identification.

17.8.1 Functions of the post-mortem team

- The post-mortem team comprises members of the various units forming the mortuary documentation team, together with the pathologist(s), who will perform post-mortem examinations, and the odontologist(s) responsible for dental comparison.

- The mortuary documentation officer will be responsible for compiling a file in respect of each body for comparison purposes and for the information of the coroner.

- Post-mortem data will be recorded on the pink Interpol DVI 'Dead Body' form and should contain all available information and be forwarded to the Identification Commission for comparison with the ante-mortem file.

17.8.2   Functions of the Ante-mortem team

- Determine a list of missing persons believed to have been involved in the disaster.

- Establish evidence that these missing persons were likely to be involved.

- Complete yellow victim identification forms in respect of each victim.

- Prepare a file for comparison purposes using the information gathered for deliberation by the Identification Commission and presentation to the coroner, subject to his/her identification requirements.

- Inform the next of kin through the family liaison coordinator when all identifications have been completed.

17.8.3   Identification commission functions

The Identification Commission functions as a matching centre. It assesses the details of missing persons provided by the casualty bureau, together with data obtained during ante-mortem and post-mortem procedures. A four-stage commission procedure is used.

Membership of the Identification Commission may include:

- the coroner or the procurator fiscal (chair)

- the coroner's officer or the procurator fiscal's officer (secretary of meeting)

- the reconciliation manager (reconciliation is the process by which data, collected during ante-mortem procedures is analysed against the data collected during post-mortem procedures, in order to identify the deceased and reunite dismembered parts of the same human body)

- the SIM

- the SIO (or representative)

- the family liaison co-ordinator

- the ante-mortem data co-ordinator

- the post-mortem data co-ordinator

- the lead forensic pathologist

- the presenting officer

- other relevant specialists (e.g. odontologist, fingerprint expert).

17.8.4 Commission procedure

The commission procedure comprises four stages:

- *Stage 1*: The post-mortem data found on the deceased is associated with the name and details of a missing person provided by the ante-mortem process.

- *Stage 2*: The post-mortem data suggests there is possibly a match between a deceased person and the name and details of a missing person provided by secondary identifier evidence obtained by the ante-mortem process.

- *Stage 3*: The post-mortem data suggests there is a probable match between a deceased person and the name and details of a missing person provided by primary identifier evidence obtained by the ante-mortem process.

- *Stage 4*: A match is made between a deceased person and the name and details of a missing person provided by the ante-mortem process.
    - The certification form is used and each relevant forensic expert signs to indicate that identification is possible, probable, established or not made. If established, the identification is certified by the chair of the Identification Commission.
    - Only after Stage 4 and formal identification by the Identification Commission should the family liaison officer be notified and the bereaved informed of the identification.
    - At Stage 4, the coroner or procurator fiscal publicly opens an inquest in respect of each of the deceased and hears evidence to confirm the identity of the deceased person(s). The coroner or procurator fiscal may then consider releasing the deceased to their next of kin for burial or cremation, and issue the necessary authority for this.

17.9 Practical procedures for identification

In any mass incident, it is vital to carry out the correct procedures to enable the best chance for correct identification from the very beginning when the bodies are first found and need to be recovered.

The location of the body must be recorded and its relationship with its surroundings and other deceased, as one would do in any crime scene. Good aerial photography to show the position of bodies on open land gives a view of the overall scene and allows the investigator to visualise the extent of the disaster and obtain clues as to how bodies were located in the positions in which they were found.

In addition to a full-length photograph of the body in situ, each one must have a label with a unique number determined using a clear unambiguous system, and be placed in a waterproof bag, which in turn should be placed in a labelled body bag. Different labels or numbering systems given to the same body will only cause confusion and most probably lead to misidentification.

Bodies are then transported to the body-holding area with onward travel to a temporary mortuary once it has been designated. At the autopsy, the property on the body should first be processed, including the associated property and clothing, then stored. The body should then be examined both externally and internally, and documented to record medical/dental details. Once the autopsy has been completed the body should be stored until identification is complete and it is ready to be released to the family.

It should be appreciated that with such mass incidents, the state of bodies may vary within the same disaster or bodies may be in a broadly similar condition, depending on the nature of the incident. The deceased will frequently not be in a fresh undamaged state but may be severely traumatised, incomplete, mutilated, and/or decomposed. Some human remains may be tissue of varying sizes which need to be assessed and associated with larger body parts where appropriate.

Below are presented four case studies of recent disasters. The Grenfell fire in London in 2017 is alluded to in Chapter 15.

Case Study 17.1 The Deal Barracks bombing

At 8:27 a.m. on 22 September 1989, a 15 lb time-bomb detonated in the recreational centre changing room at the Royal Marines School of Music (Figure 17.2). The blast destroyed the recreational centre, levelled the three-story accommodation building next to it, and caused extensive damage to the rest of the base and nearby civilian homes. Most of the personnel who used the building as a barracks had already risen and were practising marching on the parade ground when the blast occurred. Some marines had remained behind in the building, and thus

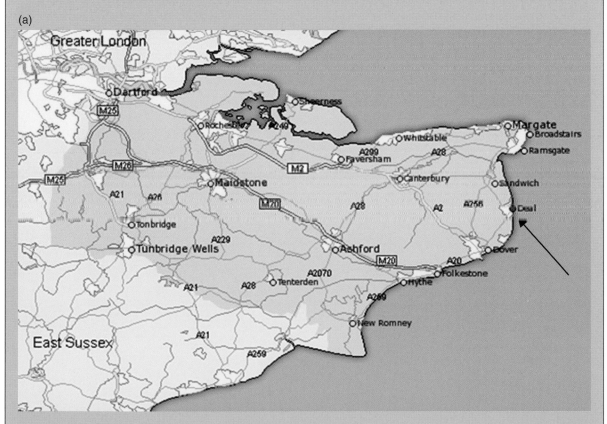

Figure 17.2 The bomb explosion at the Royal Marines School of Music. (a) Map of Kent showing the town of Deal (arrow) (Google maps). (b) Aerial view of the barracks recreation centre destroyed by the explosion (www.kentonline. co.uk/deal/news/deal-remembers-bomb-victims-20042). (c) Rescue team recovering the victims.

(b)

(c)

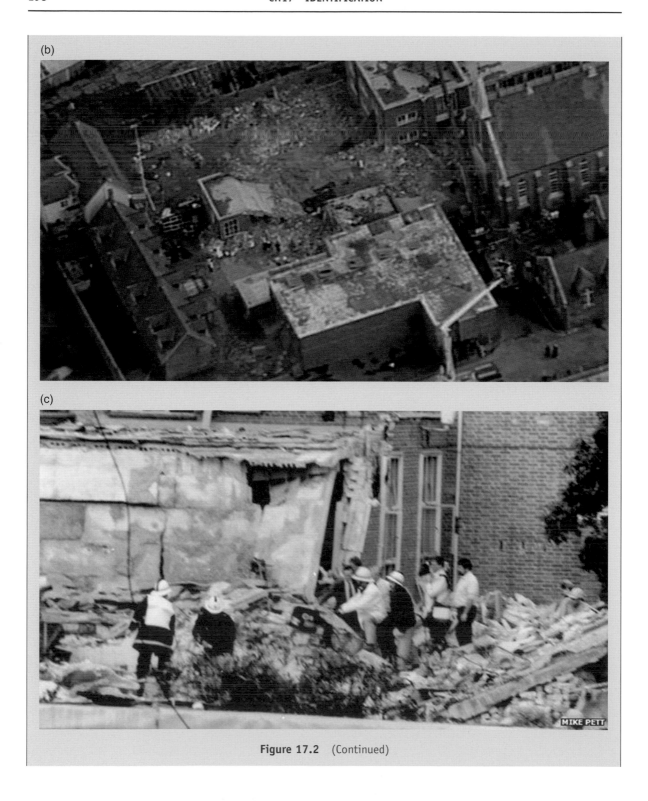

Figure 17.2   (Continued)

received the full force of the explosion. Many were trapped in the rubble for hours and military heavy lifting equipment was needed to clear much of it. Ten marines died at the scene, with most trapped in the collapsed building, although one body was later found on the roof of a nearby house. Another 21 marines were seriously injured and received treatment at local hospitals.

The Deal barracks bombing was an attack by the Provisional Irish Republican Army (IRA), who claimed responsibility.

Case Study 17.2 Chinook Helicopter crash

This crash occurred on 2 June 1994 at about 18:00 hours when a Royal Air Force (RAF) Chinook helicopter crashed on the Mull of Kintyre, Scotland, killing all 25 passengers and four crew on board. Amongst the passengers were almost all the UK's senior Northern Ireland intelligence experts. It was the RAF's worst peacetime disaster (Figure 17.3).

An RAF board of inquiry in 1995 ruled that it was impossible to establish the exact cause of the crash. This ruling was subsequently overturned by two senior reviewing officers who said the pilots were guilty of gross negligence for flying too fast and too low in thick fog. This finding proved to be controversial, especially in light of irregularities and technical issues surrounding the then-new Chinook HC.2 variant which were uncovered.

A Parliamentary inquiry conducted in 2001 found the previous verdict of gross negligence on the part of the crew to be 'unjustified'. In 2011, an independent review of the crash cleared the crew of negligence.

(a)

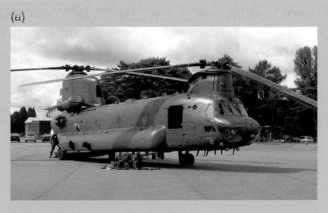

Figure 17.3 Chinook helicopter crash. (a) A Chinook helicopter similar to the crashed aircraft. Source: Original photo by Adrian Pingstone. (b) Crash site at the Mull of Kintyre. Source: *The Scotsman* newspaper. (c) Deceased neatly laid out in holding area prior to examination. (d) Temporary mortuary examination room.

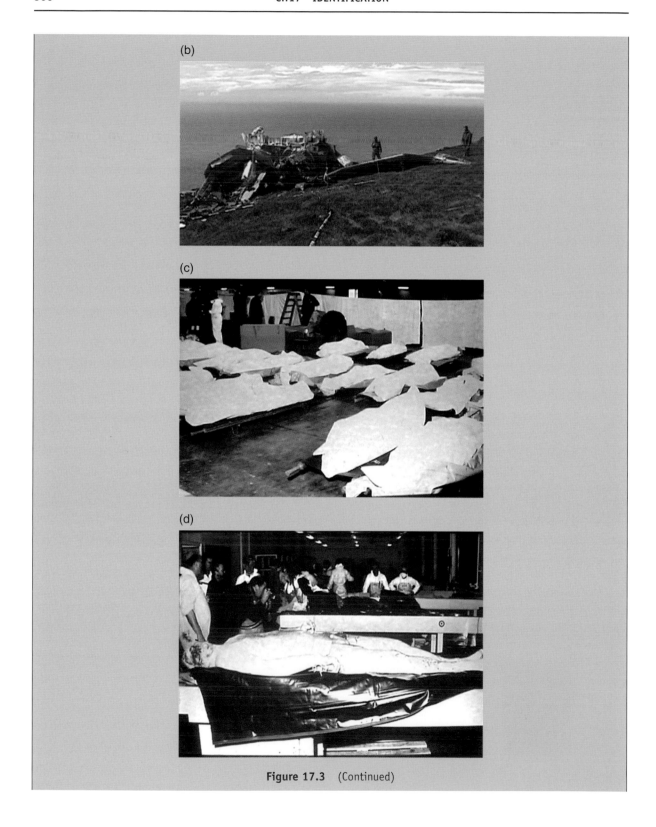

(b)

(c)

(d)

Figure 17.3 (Continued)

The Post-mortem examination and identification

There was an initial briefing between lead pathologist, the procurator fiscal, the police and RAF representatives on the evening of the crash. Macrahanish Hangar was adapted to serve as a temporary mortuary.

A team from Glasgow and the RAF comprised pathologists, odontologist, anatomic pathology technicians, photographers, exhibits officers, professional repatriation funeral services.

Post-mortems and identification work started the day following the crash (3 June) and was completed on all 29 victims by 5 June, with repatriations carried out that week. Identification was achieved by a combination of visual means, odontology, and personal property.

Case Study 17.3 King's Cross fire

The King's Cross fire broke out on Wednesday 18 November 1987 at approximately 19:30 at King's Cross St. Pancras tube station, a major interchange on the London Underground. Thirty-one people were killed and 100 were injured. As well as the mainline railway stations above ground and subsurface platforms for the Metropolitan lines, there were platforms deeper underground for the Northern, Piccadilly, and Victoria lines (Figure 17.4).

The fire started on an escalator serving the Piccadilly line and 15 minutes after being reported, as the first members of the London Fire Brigade were investigating, the fire flashed over, filling the underground ticket office with heat and smoke.

The public inquiry that followed found that the fire had started from a lit match being dropped onto the escalator, with the ensuing conflagration increasing in intensity due to a previously unknown trench effect. As a result, London Underground were strongly criticised for their attitude towards fires. Staff were complacent because there had never been a fatal fire on the Underground, and they had been given little or no training to deal with fires or evacuation. The publication of the report led to the introduction of new fire safety regulations.

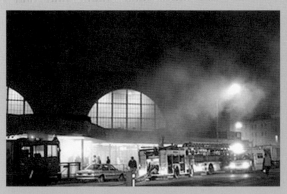
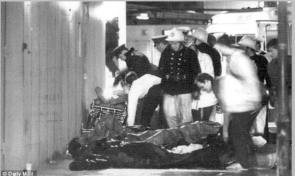

Figure 17.4 Scenes from the Kings Cross Fire. *Source:* www.strol.com (left image) and www.dailymail.co.uk (right image).

Case Study 17.4 11 September 2001 terrorist attacks

There were four coordinated terrorist attacks by the Islamic terrorist group al-Qaeda on the USA on the morning of Tuesday 11 September 2001. Four passenger airliners – which all departed from airports on the US East Coast bound for California – were hijacked by 19 al-Qaeda terrorists to be flown into buildings. Two of the planes, American Airlines Flight 11 and United Airlines Flight 175, were crashed into the North and South towers, respectively, of the World Trade Centre complex in New York City (Figure 17.5). Within 1 hour and 42 minutes, both 110-story towers collapsed, with debris and the resulting fires causing partial or complete collapse of all other buildings in the World Trade Centre complex, as well as significant damage to ten other large surrounding structures (Figure 17.6).

A third plane, American Airlines Flight 77, was crashed into the Pentagon, leading to a partial collapse in the Pentagon's western side. The fourth plane, United Airlines Flight 93, initially was steered towards Washington, DC, but crashed into a field near Shanksville, Pennsylvania after its passengers tried to overcome the hijackers. In total, the attacks claimed the lives of 2996 people (including the 19 hijackers) and caused property and infrastructure damage of at least US$10 billion and $3 trillion in total costs. It was the deadliest incident for firefighters and law enforcement officers in the history of the USA, with 343 and 72 killed, respectively.

Investigation by the Office of the Chief Medical Examiner: Recovery and processing of remains

The major goals of the Office of the Chief Medical Examiner (OCME) were to accurately identify the decedents and to promptly issue death certificates. As of September 2005, there were 1594 identifications of a total of 2749 people reported missing. Of these, 976 were identified by a single means, which included DNA analysis in 852 of the victims. On June 11 2019, CNN World reported the identification of another victim and brought the number of identifications to 1,643 (CNN 2019).

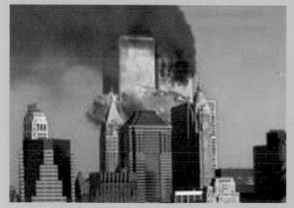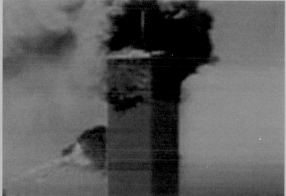

Figure 17.5   Destruction of the Twin Towers (World Trade Centre), New York, 11 September 2001 (various television networks).

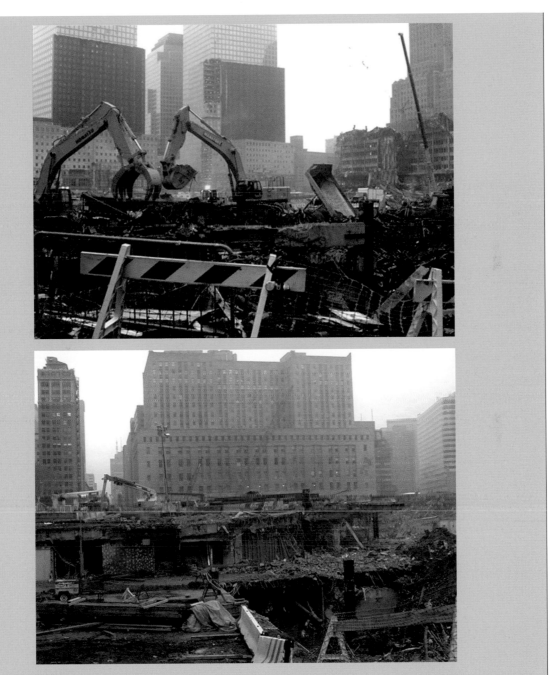

Figure 17.6 Views of 'Ground Zero' three months after the destruction of the World Trade Centre. Courtesy P.Vanezis.

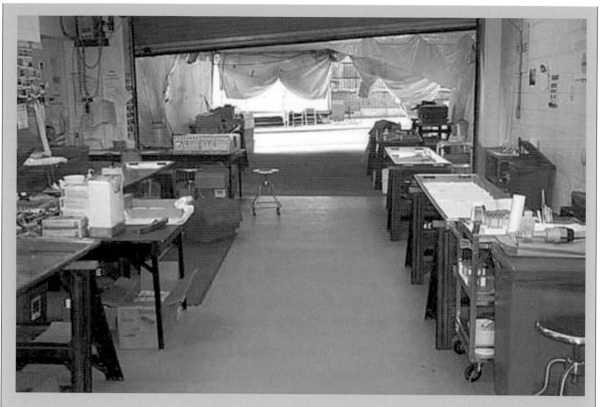

Figure 17.7 The temporary examination area at the New York City OCME. Source: Courtesy of OCME, New York.

Temporary mortuary facilities (Figures 17.7 and 17.8) were set up adjacent to the Manhattan OCME, with a multidisciplinary team of medical examiners, forensic anthropologists, medico-legal investigators, forensic biologists, odontologists, and other support staff working closely together.

Such was the extent of the disaster that a huge number of personnel were required, including 30 medical examiners, more than 200 New York Police Department (NYPD) general personnel, 5 NYPD print examiners, 265 forensic dentists, and more than 100 photographers and radiology and laboratory technicians. Other ancillary staff included representatives from the FBI Disaster Mortuary, the Operational Response Team, the New York Fire Department, the New York Department of Corrections, police officers from adjacent counties and states, medical students from New York University and Columbia, and the Salvation Army.

Forensic anthropologists triaged the remains, which were then examined by a medical examiner. Each identification station consisted of a medical examiner, a DNA technician, a missing persons' detective, a property clerk, and a scribe (medical students or physician volunteers). Remains were described and photographed. Personal effects were logged and secured. Samples of tissue for DNA were taken from each of the remains. The recovery time and environmental conditions affected the ability to collect non-degraded DNA.

During the prolonged recovery effort, the remains underwent the usual post-mortem decomposition changes with the addition of heat and fire. Eventually, bony remains became the norm. Depending on the type and condition of the remains, they were examined by radiography, fingerprint teams, and/or dentists. There were 288 intact bodies that were externally examined. No internal examinations were performed.

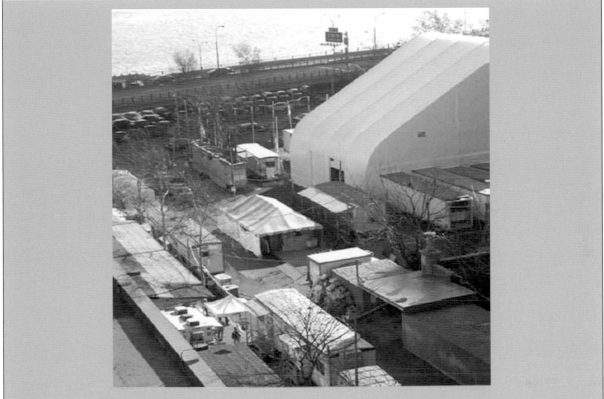

Figure 17.8 Memorial Park (white tent with refrigerated tractor trailers), where the remains were kept, and other temporary supply and staff support buildings along East 30th Street. Source: Courtesy OCME, New York.

17.10   Identification of buried human remains

Details of the procedure for the investigation of such cases is dealt with in Chapters 5 and 11.

17.11   The use of fingerprints in identification

17.11.1   Introduction

A fingerprint is formed from the ridge pattern of a finger coming into contact with a surface. They are easily deposited on various surfaces by the natural secretions of sweat glands (usually eccrine) and sebaceous glands that are present in epidermal ridges. Ridges begin forming in the foetus at 10–11 weeks, and around 14 weeks sweat glands appear at uniform intervals along the ridges. At 24 weeks, the epidermal ridge system has an adult morphology.

Fingerprints are said to be unique from empirical observation (although it cannot be proven) and thus have been in use as a method of identification for centuries. The Babylonians were one of the first to use them by pressing their fingers into clay as part of a business transaction. The practice was also carried out by the Chinese using inked marks on paper. The Chinese later also used them for burglary investigations.

However, it is only since the latter part of the nineteenth century that fingerprint analysis has been developed through classification and population databases, and supported by scientific study.

Sir William Herschel (1833–1917), a magistrate in colonial India, is credited with being the first European to recognise the value of fingerprints for identification purposes. From 1878 government pensioners in his region signed for their monthly payments with fingerprints. At the registry of deeds, landowners impressed fingerprints to authenticate their transactions. At the courthouse, convicts were forced to fingerprint their jail warrants so hired substitutes could not take their place in prison. Around the same time, Sir Henry Faulds, a Scottish physician working as a missionary in Japan, discovered fingerprints on ancient pottery and as a result carried out work to show their permanence and whether or not they might be unique. He is the first European to publish an article suggesting that fingerprints may assist crime investigations. A little later, in 1892, Sir Francis Galton published the book *Finger Prints* and in so doing significantly advanced the science of fingerprint identification. Juan Vucetich, an Argentine anthropologist, prompted by Galton's experiments with fingerprints, started to collect fingerprints to include with the anthropometric measurements he took from arrested men. He devised his own fingerprint classification method and in 1892 made the first positive identification of a criminal in a case where Francisca Rojas had killed her two sons and then cut her throat, trying to put the blame on an outside attacker. A bloody print identified her as the killer.

Sir Edward Henry, who was Inspector General of Police for Bengal Province in India assigned Azizul Haque to study the classification problem. Haque was successful in devising and setting up a classification system which was officially adopted by British India in 1897. As a result, in England the Belper Committee recommended that the fingerprints of criminals be taken and classified by the Indian System. In May 1901, Henry was made Assistant Commissioner of Police in charge of Criminal Identification at New Scotland Yard. In 1903, Henry became Commissioner of Police.

17.11.2   Current techniques in fingerprint analysis

Human fingerprints may be deposited and present in the following ways:

1. as patent prints: these are visible to the naked eye on a surface and may have been transferred there through different contaminants such as ink, paint or blood

2. as plastic prints: these are often visible and occur on soft deformable surfaces such as on putty or clay, leaving a three-dimensional impression

3. as latent prints: these are the most common type and are invisible to the naked eye. They leave secretions from sweat and sebaceous glands as well as other residues on the fingers and can be detected and developed by a number of techniques.

The initial, non-destructive examination of prints is by visual examination in natural light, white light, and by fluorescence examination, before any chemical enhancement is carried out.

The lifting and development of prints using chemical and physical procedures is multifactorial and which process is used will depend on environmental factors such as humidity, airflow, atmospheric pollutants, type of surface on which the print is found (whether a porous surface such as cardboard or a less porous smooth surface), and consideration of secretion from the fingers. Children have few sebaceous glands and numbers fall after the age of 50.

17.11.3 Classification and matching

Fingerprint matching can be carried out by comparing an individual's prints, either deceased or alive, with prints found at a scene, e.g. of a crime, or, in the case of an unknown perpetrator of a crime, against a database. Before computerisation, manual filing systems were used. They were based on the general ridge patterns of several or all fingers. In the Henry system of classification, there are three basic fingerprint patterns: loop, whorl, and arch. There are also more complex classification systems that break down patterns even further into plain arches or tented arches, and loops. There are regions where ridgelines make different shapes called singularities, which include loop, core and delta (Figure 17.9).

17.11.4 The process of identification

It should be appreciated that fingerprint examination is best described as a cognitive process which relies on the ability of a competent individual to analyse and compare areas of friction ridge detail and arrive at a decision as to whether they originate from the same person or not. In arriving at this decision, fingerprint examiners will assess the pattern, ridge flow features, and characteristic minutiae of the fingerprint (Figure 17.10). It is the convention in fingerprint examination to consider in a strict hierarchical manner first-, second- and third-level detail. These can be described as overall pattern (first level), characteristics such as ridge endings or bifurcations in ridges (second level), and detail within the ridge structure such as pores and ridge shape (third level). Each level of detail is considered in succession from first to third. It follows that if a difference is found at first or second level detail then further levels of detail would not be considered and could not be used to make an identification. To arrive at a definitive decision a fingerprint examiner should be able to demonstrate that the match or identification shows a coincident sequence of characteristics and that there are no unexplained differences.

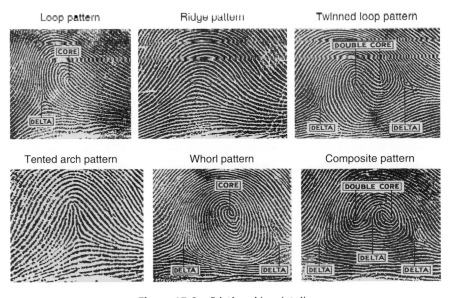

Figure 17.9 Friction ridge detail.

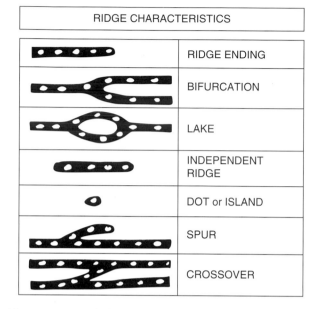

Figure 17.10   Friction ridge detail: minutiae – ridge features.

Table 17.1   ACE-V fingerprint system of scientific of identification.

Analysis (collect intelligence): the qualitative and quantitative assessment of Level 1, 2 and 3 details to determine their proportion, interrelationship, and value to individualise.
Comparison (use intelligence): to examine the attributes observed during analysis in order to determine agreement or discrepancies between two friction ridge impressions.
Evaluation (form an opinion): the cyclical procedure of comparison between two friction ridge impressions to effect a decision, i.e. made by the same friction skin, not made by the same friction skin, or insufficient detail to form a conclusive decision.
Verification: an independent analysis, comparison, and evaluation by a second qualified examiner of the friction ridge impressions.

A methodology referred to as analysis, comparison, evaluation, and verification (ACE-V) has been widely adopted in many countries, including the UK, for fingerprint examination (Table 17.1). This provides a broad, structured approach to fingerprint examination and a basis for developing technical procedures. If the ACE-V methodology is followed, particularly in relation to analysis and verification, it provides some degree of safeguard against errors and incorrect results. Within the current processes in the criminal justice system, where a fingerprint examiner makes a definitive decision, it is usual to have a verification process involving at least two further competent fingerprint examiners who must also make a definitive decision.

17.11.5   Recent developments

The Home Office has overseen a radical overhaul of their manual of fingerprint development techniques by the Centre of Applied Science and Technology to take into account changes in police laboratory operations and to implement mandatory standards. Emphasis is now placed on integrating forensic practice and the competency of the practitioner. Such developments include:

- live-scan fingerprinting, which captures finger and palm prints electronically and obviates the need for ink and paper

- transmitting crime scene prints from the scene to the bureau

- transmitting fingerprints from a remote location to the bureau

- automatic fingerprint recognition systems, which have been in existence for many years and have recently been expanded to include multimodal biometric identifiers, including iris scans, palm prints, and face recognition photos

- three-dimensional imaging of prints

- improved development techniques: a good example is the use of new fluorescent small-particle reagent methods based on zinc carbonate in prints exposed to extremes of heat, as in arson.

17.11.6   Recent legal developments

Until recently, fingerprint evidence was regarded as infallible and was not open to serious challenge in the courts. It has been demonstrated, however, that far from being an infallible method of identification, it is basically subjective, opinion evidence that relies heavily on the judgement and interpretation of the fingerprint practitioner. There have been a number of reports and enquiries which have identified significant problems with the methodology. The most prominent in the UK is the Fingerprint Inquiry Report, published in 2011 in response to controversy surrounding a Scottish case where a police officer was alleged to have left her fingerprint at the crime scene of a murder case. Although the thumbprint found at the scene was identified as the officer's at the murder trial, she denied that she was ever inside the crime scene and could not therefore have left her print there. She was prosecuted for perjury. Following evidence from independent experts that it was not her print, she was exonerated. It was later concluded at appeal that another print said to have been produced by the accused had been misidentified and his conviction was quashed. Amongst the 86 recommendations the report made, was the proposal that 'fingerprint evidence should be recognized as opinion evidence, not fact' and that it cannot be treated with '100% certainty or on any other basis to suggest that it is infallible'.

Fingerprint identity in the UK relied for many years on finding 16 points of similarity between prints. A Project Board was set up in the UK in 1996 by the Association of Chief Police Officers (ACPO) to examine the validity of the 16-point standard. They agreed that there was no scientific, moral or logical reason for retaining it, and it naturally followed that no such reasons could be found to support any other fingerprint standard applying a specific number of characteristics. They recommended that in future evidence of fingerprint identification should be presented before the courts without the need for a minimum number of matching characteristics. Providing that each identification was checked according to ACPO and Home Office guidelines (i.e. each identification must be checked by a minimum of three independent examiners), such evidence would be made available to the police and the judicial system.

Since the 16-point standard for identification was abolished, fingerprint experts have used a non-numeric scale. They use their experience, opinion, and a certain number of matching characteristics to present fingerprint identification evidence in court. How many characteristics are deemed sufficient for an identification will depend on a number of factors, including, for example, the clarity of the mark and the spatial relationship of other connected marks.

References

Bertillon, A. (1893). *Identification Anthropométrique*. Instructions Signalétiques. Melun: Imprimerie Administrative.

Black, S., Aggrawal, A., and Payne-James, J. (2010). *Age Estimation in the Living: The Practitioners Guide*. Wiley-Blackwell.

Brogdon, B.G. (ed.) (1998). Radiological identification of individual remains. In: *Forensic Radiology*. CRC Press. pp 149–187.

Civil Contingenies Act 2004. www.legislation.gov.uk

CNN World (2019). www.edition-m.cnn.com/2019/06/10/us/

Dealing with Disasters, 3rd Edition, 2003. www.ukresilience.gov.uk (Accessed March 2017).

Emergency response and recovery. Cabinet Emergencies: preparation, response and recovery Gov.UK 2013. http://www.gov.uk/guidance/emergency-response-and-recovery (accessed March 2017).

Fernandes CL. (2018). The paranasal sinuses in the human. PhD, Queen Mary University of London.

France, D.L., Griffin, T.J., Swanburg, J.G. et al. (1992). A multidisciplinary approach to the detection of clandestine graves. *J. Forensic Sci.* 37: 1445–1458.

Gatliff, B.P. and Snow, C.C. (1979). From skull to visage. *J. Biocommun.* 6: 27–30.

Home Office Communication Directorate (2004). Guidance on dealing with fatalities in emergencies. Joint publication with the Cabinet Office. http://www.gov.uk/government/uploads/system/uploads/attachment_data/file/61191/fatalities.pdf. (Accessed March 2017).

Isçan, M.Y. and Helmer, R.P. (eds.) (1993). *Forensic Analysis of the Skull*. New York: Wiley Liss.

Krogman, W.M. and Iscan, Y.M. (1986). *The Human Skeleton in Forensic Medicine*, 2e. Springfield: Charles C Thomas.

National Law Enforcement Museum Newsletter November 2011 Volume 3, Issue 9. Washington, DC 20004-2025 www.museum@nleomf.org (accessed 08/2018).

Quatrehomme, G., Fronty, P., Sapanet, M. et al. (1996). Identification by frontal sinus pattern in forensic anthropology. *Forensic Sci. Int.* 83: 147–153.

Rhine, S. and Sperry, K. (1991). Radiographic identification by mastoid sinus and arterial pattern. *J. Forensic Sci.* 36: 272–279.

Rogers, T.L. and Allard, T.T. (2004). Expert testimony and positive identification of human remains through cranial suture patterns. *J. Forensic Sci.* 49 (2): 203–207.

Scott, A.L., Congram, D., Sweet, D. et al. (2010). Anthropological and radiographic comparison of ante mortem surgical records for identification of skeletal remains. *J. Forensic Sci.* 55: 241–244.

Trotter, M. and Gleser, G.C. (1958). A re-evaluation of estimation of stature based on measurements of stature taken during life and of long bones after death. *Am. J. Phys. Anthropol.* 16: 79–123.

Vanezis, P., Blowes, R.W., Linney, A.D. et al. (1989). Application of 3-D computer graphics for facial reconstruction and comparison with sculpting techniques. *Forensic Sci. Int.* 42: 69–84.

Vanezis, M. and Vanezis, P. (2000). Cranio-facial reconstruction in forensic identification – historical development and a review of current practice. *Med. Sci. Law* 40: 197–205.

18
Use of DNA in Human Identification

Denise Syndercombe Court

Department of Analytical, Environmental and Forensic Sciences, King's College London, London, UK

18.1   DNA fingerprint discovery

In 1984 Alec Jeffreys discovered a minisatellite in myoglobin using seal meat. Using the myoglobin minisatellite he and his team were able to discover a repeated core sequence. This is a piece of DNA that is found to be similar in many different minisatellites. They used the core as a radioactive 'probe' to identify other minisatellites in the genome. The original method used by Sir Alec Jeffreys for profiling involved restriction fragment length polymorphism (RFLP) analysis. This is the difference in homologous DNA sequences that can be detected by the presence of fragments of different lengths after digestion of the DNA samples in question, with specific restriction enzymes. RFLP as a molecular marker is specific to a single clone/restriction enzyme combination. This generates thousands of DNA fragments of differing sizes as a consequence of variations between DNA sequences of different individuals. The fragments are separated on the basis of size using gel electrophoresis. The separated fragments are then transferred to a nitrocellulose or nylon filter; this procedure is called a Southern blot. The DNA fragments within the blot are permanently fixed to the filter, and the DNA strands are denatured. Radiolabelled probe molecules are then added that are complementary to sequences in the genome that contain repeat sequences. These repeat sequences tend to vary in length amongst different individuals and are called variable number tandem repeat sequences (VNTRs). The probe molecules hybridise to DNA fragments containing the repeat sequences and excess probe molecules are washed away. The blot is then exposed to an X-ray film. Fragments of DNA that have bound to the probe molecules appear as dark bands on the film (Figure 18.1).

Essential Forensic Medicine, First Edition. Edited by Peter Vanezis.
© 2020 John Wiley & Sons Ltd. Published 2020 by John Wiley & Sons Ltd.

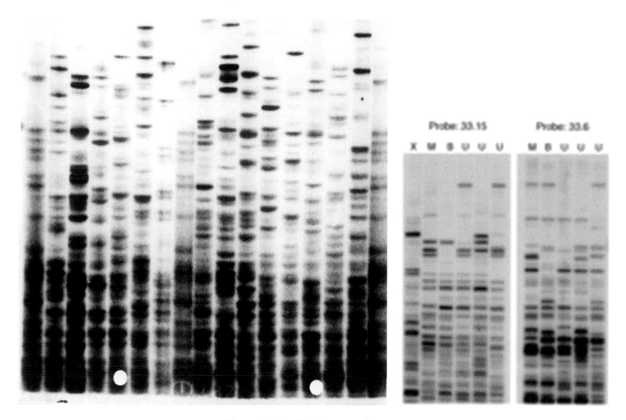

Figure 18.1   Multilocus probe test.

In a typical picture it can be very difficult to see if bands in one lane match those in another because of the difference in intensity. Intensity doesn't matter – only the position of the band.

18.2   Identification using DNA

18.2.1   DNA in human identification

The introduction of DNA for human identification has vastly improved the ability to identify both living and deceased persons. The forensic application of DNA has revolutionised the ability to bring perpetrators of crimes to justice, resolve immigration arguments, and clarify paternity issues.

Before the discovery of DNA typing methodologies, identification of remains in disasters was effectively limited to dental records and body-associated artefacts. Even the early DNA finger-printing invented by Jeffreys in 1984 (Jeffreys et al. 1985), which examined long stretches (several kilobases) of DNA looking for RFLPs, proved of little value when looking at tissues that were often fragmented and decaying. It was the invention of the polymerase chain reaction (PCR) by Kary Mullis (Mullis et al. 1986) that revolutionised forensic identification through its ability to make millions of copies of targeted sequences of DNA via a thermal cycling process, allowing scientists to examine small and degraded material that is typically found in mass disasters.

18.2.2 The human genome

The human genome consists of pairs of chromosomes (Figure 18.2), one of each pair being inherited from each parent. There are three billion bases in a single copy; only about 2% codes for proteins while the remaining is termed non-coding yet includes a variety of regions that regulate chromosome structure and control gene expression. It is the non-coding DNA that is normally used in forensic analysis.

The DNA in each chromosome consists of sequences of purine or pyrimidine nucleotides bound covalently to a sugar phosphate background. A second strand consists of a complementary sequence with adenine (A) and thymine (T), and guanine (G) and cytosine (C) paired and held together with hydrogen bonds (Figure 18.3). The configuration of the bonding provides the helical structure of

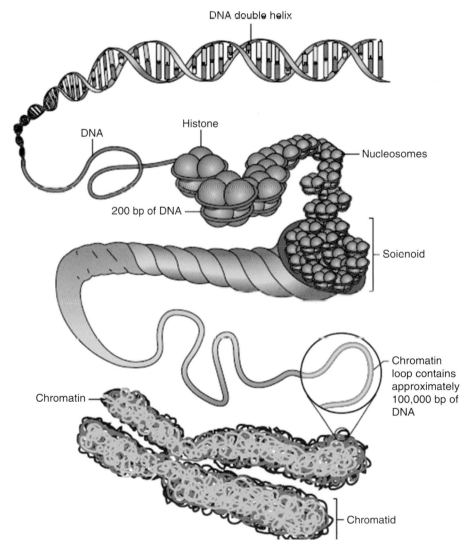

Figure 18.2 Unpacking a chromosome.

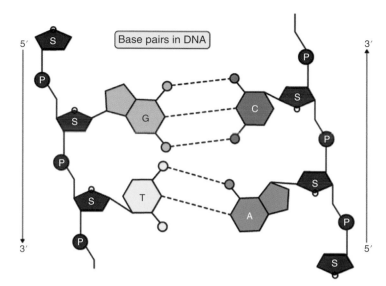

Figure 18.3   Unpacking the double helix.

the molecule. In its natural state in the cell, DNA is almost always double-stranded, but it can be separated by enzymes *in vivo*, and this is necessary for replication to occur. Separation of the strands exposes the bases and these can then act as a template for the formation of a new strand from more nucleotide subunits. Separation of the strands can also be facilitated *in vitro* by an increase in temperature, for example, and it is this process that is utilised in the polymerase chain reaction (PCR) process, enabling areas of DNA to be copied.

18.2.3   PCR analysis

PCR has enabled a hundredfold reduction in the amount of extracted DNA that can be analysed, in comparison with Jeffreys' RFLP method. The PCR amplification process involves primers, short oligonucleotide sequences (required as a starting point for DNA synthesis), and binding to a single-stranded DNA template, which then provides a location for DNA polymerase to produce a copy of the opposite strand. The process repeats in a three-stage cycle of DNA denaturation, primer annealing, and extension. Each cycle generates a twofold increase in the target DNA. PCR mimics the biological process of DNA replication, but only to specific, and relatively short, DNA sequences of interest, typically up to 500 base pairs in length, defined by the primers used..

18.2.4   STR analysis

A large proportion of the DNA molecule consists of repeated sequences of variable lengths. Of particular interest in forensic analysis, because the sequences are short (commonly four nucleotide bases – tetranucleotides), are regions of the genetic sequence called short tandem repeats (STRs) in which the blocks of sequences are repeated one after the other (in tandem) (Figure 18.3). STRs for forensic analysis are also chosen because they are polymorphic in all populations, inherited independently (normally on different chromosomes, or perhaps on different arms of the same chromosome), robust when being multiplied, able to be multiplexed with other loci, display limited

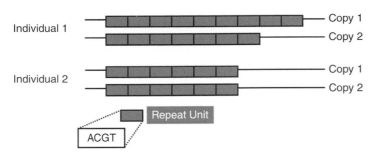

Figure 18.4 Short tandem repeat.

copy artefacts, and have a low mutation rate (Butler 2006). Although there may also be some sequence variation within repeat regions, the different polymorphic types (alleles) are named after the number of repeat blocks. For example, the genotype at the region of the DNA illustrated in Figure 18.4 in Individual 1 has alleles 7 and 9, and is said to be heterozygous at this locus, whereas Individual 2 appears to have inherited the 6 allele from each parent, and is said to be homozygous. Sequence variation between alleles is beginning to be exploited in new multiple parallel sequencing techniques that are entering the forensic arena.

The set of alleles from an individual derived from different defined chromosome locations (loci) is called a DNA profile (differentiating this from the DNA fingerprint developed by Jeffreys). Copying a target length of DNA through the polymerase enzyme is not always a perfect process and sometimes the enzyme appears to slip along the strand that is being copied, resulting in the production of a small amount of DNA produce that is, generally, one repeat shorter, producing a small stutter allele. For example, if the allele has ten repeats, we expect to see a small stutter allele 9, typically under 15% of the height of the 10 allele. Sometimes over-stutter can also be observed

These STR loci (locations on a chromosome) are targeted with sequence-specific primers and amplified using PCR. The DNA fragments that result are then separated and detected using electrophoresis. There are two common methods of separation and detection: capillary electrophoresis (CE) and gel electrophoresis. The former is commonly used today as it is more sensitive, enabling the differentiation of fragments that differ by only one base pair (bp). Using Figure 18.4 as an example, it is important to be able to detect if a single one of these repeat units only has three nucleotide bases, rather than four.

Essential to the analytical process is the ability to visualise the results of the PCR targeted amplification. This is facilitated through incorporation of different fluorescent dyes into the primers, which are then multiplied up along with the target DNA and can be detected electronically within an instrument. Fluorescently labelled target amplicons of varying lengths are separated by electrokinetic injection (because DNA molecules are charged) as they move through a very fine long glass capillary (about 50 cm in length and around the width of a human hair). An argon ion laser detector excites the fluorescent dye as it passes through a point in the capillary and the instrument collects information about the time of detection (which is proportional to the length of the fragment being detected) and the wavelength of the fluorescence, which identifies the dye and therefore also the sequence being targeted (Butler 2010).

The ability to manipulate the time of detection through primer design and being able to detect different targets simultaneously, through the use of different fluorescent dyes, means that a large number of targeted areas of the DNA molecule can be analysed at the same time (*multiplexed*). Addition of known DNA fragments, labelled with a different dye, in the form of a size standard into each sample, allows calibration of the output to provide the fragment size in base pairs (bp), and running standard samples alongside one that contains all of the known allelic variants (an allelic ladder, Figure 18.5) facilitates the conversion of the targeted amplicon into an output with the detected alleles named in the form of an *electropherogram*.

Typically each STR allele will be shared by around 5–20% of individuals. The power of STR analysis comes from looking at multiple STR loci simultaneously. The more STR regions that are tested in an individual the more discriminating the test becomes. Typically, a full DNA profile (from at least ten selected loci) will be shared by less than one in a billion individuals and so provides a very powerful identification tool.

In 2014 England and Wales moved to a new multiplex, known as DNA17, which added loci recommended by the European Union to the current SGMPlus multiplex currently used in the National DNA Database (NDNAD). DNA17 multiplexes are manufactured by several commercial suppliers. Figure 18.6 depicts a DNA17 profile. Five dyes are used, four being associated with the loci and a fifth (not shown) to provide the size standard for each sample. Other parts of the UK have chosen different a different set, consisting of even more loci, but all contain the core set of loci used in England and Wales.

Alleles at each locus are depicted by the coloured peaks, which are separated by size, the larger fragments being shown on the right of the graph. All individuals inherit an allele at each locus from their parents and so, typically, two peaks are seen; where only one peak is present at a locus that implies that the individual has inherited the same allele from both parents. In addition to the STR loci most DNA multiplexes also target an area on the amelogenin gene.

The amelogenin gene is found on the X chromosome, with a single copy on the Y chromosome. The intron on the X chromosome has a 6 bp deletion and this facilitates determination of sex in the STR analysis, which is revealed by two peaks for males and a single peak for females. This is seen in Figure 18.5 with the peaks in the top left corner indicating that the profile is from a male individual.

18.3   The National DNA database

The UK NDNAD was set up in 1995 and holds profiles of every arrested individual for comparison with DNA recovered from crime scenes. The database is interrogated on a daily basis, and matches and partial matches are reported to the police force that deposits the information.

Until relatively recently profiles of all named individuals entered on to the database were retained, even if the individual was never charged. An application to the European Court of Human Rights by Child S (charged and acquitted of attempted robbery) and Michael Marper (charged with harassment against his partner, subsequently dropped) to have their profiles removed from the database (S and Marper v United Kingdom ECHR 1581, 2008) led to a judgement that Article 8 of the UN Convention on the Rights of the Child had been violated. The UK Government responded with the Protection of Freedoms Act (2012), which enforces the removal of profiles from innocents and children from the database, and sets down the rules that govern profile retention. DNA samples from named individuals, regardless of conviction, are now destroyed within six months of being taken.

Profiles held in relation to missing persons, or from individuals at risk of harm, are have also been removed from the database and these are now held separately on the Missing Persons DNA Database, which also holds profiles from bodies of unidentified people, or the Vulnerable Persons DNA Database.

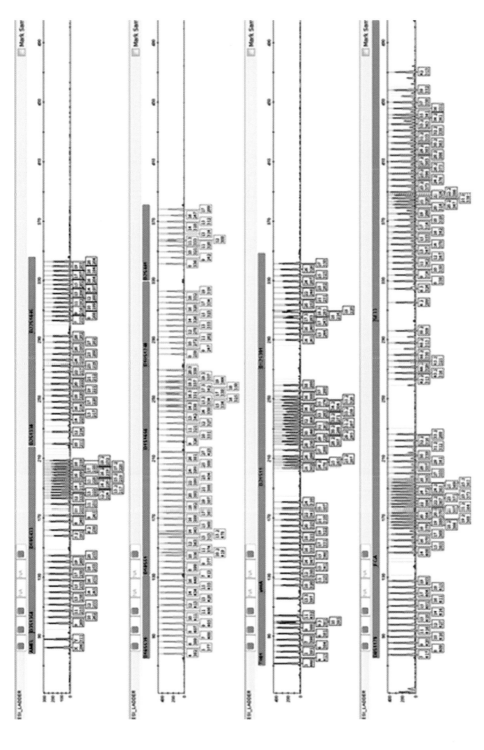

Figure 18.5 An electropherogram of an allelic ladder, showing all the common STR alleles in a DNA17 multiplex. Note: There are many multiplexes of STRs used worldwide. STRBase (http://www.cstl.nist.gov/biotech/strbase) provides a dynamic resource of information about the loci used in forensic science.

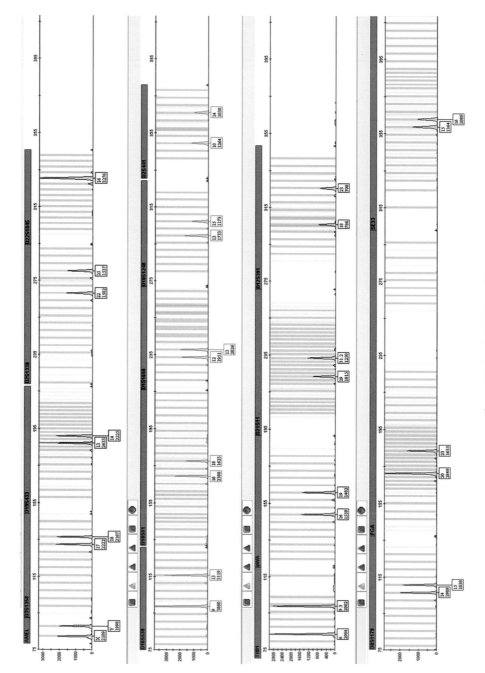

Figure 18.6 A DNA17 profile.

About 5.7 million DNA profiles remained present on the database in 2014, reduced from over 7.1 million before the Act. The large size of the database has meant that in over 60% of crimes where a DNA profile has been recovered, a DNA match provides the police with the name of a possible suspect.

18.4 Forensic analysis

The nature of crime means that deposits of human cellular material at a scene are complex in nature, often being present in mixtures of individuals in differing amounts, sometimes consisting only of a handful of cells, that may have been exposed to environmental insults, both natural and chemical, that can damage the cells and the DNA within.

18.4.1 DNA inhibition

PCR amplification can be affected by chemical inhibitors that may be extracted from material at a crime scene along with the body cell material of interest. Environmental substances that may be found in inorganic and organic chemicals can interfere with cell lysis, may degrade or chemically alter the DNA molecule, or may interfere with the polymerase enzyme used in the amplification. Table 18.1 lists some well-known inhibitors. Various techniques are used within the laboratory to limit the effect of these inhibitors, such as diluting the sample (and therefore also the inhibitor), changing the polymerase, chemical neutralisation of the inhibitors, and the use of various filtration devices prior to PCR.

18.4.2 DNA degradation

DNA degrades through a variety of enzymatic and chemical processes. On cellular death body enzymic processes result in cell lysis; this process can be amplified in the presence of bacterial, fungal, and insect growth. UV light, from sunlight, can lead to adjacent thymine (T) bases cross-linking, which interferes with the polymerase enzyme as it progresses along the DNA strand.

The DNA strand can also be affected by oxidative damage to the bases, which can make the detection and amplification of the target DNA molecule difficult. The damage leads to hydrolytic

Table 18.1 DNA inhibitors and their possible source.

Inhibitor	Potential source
Bile salts	Faeces
Calcium	Bone
Collagen	Body tissue
Heme	Blood
Humic acid	Soil
Indigo dye	Clothing
Melanin	Hair
Myoglobin	Muscle
Polysaccharides	Faeces and plant material

cleavage of the glycosidic base–sugar bond: the nucleobase is lost from the strand and this results in a break in the DNA strand sequence. Heat and humidity in particular increase this hydrolytic damage, which occurs randomly along the DNA strand.

The targeted amplified material we are aiming to analyse consists of lengths of DNA, typically between 100 and 500 bp. The larger the target molecule, the greater the chance that hydrolytic damage will break the strand, leading to an inability to detect that fragment. Typically, within a multiplex PCR this is seen in an electropherogram through the complete loss of alleles above a certain fragment length size (Figure 18.7).

STR kit manufacturers have responded to the problems associated with DNA degradation by developing sets of *miniSTRs*, which have a reduced size PCR product (under 250 bp). Packing sufficient markers into a much smaller space is problematic but use of six dye chemistries has helped. It is likely that, in the future, more dyes will be utilised in order to increase the capacity of forensic multiplexes.

18.4.3   Low-level DNA

DNA analysis from a few cells (low-level DNA), such as might be deposited through touch, provides its own challenges due to stochastic effects which lead to loss of alleles from a profile. These effects are more pronounced when the numbers of cells available to be amplified are at a very low level and there is unequal sampling of the alleles in the early part of the PCR process, resulting in some alleles being over-represented and others being under-represented. This produces locus imbalance or total loss of the allele (Figure 18.8), the latter being known as *drop-out*.

Historically, scientists dealt with the problem of limited DNA by increasing the amplification cycles in a process known as low copy number (LCN). While this increases the chance of an individual allele being amplified and therefore detected, it does not overcome the stochastic effects, which can become exaggerated. The resultant imbalanced loci and exaggerated stutter can lead to interpretation problems in understanding whether a mixture is present, and the ability to differentiate alleles from stutter artefact.

LCN was criticised heavily in the Omagh bombing trial. In a subsequent review of the procedure the Caddy Report (Caddy 2008) recommended that DNA be quantified so that stochastic processes can be limited in the subsequent analysis. The Appeal Court in R v Reed (R v Reed, Reed, R v Garmson [2009] 2698) suggested that LCN could be reliably interpreted when the amount of DNA used was greater than somewhere between 100 and 200 pg.

Changes in the chemistry of commercial multiplexes has increased the sensitivity of DNA amplification such that today there is little need to employ increased amplification cycles or to use the variety of other techniques, such as nested PCR, reduced volume PCR, increased capillary electrophoretic injection, and post-PCR purification, that were developed to deal with low-level DNA.

18.4.4   DNA contamination

Contamination of a DNA sample with DNA from another source is obviously problematic and may be overt or seen only at a very low level within an analysis. The high sensitivity of DNA

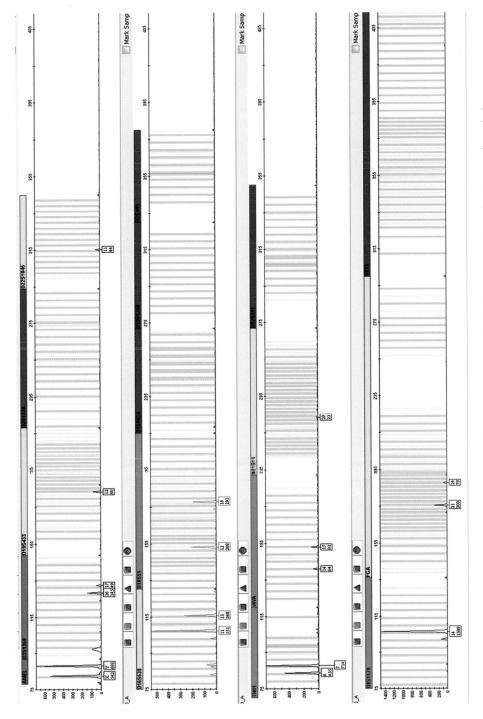

Figure 18.7 An electropherogram of a DNA profile in which alleles have been lost due to DNA degradation.

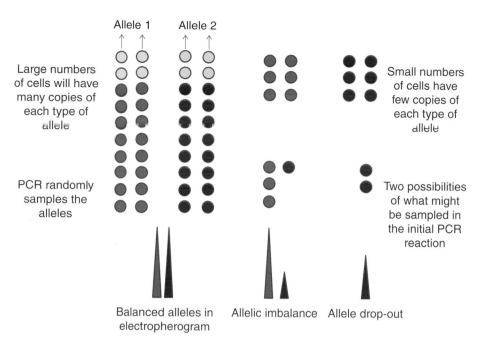

Figure 18.8   Stochastic variation.

analysis today means that the unwanted presence of only a few cells from another source can be detected, producing an apparent mixture within a sample. Being able to differentiate this contamination from a true mixture is important and measures to avoid potential contamination are vital.

The ease with which contamination, particularly that found at a low level, can occur has led to quality measures being adopted within laboratories, including the use of disposable gowns, gloves, head, face, and foot coverings, and associated strict processes. Laboratory spaces are restricted to registered personnel and will often be supplied with positive air-flow. Different areas are designated to pre-PCR and post-PCR, with a one-way flow of material to avoid contamination. Regular cleaning processes (before and after every process) and regular monitoring of the environment are undertaken as checks. The DNA profiles of all staff are stored on an elimination database so that the source of any contamination can be determined.

In order to ensure that DNA contaminants are not introduced in the process, controls are included as part of each analysis; sample extraction and amplification negative controls use all of the chemicals in the process in the absence of any known DNA samples to be analysed. Low-level DNA analysis is particularly vulnerable and often analysts will produce duplicated or triplicated analyses, recording only those alleles that have been detected on more than one occasion (see the section on the murder of Meredith Kercher, below). This will also deal with the problem of chance contamination of a single plastic consumable that would not otherwise be detected in batch tests.

While DNA analysts may take enormous care to avoid contamination and transfer events within the laboratory, they cannot control what has happened before the sample has been received, and processes to avoid potential contamination at the crime scene are equally important.

Case Study 18.1 The murder of Meredith Kercher

Meredith Kercher was murdered on 1 November 2007 in Perugia, Italy. Rudy Guede, Raffaele Solliecito, and his girlfriend at the time, Amanda Knox, were suspected of the crime. After his fingerprints were found at the scene, stained with blood matching Kercher, Guede was convicted of her murder in 2008. In 2009 Sollecito and Knox were also convicted. A successful appeal led to their acquittal in 2011 but the prosecution successfully argued for a second trial and both were again acquitted in 2015.

The evidence against Sollecito related to a bra found at the scene. Low-level DNA, said to be consistent with originating from Kercher and Sollecito, was found on the bra clasp. However, there was also, apparently, DNA present from at least one other in the mixture. There were several criticisms of the evidence: the bra was not recovered from the scene for 46 days. In the intervening time, photographs showed that it had moved locations and the scene had showed considerable disruption. There was criticism over the interpretation of the findings and a suggestion that international protocols had not been followed. Overall, environmental or handling contamination could not be ruled out.

The evidence against Knox related to a knife found in Sollecito's flat. There was no suggestion that this was the murder weapon and no blood was detected on the knife. DNA matching Knox was found on the handle, and a very poor profile matching Kercher found on the blade. There was poor information about how the knife was recovered and packaged, and it could have been handled by individuals who may have examined other items from Kercher within the laboratory. The analysis was not repeated and there was no evidence that negative controls had been run. The poor control associated with the item and its examination meant that inadvertent transfer could not be ruled out.

More overt contamination has been detected in a number of cases and these are generally associated with a lack of appropriate quality control or the failure to follow standard operating procedures designed to avoid contamination. Two examples illustrate this: the phantom of Heilbronn and the case of Adam Scott.

Case Study 18.2 The phantom of Heilbronn

An intensive forensic investigation took place in 2007 after a female police officer was murdered in Germany. A DNA profile from a female was found and linked with around 40 crimes, including six murders, burglary, and car thieving in Germany, Austria, and France, going back to 1993. An intensive search involving more than 16000 police hours were spent investigating this apparent serial killer. No witnesses had described a female suspect and a photofit of an apparent male was produced, with the suggested implication that the culprit could be a transsexual individual. It was only when the same profile was found associated with fingerprints from a missing male that police realised that something was seriously wrong with the evidence and the profile was traced back to a female worker engaged in making DNA swabs that had been distributed from the manufacturers across Europe. At the time it was not understood that standard sterilisation processes would not destroy DNA.

Case Study 18.3 Adam Scott

Adam Scott was charged with a rape in Manchester in October 2011. He lived in Exeter and denied ever being in Manchester and there was no evidence that he had been there at the time, yet his DNA had been found in association with a vaginal swab from the female complainant who thought she might have been raped.

Adam Scott had been identified because he was on the DNA database. He had, reportedly, spat at a police officer in the west of England, and the saliva had been submitted to the forensic laboratory to confirm that it was his a short time before the rape investigation. Material for forensic analysis is loaded into wells within disposable plastic plates and robots take out the material to extract the DNA. The protocol states that the plate must then be disposed of but in this instance it was not. The plate would have appeared clean and it was used again in error. The well, still containing the remnants of high-level DNA saliva from Adam Scott, was then loaded with a vaginal swab extract from the victim in the Manchester rape. A defence-initiated investigation led to a repeat examination from the original swab and the contamination was revealed – a clear failure to follow standard operating procedures.

18.5   DNA mixtures

True DNA mixtures are of interest to the scientist. When material is collected from a crime scene, often by swabbing or using sticky tape to collect any human cellular material, the aim is to find DNA profiles of interest to the police. Inevitably that may also include DNA from innocent people who may have left their cells on a surface or item being investigated and adventitious transfer from innocents must always be considered when interpreting the data.

The attribution of DNA components to a particular individual can sometimes be problematic. Figures 18.9 and 18.10 show two examples of mixtures, typical of the casework that a scientist will be asked to interpret.

In Figure 18.9 the mixture is recognised by the presence of more than two alleles at any one locus (one individual can provide a maximum of two alleles), and the very unbalanced pairs of loci in some others. It is not possible to say that there is DNA from only two people in the mixture because more people could have provided the same alleles and their individual contribution will be hidden under the peak. (New sequencing technologies that are now being employed will often reveal such mixtures within an allele). Examination of the profile, however, reveals some components that stand out in the mixture and it may be possible to be confident that these prominent components originate from one individual. In this case the main contributor to the sample is likely to be from a female: this can be seen from examination of the amelogenin locus where the X component is very strong and the male Y component only at a low level.

In contrast, in Figure 18.10 the mixture is much more complex and it is not possible to deconvolute the mixture to determine which components come from a particular individual and simply matching the profile of the suspect to the mixture is dangerous (but see R v Dlugosz below). Here the Y component is at least as strong as the X component, suggesting that the mixture may just be of males, but that can never be certain as a female may provide only a small contribution to the mixture and not be detected by an increase in X. Here the X and Y are unbalanced presumably due

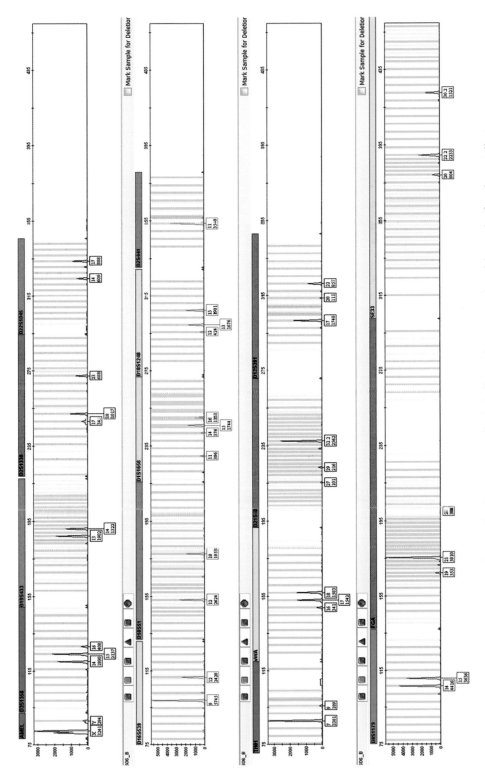

Figure 18.9 DNA mixture of ≥ least two people, including at least one male, with a major female contributor.

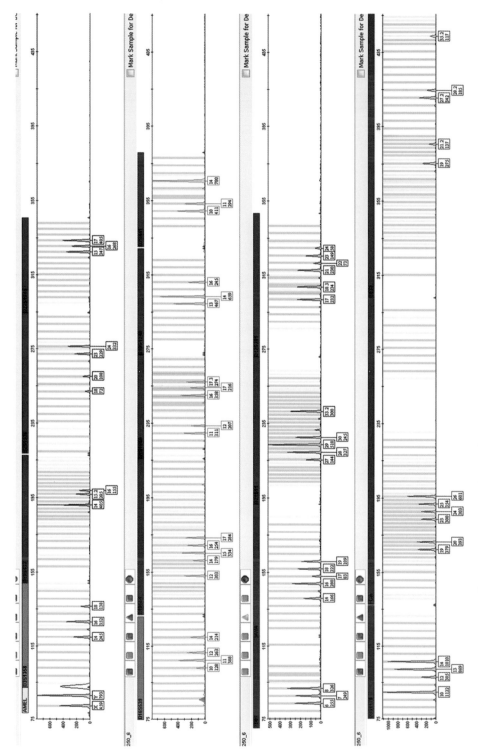

Figure 18.10 DNA mixture of at least three people with at least one male contributor.

to stochastic effects – one would expect a mixture of males to provide a balanced X and Y. Counting the alleles at each locus reveals six in some areas and so one can say that this mixture is of at least three individuals. While virtually all three-person mixtures will be detected as coming from three people, about 70% of four-person mixtures, 40% of five-person mixtures, and 14% of six-person mixtures will look like a three-person mixture.

If a profile from a single person can be safely determined from a mixture, such as possibly in Figure 18.9, the scientist can determine a *match probability*. The match probability simply records the chance that the matching profile would be seen within unrelated individuals within the population – 0.000000001 or 1 in 1 billion for a full matching SGMPlus profile. This process does not help in the assessment of the minor components in Figure 18.9, nor any of the components in Figure 18.10.

Without certainty of a clear profile, a match probability cannot be assessed and instead an assessment of the evidence is made in the form of a likelihood ratio (LR) that contrasts two hypotheses:

- The probability (p) of the evidence (E) (a DNA match) given the prosecution hypothesis (Hp) that the suspect has left the DNA – certainty.

- The probability of the evidence (a DNA match) given the defence hypothesis (Hd) that another, unrelated person has left the DNA – how common the profile is in the population.

This can be formalised as:

$$LR = \frac{p(E)|Hp}{p(E)|Hd}$$

This can be simply calculated, in the case of a single profile, as:

$$LR = \frac{1}{0.000000001} = 1\,billion$$

The evidence is thus one billion times more likely if the prosecution hypothesis was true, rather than the defence hypothesis.

Note that this does not answer the jury question of innocence or guilt: what is the probability that the suspect is guilty, given the evidence? The jury also needs to consider non-genetic evidence in the case:

$$\frac{p(Hp)|E}{p(Hd)|E} = \frac{p(E)|Hp}{p(E)|Hd} \times \frac{p(Hp)}{p(Hd)}$$

This can be more simply stated as:

$$odds\ of\ guilt = genetic\ evidence \times non\text{-}genetic\ evidence$$

The jury considers the answer to the question on the left of the equation. The scientist provides the genetic evidence; the jury will be presented with the non-genetic evidence, which they must consider. For example, if they are sure that the defendant could not have committed the crime (perhaps because he or she was in prison), then the term to the right would be zero, effectively nullifying any genetic evidence.

Regardless of the responsibility of the jury, the scientist is tasked with providing a likelihood ratio representing the genetic evidence, and that is not simple, as we have seen when looking at the minor contributions to profiles such as those seen in Figure 18.9.

Many different strategies have been proposed to interpret mixtures. One commonly used series of steps involves identifying that a mixture is present, designating the alleles, identifying the number of potential contributors, estimating the ratio of individuals' contributions to the mixture, considering all possible genotype combinations, comparing with reference profiles, and finally determining the weight of evidence (Clayton et al. 1998). In the absence of a major profile, using these methods when the mixture contains, or may contain, material from more than two individuals is problematic and a recent appeal court judgement (R v Dlugosz [2013] EWCA Crim 2) stated that:

> An expert who spends years studying this kind of comparison can properly form a judgment as to the significance of what he has found in any particular case. It is a judgment based on his experience. A jury is entitled to be informed of his assessment.

This judgement has been questioned by forensic statisticians, who suggest that this could inappropriately bias a jury who might think, on learning that a large number of alleles within the mixture are also seen in the defendant's profile, that the defendant's DNA is present in the mixture.

In response to the problems increasingly facing analysts with more sensitive DNA tests, forensic statisticians have provided software solutions, both commercial and non-commercial, using probabilistic approaches. Two iexamples of readily available open-source software to interpret complex mixtures are LRMix (Gill and Haned 2013) and EuroForMix (Bleka, Storvik and Gill 2015).

18.6   Lineage markers

Standard STR DNA analysis looks at autosomes. Lineage markers are those passed down intact from generation to generation. Paternal lineages can be tracked thought the Y chromosome and maternal lineages through mitochondrial DNA sequences; markers on the X chromosome also have some more limited applicability.

18.6.1   Y Chromosome analysis

The Y male sex-determining chromosome, as it is inherited only by males from their fathers, is almost identical down the patrilineal line (assuming intact paternity) and as a result leads to a less precise analysis than if autosomal chromosomes were being tested because of, in the latter, the random exchange that occurs between pairs of chromosomes as zygotes are being made. Nevertheless, analysis of STRs on the Y chromosome has an important role in both forensic and kinship analysis.

Its primary use in forensic examination (Roewer 2009) is in sexual assault, particularly in cases where there has been no ejaculation or in azoospermic males in which plentiful DNA from the female overwhelms autosomal STR profiles, whereas analysis of the Y chromosome can occur without any inhibition from the female material. It can also assist in deciphering the number of males participating in a 'gang rape'. Because the set of Y STRs originates from a single chromosome, the resulting profile is known as a *haplotype*.

In addition to its use in historical human migration and genealogical questions, familial searches, and deficient paternity tests (where the father is not available), Y chromosome analysis can be particularly helpful in missing person investigations and mass disaster identification.

Several manufacturers have produced Y chromosome multiplexes: GlobalFiler, PowerPlex Fusion and PowerPlex 23 are recently developed sets. Rapidly mutating Y STRs can also be useful to increase the chance of distinguishing close relatives. The YHRD database (https://yhrd.org) maintains a collection of forensically validated haplotypes and can be used to estimate the frequency of a particular haplotype.

18.6.2   X Chromosome analysis

X chromosomes are more complex than other lineage markers. Normal males have one X chromosome and so will pass this to their daughters only. Females will pass one of their two X chromosomes to all of their children. There are, therefore, some family relationships where X chromosome analysis can be useful: mother–son, mother–daughter, father–daughter, paternal grandmother–granddaughter. X chromosome analysis is not often undertaken but it is particularly useful in some circumstances where one of the parents is not available, and in missing persons and disaster victim identification (DVI).

18.7   Mitochondrial analysis

Most of the human genome is located within the cell nucleus. However, within the cytoplasm lies a small circular genome found within organelles known as mitochondria. The majority of these organelles have originated from the mother because it is she who donates the egg; the sperm, fertilising the egg, donates mainly nuclear DNA within the sperm head.

Mitochondria are dedicated to produce energy within the cell and, on average, cells contain around 500 mitochondria. The large number of mitochondrial genomes, in comparison with nuclear genomes, means that in situations where nuclear DNA analysis is not possible because of damage or degradation, such as in ancient remains, or in single hairs where there is no root present, mitochondrial sequence analysis can be successful.

The circular molecule consists of about 16,539 base pairs which transcribe 37 genes within a coding region and a 1122 bp control region or D-loop (Figure 18.11). The D-loop is more variable (because it does not code for important genes) and is the region which is targeted in forensic analysis. Historically scientists would sequence two hypervariable areas, known as HVS I and HVS II, but increasingly the whole of the control region is targeted. Bases are numbered from a particular position within the control region (lying between HVS I and HVS II) and base changes that differ from the revised Cambridge Reference Sequence (rCRS) are recorded in forensic casework.

Mitochondrial DNA (mtDNA) analysis is also useful in DVI and has been used in a number of high-profile human remains cases, including the identification of the remains of the Russian Romanov family (Gill et al. 1994).

Concerns have been raised in relation to mtDNA databases, many of which have been shown to contain errors. These errors include clerical errors, sample mix-up, contamination, and incorrect

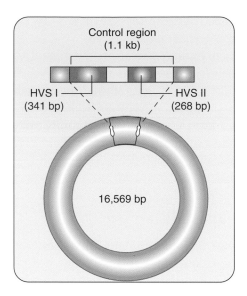

Figure 18.11   Diagram of the mitochondrial genome illustrating the area of interest to forensic scientists.

nomenclature. The European forensic mitochondrial population database project (EMPOP; http://empop.online) was initiated in 2006 to provide the forensic community with a high-quality database.

18.8   Kinship testing

Using PCR technology, DNA analysis is widely applied to determine genetic family relationships such as paternity, maternity, siblingship, and other kinships and is key to DVI. In crime, familial searches are only used in relation to the most serious crimes and each search requires the approval of the DNA Strategy Board.

There are predictable inheritance patterns at certain loci in the human genome, which have been found to be useful in determining both identity and biological relationships. In a routine DNA paternity test, the markers used are STRs. If there are markers shared amongst the tested individuals, the probability of biological relationship is calculated to determine how likely it is the tested individuals share the same markers due to a familial relationship. Parents and children share half of their DNA; chance transmission means that sharing between full siblings is 50% only on average, reducing to 25% on average for grandparent–grandchild, half sibling and avuncular relationships. In addition, because most STR alleles are found in about 15–40% of the population, many can be shared by chance (*identical by state, ibs*) rather than shared because individuals are related (*identical by descent, ibd*) and this means that proof of a relationship beyond the direct parent–child can be difficult.

18.9   Missing persons investigations

Tens of thousands of individuals are reported missing annually and a similar number of unidentified remains are recovered. The latter normally consist of skeletal remains: bones, teeth or tissue. Much is highly degraded and mtDNA sequences may provide the only information as to the identity of the remains. Reference material from people who report missing relatives is provided in two forms: direct reference material, such a Guthrie card from newborn screening, biopsy samples, and personal effects such as a toothbrush, or indirect reference material from close relatives or from more distant relatives where direct maternal or paternal relationships can help.

The UK Missing Persons Bureau is focused exclusively on missing people and serves UK and overseas police forces, maintaining a central national database.

18.10   Disaster victim identification

Mass disasters, natural or man-made, can result in the death of many victims in closed or open incidents. In a closed system, such as an airline crash, the victims are potentially all known. In an open system, such as a natural disaster, knowledge of the total number of victims may never be known. The efforts that scientists worldwide go to identify the victims is known as DVI.

The use of fingerprints and dental examinations play an important part in identification but these rely on archived fingerprints and dental records being available. DNA has a major advantage because it can be used on all recovered tissue provided sufficient material is available and there is reference material available. Sometimes, however, the human remains may be virtually destroyed or burnt, very fragmented or comingled with other remains.

DVI always involves a comparison of post-mortem remains with ante-mortem reference data and the analysis is much more complex than parentage testing because of the large number of potential comparisons and the potentially limited amount of genetic information obtained from the degraded material. Two historic DVI examples are described below.

The international community has made recommendations in relation to the role of forensic genetics in DVI (Prinz et al. 2007). These are summarised below:

Recommendation 1: Genetics laboratories should contact relevant authorities dealing with emergency response and establish their involvement in a possible mass fatality. If a laboratory is going to be involved it will need to have an internal plan with named responsible and fully trained individuals.

Recommendation 2: The internal plan must address throughput capacity and sample tracking. Named responsible people must be kept updated.

Recommendation 3: Several sample types should be taken as soon as possible, even if identity is already established. Traceability must be guaranteed and proper storage assured. The selected sample collection depends on the condition of the body:

- whole body, not decomposed – blood (on FTA (Flinders Technology Associates) cards or swabs) and mouth swabs

- fragmented body, not decomposed – blood, if available, and deep red muscle tissue (approximately 1 g)

- decomposed whole bodies and remains – long compact bone (4–6 cm with a window cut) and/ or healthy teeth (no fillings, preferably molars) and/or any available bone (dense cortical 10 g if possible)

- severely burnt bodies – any of the above, or swabs from the urinary bladder.

Sample collection must be properly documented. In the absence of freezers, appropriate preservatives should be used (not formalin). In addition to various commercial solutions, salt, dimethyl suplphoxide (DMSO), and ethanol have proven to be useful.

Recommendation 4: Multiple direct references should be collected from first-degree relatives for each missing person. Scientists with knowledge of genetics should be available for training and family liaison. Family references should be collected as soon as possible and family trees drawn up. If there are no first-degree relatives, multiple distant relative samples should be collected from grandparents, aunts, uncles, siblings, and half siblings. Advice should be given to families on suitable direct reference materials. Good sources of DNA in particular are toothbrushes, razors, hairbrushes, and combs. Searches for other reference material that may be present in medical facilities may be worthwhile.

Recommendation 5: DVI DNA testing should only be undertaken by laboratories that have demonstrated capability and experience with the sample types. Experience with extraction of degraded bone is one of the most important capabilities.

Recommendation 6: The STR loci used should be agreed between the countries and a minimum of 12 independent loci used as a standard.

Recommendation 7: All allele calls and matches must be thoroughly reviewed. Duplication should be used whenever possible, checking for consistency against the family references. For postmortem tissues two extractions, or concordant results from two specimens from the same body part should be undertaken.

Recommendation 8: If STRs fail, mtDNA, Y STRs or single-nucleotide polymorphisms should be employed.

Recommendation 9: A central database must be used for data comparison and electronic transmission used to avoid transcription errors.

Recommendation 10: DNA-based identification should be accompanied by another form of identification or multiple DNA references. Care must be taken to consider matching problems associated with mutations and null alleles, and allowance incorporated into matching software.

Case Study 18.4 Waco Branch Davidian Fire

This was an early example of DVI in which over 80 members of the Branch Davidian sect in Waco, Texas died in a fire after a FBI siege in 1993. About half of the victims were identified by non-DNA methods. Twenty-six individuals were further identified using relative references and family trees but a shortage of reference samples prevented further identification.

Case Study 18.5 11 September 2001

Over 2000 people died as a result of terrorist attacks on the United States that occurred simultaneously on the Pentagon and the World Trade Centre, and as a result of a plane crashing a field in Pennsylvania,.

At the Pentagon, 188 people died and a variety of DNA, dental records, and fingerprints were used to identify all except five individuals. A further five unidentified individuals were revealed to have near-east mtDNA haplotypes that presumably originated from the terrorists.

All 40 people who died when Flight 93 was forced to crash in Pennsylvania were similarly identified from a total of 1319 remains. Four unidentified males, presumed terrorists, were also shown to have near-east mtDNA haplotypes.

Death certificates have been issued for 2753 individuals in relation to the attack on the World Trade Centre. Up until 2018, 1642 individuals had been identified from more than 21 000 tissue remains. DNA was the most important source of identification information, using STRs, mtDNA and SNPs.

References

Bleka, Ø., Storvik, G., Gill, P (2016). EuroForMix: An open source software based on a continuous model to evaluate STR DNA profiles from a mixture of contributors with artefacts. *Forensic Science International Genetics* 25: 35–44

Butler, J.M. (2006). Genetics and genomics of core short tandem repeat loci used in human identity testing. *Journal of Forensic Sciences* 51: 253–265.

Butler, J.M. (2010). Fundamentals of DNA separation and detection. In: *Fundamentals of Forensic DNA Typing*, 175–203. San Diego: Elsevier Academic Press.

Caddy B (2008). Review of the science of low template DNA analysis. http://tna.europarchive.org/20100419081706/ http:/www.police.homeoffice.gov.uk/publications/operational-policing/Review_of_Low_Template_DNA_1.pdf.

Clayton, T.M., Whitaker, J.P., Sparkes, R., and Gill, P. (1998). Analysis and interpretation of mixed forensic stains using DNA STR profiling. *Forensic Science International* 91: 55–70.

Gill, P. and Haned, H. (2013). A new methodological framework to interpret complex DNA profiles using likelihood ratios. *Forensic Science International: Genetics* 7: 251–263.

Gill, P., Ivanov, P.L., Kimpton, C. et al. (1994). Identification of the remains of the Romanov family by DNA analysis. *Nature Genetics* 6: 130–135.

Jeffreys, A., Wilson, V., and Thein, S.L. (1985). Individual-specific 'fingerprints' of human DNA. *Nature* 316: 76–79.

Mullis, K., Faloona, F., Scharf, S. et al. (1986). Specific enzymatic amplification of DNA in vitro: the polymerase chain reaction. *Cold Spring Harbor Symposium on Quantitative Biology* 51: 263–273.

Prinz, M., Carracedo, A., Mayr, W.R. et al. (2007). International Society for Forensic Genetics. DNA Commission of the International Society for forensic genetics (ISFG): recommendations regarding the role of forensic genetics for disaster victim identification (DVI). *Forensic Science International: Genetics* 1: 3–12.

Roewer, L. (2009). Y chromosome STR typing in crime casework. *Forensic Science, Medicine and Pathology* 5: 77–84.

19
Forensic Odontology and Human Identification

Philip Marsden
Consultant Forensic Odontologist, London, UK

Forensic odontology is the application of dentistry in relation to the law. Worldwide, dental identification along with bite mark analysis are probably the most widely used subdivisions of forensic odontology.

In the UK, in common with the majority of countries in the world, there is a legal requirement to identify the dead. The specific responsibility for the identification of the deceased in England and Wales lies with Her Majesty's Coroner under section 5(1)(a) of the Coroners and Justice Act 2009 (Coroners 2009) which came into force on 25 July 2013. The work of the forensic odontologist in human identification is thus to assist the coroner in their statutory duty.

Dental identification is classed as one of the primary methods of identification and where the dental evidence is of sufficient quality and quantity, it can stand alone. It is always good practice, however, to have additional primary and/or supporting evidence for every identification. It is stated in the Interpol DVI Guide 2009 (DVI Guide 2009) that 'The primary and most reliable means of identification are fingerprint analysis, comparative dental analysis and DNA analysis.'

19.1 The human dentition

Teeth are composed of the hardest tissues in the human body. They can survive a large number of insults, including the passage of time, emersion in water, and, to a certain degree, thermal exposure. It is this resilience that allows them to outlast any other body tissue. The properties and variability of human dentitions lend themselves to being used for identification purposes. This is enhanced by

Essential Forensic Medicine, First Edition. Edited by Peter Vanezis.
© 2020 John Wiley & Sons Ltd. Published 2020 by John Wiley & Sons Ltd.

the intervention of dentistry, which leaves permanent changes to the dentition. These intentional changes are often recorded in dental records and can thus provide useful ante-mortem data.

The human dentition is composed of two complete sets of teeth (Diphyodontism). These are the deciduous or milk teeth and the permanent or adult teeth. They have chronologically overlapping developmental periods, which begin at about week 6 intra-uterine, up to 14 years and beyond. At birth, all 20 of the deciduous dentition have started to calcify within the upper and lower jaws, along with a small part of each of the four adult first molars. The deciduous teeth will tend to emerge into the mouth cavity during the period between the ages of 6 months and 2½ years. The adult teeth will emerge from about 6 years of age, gradually replacing the deciduous teeth up to about the age of 12 years. The last adult teeth which may emerge are the four wisdom teeth (third molars). These teeth are very variable but are commonly stated to emerge at about the age of 18–21 years. There are potentially 32 adult teeth in the normal human dentition.

19.2   The dental identification process

The odontologist is unusual within human identification in potentially being involved at each stage of the process, from initial body recovery to the ante-mortem (AM) and post-mortem (PM) phases, through reconciliation to the final identification. Each of these stages occurs whether there is a single body situation or a multiple fatality mass disaster.

Although not a frequent requirement, there are occasions when an odontologist may be called to the scene where human remains are found in order to assist in the recovery of dental evidence. Examples of when this may be required include recovery of teeth where animals have dispersed skeletal remains or in the event of severe fire damage where burnt jaws and teeth may be extremely fragile and if handled incorrectly important evidence may potentially be lost. It is good practice to either place the head area in a plastic bag or wrap it in bubble-wrap to preserve evidence with severely burned remains.

19.2.1   Dental records

Generally, human identification involves the comparison of AM and PM information. A written record of treatment provided by the dentist is most frequently recorded in the UK on a record card or envelope known as an FP25a (for NHS patients) or a PP25A (for private patients). Increasingly, dental records are being recorded using various computer programs. There is no central record of treatments carried out under private contract, the records being retained within the individual dental practice. However, dental treatment carried out under the NHS is recorded both at the individual dental practice and centrally by the Business Services Authority (BSA) (Business Services Authority 2014). The BSA retain this information for a limited time. On the record card, there is a graphical representation, called an odontogram, of each of the 32 adult teeth, which allows any work carried out to be recorded. It includes which tooth and which tooth surfaces have been treated. Ideally, a full charting should be made of all the dental work that is present in the mouth when a patient is seen for the first time. It is a legal requirement to make such a record in some countries but currently not in the UK, although obviously it is good clinical practice. There are many different styles of odontogram throughout the world, but all are designed to record the same information.

In England and Wales, dental treatment can be provided either under the National Health Service (NHS) (National Health Service 1977, 2005(a, b), 2006(a, b)) or increasingly under private contract. Dental records of patients treated under private contract are the property of the dental practice, whilst those under NHS regulations are covered by the Public Records Acts of 1958 and 1967 (Public Records Acts 1958, 1967) and by Department of Health guidelines. NHS records are owned by the Secretary of State. These records must be kept for a minimum of 11 years or up to the 25th birthday if this is longer. Permanent retention of dental records is to be commended.

Both private and NHS records are confidential. This raises an issue when they are required for identification purposes, since normally the consent of the individual to whom they relate is required in order to release them to a third party. Clearly, if the person is dead, then they cannot consent but the records are needed to confirm that they are dead; it is thus a Catch 22 situation. The various Dental Defence Unions in the UK will advise dental practitioners that, provided there is reasonable evidence that the individual is deceased and the request comes from an official source, such as the police or the coroner, then the release of the records is justified for the greater good. It is prudent for the practitioner to retain a copy of any records released, since the odontologist will want the originals.

Items that may be contained in the dental records include clinical photographs, stone models (casts), and old dental appliances such as dentures or bleaching trays/night guards, which can be compared directly with the remains. Personal photographs showing the individual smiling may also prove helpful for comparison of the anterior teeth and photographic superimposition can be employed. There may be letters of referral to a number of different specialists within the field of dentistry, which may lead to the acquisition of further AM information and radiographs.

19.2.2 Radiographs

It is very common for radiographs of the teeth to be taken during the course of dental treatment and these can be extremely valuable for dental identification, especially where the written record is suboptimal. Other forms of radiograph of the head and neck from medical or hospital records may also show dental structures and can give valuable information. These may have been taken for reasons not related to teeth, such as head trauma. The advantage of AM radiographs for identification purposes is that each one contains a great deal of information, ranging from the morphology of anatomical structures to the presence and extent of any dental restorations. The combined weight of these features, many of which would be unique to the individual, means that it *may* be possible to confirm identity from a single radiograph, provided there are sufficient individual characteristics to compare with an equivalent PM image. This may be particularly valuable where records written in a foreign language are received and translation facilities are not readily available. Due to advances in preventative dentistry and improved oral health, there is a reduction in the number of fillings etc. being placed. This is likely to make the importance of AM radiographs even greater in the future.

The most commonly taken dental radiographs in clinical practice are called bitewings, which show the crowns of the upper and lower posterior teeth.

They tend to be taken as a regular check for decay and are usually found in pairs (right and left sides). A small selection of adjacent teeth can be visualised with a peri-apical radiograph, which also shows the root ends or apices. The third most common type of dental film is the panoramic radiograph or orthopantomograph (frequently abbreviated to OPG or OPT). This uses rotational tomography and shows all the teeth along with the upper and lower jaws (Figure 19.1).

Alternative dental views are available but are less frequently encountered in dental records. Cone beam computed tomography (CBCT) is also increasingly used in certain specialist centres for dental assessment of dental implants and surgical patients. Standard dental images were historically

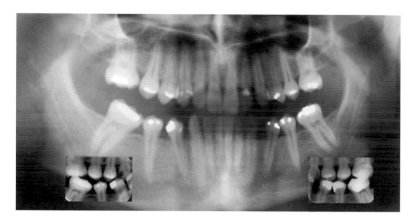

Figure 19.1   Orthopantomogram and bitewing radiographs taken 10 years apart.

always recorded on 'wet film'. This is increasingly being replaced by the use of digital radiography involving a sensor instead of film. The digital file that results is easy to manipulate and to transfer by electronic means. Where a non-digital radiograph needs to be reproduced and transmitted electronically, it can simply be photographed with a light source behind it by a digital camera. In this case, it is essential that it be photographed from the correct side. The original wet film has a raised dot, which would always face towards the viewer. The odontologist will be mindful of the possibility of image reversal when making any comparisons utilising images of radiographs.

19.3   Post-mortem procedure

The PM phase will be carried out in a mortuary. This may be an established working mortuary if the numbers involved are small or a temporary mortuary facility where the numbers are greater. The decisive factor for the established mortuary is whether it is able to deal with the increased numbers or not, whilst still being able to function with its continuing day-to-day workload.

19.3.1   Access to the mouth

During the dental PM examination the body must always be treated with dignity and respect. Gaining access in order to view the teeth should always be done in the least invasive way, consistent with the task in hand. There are a number of factors that may make access to the teeth difficult in the early stages. Rigor mortis, once established, normally affects the muscles in the body, including those keeping the jaws closed, during the first 36–48 hours PM. However, the odontologist is seldom called in during this early period and thus rigor has often worn off by the time the dental examination is needed. This means that a simple non-destructive technique can be utilised to open the mouth of the deceased in most cases. As decomposition progresses, this access becomes easier as the tissues soften. The gentle use of a mechanical mouth gag can assist in the opening of the jaws, which even though no longer in rigor mortis can still prove difficult.

One technique which can be employed and which results in no further disfigurement and at the same time gives excellent visualisation of the jaws and teeth is to continue the 'Y' incision from the standard PM examination. In this way, a full facial flap can carefully be raised, then repositioned and sutured. The face of the victim is unaffected by this approach.

Access to the teeth may be more problematic in the case of burning, where the peri-oral tissues are affected by heat and become stiff. This is one of the few occasions where there may be no alternative to an invasive approach and relieving incisions may be required at the corners of the mouth. This can sometimes be avoided by the use of high quality Computed Tomography (CT) images. In all cases, appropriate internal incision of the muscles of mastication will make access more straightforward. A further problem may be encountered in bodies that have been deep-frozen for storage and it is essential that sufficient time be allowed (1–2 days) for the body to thaw before being examined by the odontologist. Bodies that have been repatriated from abroad can also be challenging, since the embalming process required for international transportation results in considerable stiffening of the tissues, with associated access difficulties.

The purpose of the dental PM is to allow the accurate recording of the victim's dentition. This will include the teeth themselves along with any dental restorations such as fillings, crowns, bridges, and dentures. There may be characteristics of the teeth that are of racial origin, such as the prevalence of shovel-shaped incisor teeth in Mongoloids and the greater presence of the cusp of Carabelli in the upper molars of Caucasoids. Common things are common and rare things are rare, so any unusual feature may hold great significance in relation to dental identification. The features may be part of the teeth themselves or constitute part of the dental work carried out on them. Sometimes the style of dental work may suggest a country where this was carried out, which is not of course necessarily the same as the country of origin of the victim. Analysis of the composition of the materials used to restore the teeth may also indicate the country of origin of that work. This type of investigation, however, would be employed in very few cases.

Dental radiographs can be taken PM to compare to those in the AM records. If there is a putative identity, such as may occur in a house or car fire, then it is very useful to have the AM dental records available at the time of PM examination. This allows any specific radiographic views to be duplicated in both type and angulation for the best comparison. Sometimes this is not possible and often in large-scale disasters the AM records will be sent to the reconciliation centre, which may be quite remote from the temporary mortuary. In such a case, it may be decided that all bodies will have a full set of dental radiographs taken so that there is a good chance of being able to compare to any images from an AM record, regardless of which teeth they show. Hand-held digital X-ray machines such as the Nomad™ (KaVo Dental) are widely used for this process. They have become more popular due to the universal lack of dental X-ray facilities in mortuaries.

19.4 Dental ageing

Another aspect of identification in which odontology may assist is with the ageing of the deceased. Chronological age is a fundamental part of a person's identity. Dental age, which is a reflection of dental maturity, can be used to give an estimate of chronological age within an age range. In common with most forms of forensic age estimation, the results are more accurate with younger age groups and generally become less accurate for older individuals. The most useful period is whilst the teeth are actively forming. This covers the period from foetal life potentially up to the age of about 22 years (if the third molars are present). Where a disaster involves a large number of children, the ability to place them into groups of ages may be very important. An identification by age exclusion may also be possible within a closed population of victims.

Where no dental records are available, there may be other information that can be derived from the teeth. Unlike bones, once teeth have finished forming there is no turnover of minerals within the bulk of the tooth. Each tooth therefore contains a history of the minerals present when it was formed. Analysis of the stable isotopes within the tooth may thus give a clue as to the geographic location of the individual at that point in time, i.e. childhood. This could be significant, for example in a multinationality incident.

19.5 Dental reconciliation

The reconciliation phase involves the comparison of the collected PM data with the AM data of the known individual/s. This can be done by hand or with the assistance of a number of different computer software systems. DVI System International by the Danish company Plassdata (Plassdata Software 2013) is probably the most widely used identification program and was used extensively in the South-East Asian tsunami of 26 December 2004, where it evolved considerably in the field. In the United States a computer program called WinID3 (WIN ID 2014) is more widely used and was developed by Dr Jim McGivney. It is derived from the earlier Computer Assisted Post-Mortem Identification (CAPMI) system, which had itself been developed at the US Army Institute of Dental Research in the 1980s.

Both the PlassData and WinID3 programs allow any number of specific characteristics to be compared to any number of records, resulting in a list of possible matches. Although these are powerful tools, the final comparison must always be done by an odontologist. It must be remembered that the AM record (and to a lesser degree the PM record) may contain errors. These can exist for a number of reasons and the trained odontologist should be familiar with these when they occur.

19.6 Identification outcomes

The Interpol DVI guide gives the following conclusions that are available to the odontologist following comparison of PM and AM dental records:

Identification (there is absolute certainty the PM and AM records are from the same person)

Identification probable (specific characteristics correspond between PM and AM but either PM or AM data or both are minimal)

Identification possible (there is nothing that excludes the identity but either PM or AM data or both are minimal)

Identity excluded (PM and AM records are from different persons)

19.6.1 No Comparison can be Made

There is no set minimum number of concordant dental features that is required for a positive dental identification. The conclusions reached are thus subjective and must be made by the trained odontologist, taking account of the amount and quality of the features present.

Historically, dental identification has been used successfully in many single and multiple fatality incidents. It has frequently been possible to confirm an identity more quickly by dental means than by using other primary methods, which may involve a collection or processing time lag. This reduces delays for relatives and friends of the victim. The degree to which dental identification can be utilised will vary between cases and there may be situations where dentistry cannot be used.

Where the quantity and quality of AM and PM dental data is sufficient, dental identification is a very useful, rapid, and reliable method of human identification.

19.7 Bite Marks

There are some similarities between biological identification by dental means and the potential identification of an individual from a bite mark. The analysis and interpretation of a bite mark injury can be one of the most challenging for the forensic odontologist. It has two main aspects. First, the confirmation that the injury is in fact a bite mark, either human or animal, and, second, an opinion as to whether or not a specific set of teeth could have made such an injury.

There will be a range of degree of certainty for both these elements.

In relation to the question 'Is it a bite mark?' possible conclusions are:

Exclusion: the injury is not a bite mark.

Possible: an injury showing a pattern that may or may not have been caused by teeth; the injury may have been caused by other factors but biting cannot be ruled out.

Probable: the pattern of the injury strongly suggests or supports an origin from teeth but could conceivably be caused by something else.

Definite: there is no reasonable doubt that teeth created the injury.

In relation to the question 'Is this individual the biter?' it is my opinion that a cautious approach should be taken. If there are substantial differences between the features of the dentition and the pattern of injury, then it may be possible to exclude an individual. Where there are close similarities and no major discrepancies, it may not be possible to exclude that individual. Equally, there may be insufficient evidence on which to base a justifiable conclusion.

In much the same way as an incorrect human identification can have far-reaching consequences, so can errors with bite mark interpretation. Such interpretation should only be carried out by experienced odontologists or those with a suitably experienced mentor. Bite mark analysis can feature in both civil and criminal cases. It involves the comparison of the individual pattern and characteristics of the dentition in question (in the form of stone dental models created from impressions of the teeth) with the pattern and characteristics found in the bite mark injury, or an object displaying teeth marks. The latter may occur in foodstuffs, for instance.

In criminal cases in the UK, impressions of the teeth are covered under the Police and Criminal Evidence Act (PACE) and are classed as intimate samples. They can only be taken with the consent of the suspect.

Bite mark injuries can have very variable presentations, from the faintest of bruises to the complete avulsion of tissue. Scaled images of the injury are used which are reproduced either life size or some known multiple of this. Where a direct comparison technique is used, an overlay or exemplar of the biting edges of the teeth is then placed over the injury (Figure 19.2). This is usually performed using PhotoShop®.

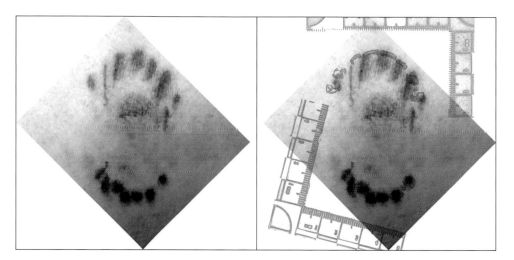

Figure 19.2   Bite marks: the figure on the right shows a scale and is overlayed with the suspect's teeth overlays.

An alternative method is a pattern-matching exercise whereby the characteristics seen in the injury are compared and contrasted to the characteristics of the dentition under investigation. This technique may be particularly useful where there is obvious distortion in the injury. Examples of distortion can be as a result of posture, movement or photographic angulation. The detailed assessment and interpretation of bite marks are beyond the scope of this chapter and the reader is directed to the standard texts of forensic odontology.

Bite mark interpretation has its limitations. However, when carried out by suitably trained and experienced individuals who are aware and mindful of these limitations, it can potentially provide vital and useful evidence.

References

Business Services Authority, Contact NHS Dental Services https://www.nhsbsa.nhs.uk/contact-nhs-dental-services Accessed 09.06.19.

Coroners and Justice Act 2009 (2009 Ch. 25) Available online at: www.legislation.gov.uk/ukpga/2009/25 Accessed 06.10.13.

DVI Guide: INTERPOL 2018 Available online at: https://www.interpol.int/How-we-work/Forensics/Disaster-Victim-Identification-DVI Accessed 09.06.19.

National Health Service (General Dental Services Contracts) Regulations 2005a[3]

National Health Service (Personal Dental Services Agreements) Regulations 2005a[4]

National Health Service (General Dental Services Contracts) (Wales) Regulations 2006a

National Health Service (Personal Dental Services Agreements) (Wales) Regulations 2006b

National Health Service Act 1977[1].

PlassData Software A/SAhlgade 17A, st.th.4300 HolbaekDenmark 2019.

KAVO DENTAL11727 Fruehauf Drive, Charlotte, NC 28273

Public Records Acts of 1958 and 1967 www.legislation.gov.uk/ukpga/Eliz2/6-7/51/enacted Accessed 26.01.14.

WIN ID http://winid.com Accessed 26.01.2014.

Further reading

Adams, C., Carabott, R., and Evans, S. (2014). *Forensic Odontology: An Essential Guide*, 1e. Wiley-Blackwell.

Black, S., Aggrawal, A., and Payne-James, J. (2011). *Age Estimation in the Living: The Practitioner's Guide*. Wiley.

Blenkin, M. (2009). *Forensic Odontology and Age Estimation: An Introduction to Concepts and Methods*. Germany: VDM Verlag, Saarbrücken.

Michael Bowers, C. (2010). *Forensic Dental Evidence: An Investigator's Handbook*, 2e. Academic Press.

Senn, D.R. and Stimson, P.G. (2010). *Forensic Dentistry*, 2e. Boca Raton: CRC Press.

Thompson, T. and Black, S. (2006). *Forensic Human Identification: An Introduction*, 1e. Boca Raton: CRC Press.

20
Crime and Mental Health/Forensic Psychiatry

Vivek Khosla and Orlando Trujillo-Bueno

Oxford Clinic Medium Secure Unit|Littlemore Mental Health Centre, Oxford Health NHS Foundation Trust, Oxford, UK

Oxford Health NHS Foundation Trust, Oxford, UK

20.1   Introduction

There were no institutional facilities available to treat and rehabilitate offenders with mental illness prior to the nineteenth century. Mentally disordered offenders were admitted to lunatic asylums, particularly individuals who had low social status, while wealthy individuals were able to afford private physicians to look after them. One notable historical example was the case of King George III, who suffered from symptoms relating to mental illness and was treated by his private physicians. However, it is said that even the King could not be offered other treatment beyond restraint. In contrast, Mr James Hadfield, who was found to be criminally insane when he tried to kill King George III, was transferred to Bethlem Hospital from prison at the beginning of the nineteenth century. Britain had at this time begun to develop specific facilities to deal with the criminally insane (Scull 1979). During the nineteenth century Broadmoor Hospital was opened and became the criminal lunatic asylum of the time. In Ireland, Dundrum Central Criminal Asylum was opened in 1850, subsequently, Rampton Criminal Lunatic Asylum (Nottinghamshire) was opened in 1912, and the amalgamation of two older hospitals, Park Lane and Moss Side, became the Ashworth Hospital in 1989. Currently Broadmoor, Rampton, and Ashworth are the three high-security hospitals in England whilst the State Hospital, Carstairs serves Scotland and Northern Ireland.

The Butler report (Kennedy 2002) gives a historical perspective of the evolution of secure psychiatric services in the UK, while Bluglass and Bowden (1990) provide an international perspective.

(For the sake of simplicity we describe legislation in England and Wales. Note that Northern Ireland (legislation.gov.uk 1986) and Scotland (legislation.gov.uk 2003) have separate legislation.

A shift in the care of the mentally ill took place in the early 1990s. Adverse media publicity of the rare events of homicide by the mentally ill, such as the murder of Jonathan Zito by Christopher Clunis in 1992 (Waterhouse and Williams 1993), and criticism of psychiatric services by subsequent independent inquiries led to concerns regarding the care of the mentally ill in the community and public safety. These concerns initiated changes in the existing services and legislation.

The outcomes of mental health assessments on individuals who suffer from mental disorders and have committed a criminal offence involve combined input from both mental health and criminal justice professionals. Both disciplines interface professionally, which in practice brings mutual benefit and a variety of challenges. One of the challenges facing professionals is to produce fair outcomes reflecting the interests of the offender and the public, whilst complying with the relevant aspects of mental health legislation and the criminal justice system.

Some mentally disordered offenders require diversion to and detention at a facility where appropriate treatment and rehabilitation are available (Reed 1992). The diversion scheme is a government policy that was introduced to divert mentally disordered offenders away from the criminal justice system to the health system. The development of this policy and court diversion schemes provides a service to offenders suffering from a mental disorder who are deemed to require mainstream health and social services input to address their needs. This enables treatment and rehabilitation of criminal offenders and improves the outcome for both the individual and overall public health (Senior et al. 2011). Diversion of mentally disordered offenders can occur at several points of the offender pathway in the criminal justice system, but culminates in a setting where the level of security is determined by a professional assessment of risk, the nature of the mental disorder, and the legal considerations.

20.2 Mental disorder

Mental disorder and mental illness are terms that are often used interchangeably. Basically, they refer to changes to an individual's mood, thoughts, feelings, and behaviour that cause distress and disruption to others and themselves. The use of the term mental illness has caused philosophical and socio-anthropological debate in the past as this term is linked to the medical model, and the connotations and views it invokes from a socio-cultural point of view (Skultans and Cox 2000). For example, in some cultures, odd human behaviour is thought to be due to the individual being possessed by supernatural forces rather than the acceptance that there is a link between odd behaviour and a brain disorder.

There are currently two widely established international systems for classifying mental disorders. The World Health Organisation (WHO) has established the International Classification of Diseases (currently, ICD-10). The American Psychiatry Association has established the Diagnostic and Statistical Manual of Mental Disorders (currently, DSM-V). The ICD-10 is widely used in Europe while the DSM is the official diagnostic system in the USA. Both systems have different ways to classify mental disorders, but broadly speaking they are comparable. Each system classifies mental disorders in a list of categories or groups and there are subcategories within each group. In general, both systems recognise that mental disorder is not an exact term, but nevertheless is widely used to cover significant sets of symptoms or behaviours that are directly linked to the individual's mental health distress, which in turns interferes with the individual's ability to relate to others and maintain day-today functioning (WHO 1992). The DSM system also notes that there are no clear boundaries or divisions within each category, in particular when it comes to applying the classification system in practice. The DSM-V published in 2013 discarded the multiaxial classification, which was still in place up to the DSM-IV version (previously, the DSM-IV organised each psychiatric diagnosis into five dimensions [axes] relating to different aspects of disorder or disability). Both classification systems have their limitations but are enormously helpful in communication between professionals and with patients, and research and service developments.

According to the international classification systems, all major diagnostic categories of mental disorders can be broadly classified as:

– *organic disorders*, such as dementia and delirium
– *substance misuse disorders*, such as alcohol and drug dependence
– *mood disorders*, such as bipolar affective disorder and depression
– *psychotic disorders*, such as schizophrenia
– *neurotic and anxiety disorders*, such as generalised anxiety disorder (GAD), obsessive compulsive disorder (OCD), post-traumatic stress disorder (PTSD), and phobias
– *personality disorders*
   disorders related to learning disability
– *disorders of a sexual nature.*

20.3 Mental Disorder and Criminal Behaviour

Violence in any form constitutes a global public health issue and as such it does concern forensic psychiatry. However, this devastating global issue, which shatters life and communities, also involves very complicated socio-economical systems in the broader sense. Violence and its prevention must be addressed globally and it is everyone's responsibility to address this regardless of socio-political, economic, religious or cultural differences. According to a report published in 2014 by WHO more than 1.3 million people die from violence each year. Furthermore, this report added that violence is the fourth cause of death globally for people between 15 and 44 years of age (WHO 2014). In addition to direct physical violence, threats to kill are also recognised as a type of non-contact violent behaviour. This report refers in detail to the different type of violence, including child abuse and neglect, youth violence, domestic violence, self-direct violence, elder abuse, and collective violence. It is very important to distinguish what is clinically pathological in terms of the individual's mental state from what is criminal behaviour in itself. Criminal and odd social behaviour cannot be assumed to be the manifestations of mental disorders, but equally criminal offences such as violence, fire setting, sexual offences, and compulsive stealing could be the manifestations of mental disorder. Overall, individuals could respond to life events based on their own perceptions and interpretations. These psychological processes are influenced by the individual's thoughts, previous experiences, personality and social factors. There are multifactorial variables involved in criminal behaviours such as gender differences in criminality and the use and abuse of alcohol and other recreational substances. It is important to understand the nature of violent behaviour, and what triggers and maintains violence. These would inform risk assessment of violent behaviour, which in turn would also inform the therapeutic focus on addressing areas of risk and the implementation of preventive measures (Gunn and Tayler 2014).

20.4   Organic disorders

Dementia, delirium, brain injury, epilepsy, and sleeping disorders should be excluded when a link between organic brain disorders and criminal offending is suspected.

20.4.1   Dementia

Dementia is a devastating organic brain disorder, usually chronic and progressive, which presents with a group of symptoms including cognitive impairment and memory loss, confusion, mood changes, and difficulty with day-to-day tasks. There are various type of dementia including Alzheimer's disease, vascular dementia, dementia with Lewy bodies, frontotemporal dementia, Creutzfeldt–Jacob dementia, Korsakoff's syndrome, and other rare causes of dementia and cognitive impairment, including HIV-related cognitive impairment (Gelder et al. 2012). Although dementia is not usually associated with violence, individuals suffering from dementia can be verbally or physically aggressive. Associations of aggressive behaviour in dementia include cognitive impairment, change in personality as a result of the brain disease, physical illness, and comorbid depression or psychosis (Hall and O'Connor 2004).

20.4.2   Delirium

Delirium is an acute state of mental confusion characterised by 'disturbances of consciousness and attention, perception, thinking, memory, psychomotor behaviour' (ICD-10). It can be caused by various organic disorders affecting the brain, such as vascular disorders, for example stroke, liver or kidney illness, exposure to high temperatures, dehydration, terminal illness, brain injury, and infections. Recent exposure to surgery and some medication side effects could also be causative factors (David et al. 2012). Delirium can be associated with agitation and aggression in some cases and it is important to prevent and treat delirium promptly (Amos and Robertson 2010).

20.4.3   Brain damage and personality change

Brain damage is associated with changes in personality. These changes could include impulsive, violent, and socially inappropriate behaviours (David et al. 2012). Studies have shown that damage to the prefrontal cortex (part of the frontal lobe) is associated with violence. The prefrontal cortex takes signals from other parts of the brain, particularly from brain areas that process emotions (amygdala) and decide what actions or behaviours to take. Organic brain damage causes disruption of the chemistry of the brain and this has been linked to aggression and violence (David et al. 2012).

20.4.4   Epilepsy and Sleeping Disorders

Epilepsy is often 'idiopathic' that is, the cause is unknown. In some cases it can occur due to brain injury, for instance at birth, head injury, infections or brain tumours. It is rarely directly associated with violence, but violent behaviour can occur in the period just before a seizure (called the prodrome) or the period after a seizure (called the post ictal phase) (Gunn and Tayler 2014). When the cause of epilepsy is a brain injury, that in itself may increase the risk of violent behaviour.

Sleep disorders and violence is not well understood, but there are psychiatric disorders associated with sleep disorders and violence (Siclari et al. 2010). Clinical criteria to establish a link between an underlying sleep disorder and violence has been proposed (Mahowald et al. 1990), and this requires an extensive forensic psychiatry assessment to be carried out.

20.5 Substance Misuse Disorders

Drug use can increase the risk of being a victim and/or perpetrator of violence (WHO 2009). Studies have shown that substance abuse on its own appears to be a major determinant of violence whether or not it concomitantly takes place within the context of mental illness (Stuart 2003). The risk of violence is higher when an individual suffering from a major mental disorder, especially schizophrenia, uses and becomes dependent on substance misuse, particularly alcohol (Soyka 2000). Epidemiologic surveys have also found that individuals with substance misuse disorders without mental disorders were more than twice as likely to exhibit violent behaviours when compared to individuals suffering from schizophrenia (Swanson et al. 1990). Combined diagnosis of substance misuse with psychotic and personality disorder is common in forensic mental health settings. Therefore, substance misuse management is central to the rehabilitation programme provided.

20.6 Mood Disorders

Disturbed mood state is the main feature involved. Affected individuals could be suffering from extreme high moods such as mania, low moods such as depression, or bipolar disorder, which is a mental disorder in which an individual experiences periods of elated mood and depression. Although mood disorders have received less attention than schizophrenia, a review published in 2009 suggested that there is an association between mood disorders and violence (Oakley et al. 2009). This association is stronger for mania, symptoms of which include elated mood, grandiosity, over-activity, and irritability. Mania is a risk factor for aggression but available research indicates that it is usually associated with minor forms of aggression rather than serious homicidal violence (Nielssen et al 2012). A recent study suggests that the risk of committing violent crime is increased in individuals suffering from depression (Fazel et al. 2015). Specific links between violence and mood disorders include depression and homicide–suicide, such as when a person kills someone and then commits suicide, and cases of depression and infanticide seen in post-natal depression (Oakley et al. 2009).

20.7 Psychotic Disorders

Psychosis is a severe mental disorder that causes individuals to lose touch with reality as affected individuals experience abnormal perception of the world and abnormal thinking. Psychotic disorders or psychotic states such as schizophrenia broadly speaking involve abnormal perceptions of the external world, such as when an individual hears voices that others around cannot hear (auditory hallucinations). For example, the individual could be hearing voices providing him/her with instructions to harm themselves or others. The individual could see things others around cannot see (visual hallucinations), which can be a terrifying experience. The individual could also have an altered interpretation of the relationship with others, such as when an individual has a fixed believe that others are intending to cause harm (paranoid delusions), believing that broadcast news contains a secret code message, believing that the individual is controlled by external forces, or having in mind a relationship that does not exist (Gelder et al. 2012). It is not too difficult therefore to imagine that the risk of violence could increase when an individual is experiencing these symptoms. However, the relationship between the individual's psychotic mental state and criminal behaviour is complex and despite the fact there is a direct association between psychosis and violence (Gulati et al. 2009 in Fazel et al. 2009), studies have shown that the absolute risk of violence as a result of mental illness is small, in other words, an individual with a mental disorder is more likely to become the victim (Walsh et al. 2003) of violence rather than the perpetrator. Studies also suggest that violence in schizophrenia and other psychoses is likely to be mediated largely by substance abuse (Fazel et al. 2009).

20.8 Neurotic and Anxiety Disorders

There is no strong evidence linking mental disorders such as GAD and OCD with offending behaviour. However, neurotic disorders could be a likely group of disorders present in those who offend (Gunn and Tayler 2014). De Coster and Heimer (2001) suggests that the link between minor mental disorders such as mild depression and crime can be influenced by previous exposure to stressful life events and socioeconomic status during the critical period of adolescence.

PTSD is an anxiety disorder triggered by previous exposure to distressing or life-threatening events, which could be linked to increase risk of offending behaviour. Typical symptoms of this condition are flashbacks and emotional blunting. Other symptoms include hyperarousal and increased vigilance (WHO 1992). A hyperarousal mental state (heightened emotional states) could trigger impulsive and violent behaviour. Hypervigilance could make the individual over-reactive and focused on identifying threatening or dangerous situations in an amplified manner. Equally, experiencing flashbacks of very distressing memories could make the individual react in an impulsive and angry way. Another contributing factor to violence in PTSD is an underlying high risk of substance abuse (Carr 2005).

20.9 Personality Disorders

The ICD-10 defines personality disorder as a severe disturbance in character and behavioural tendencies causing considerable personal and social disruption that are not the direct result of disease, organic brain damage, or another psychiatric disorder (WHO 1992). These maladaptive behavioural patterns are usually associated with exposure to traumatic early life experiences including physical, sexual, and emotional abuse. According to ICD 10, these disorders 'represent either extreme or significant deviations from the way the average individual in a given culture perceives, thinks, feels, and particularly relates to others'. Personality disorders tend to be part of the individual's personality and often become apparent in childhood and adolescence and continue into adulthood. There are types of personality disorders that are more associated with impulsive and violent behaviours, such as emotionally unstable borderline personality disorder, antisocial personality disorder, paranoid and narcissistic personality disorders. However, it is suggested that rather than keeping the focus on the diagnosis of specific types of personality disorders, it is of greater interest to assess on an individual basis what personality traits, such as impulsiveness, irritability, intolerance to frustration, and paranoid and narcissistic attributes, could potentially be contributing to a high risk of offending behaviours (Sirotich 2008).

20.10   Learning Disabilities

According to the ICD-10 definition, learning disability is 'a condition of arrested or incomplete development of the mind, which is especially characterized by impairment of skills manifested during the developmental period, skills which contribute to the overall level of intelligence'. The ICD-10 provides four levels of cognitive disability according to IQ score:[1] mild (IQ 50–69), moderate (IQ 35–49), severe (IQ 20–34), and profound mental retardation (IQ under 20). The relationship between intellectual disability and criminal offending is complex. There are several issues associated with the diagnosis of learning disability, including issues regarding the individual's disadvantages and vulnerabilities, the impact on the individual's life when a forensic label is acquired, public protection and social connotations, and the complex distinction between challenging behaviours related to learning disabilities and offending. Broadly speaking people with learning disability are more likely to become the victims of violence, and therefore are more likely to develop other mental health problems, which in turn increases the risks of violence, rather than there being a direct link between learning disability and offending behaviour (Hughes et al. 2012).

20.11   Sexual Offending and Mental Disorders

Broadly speaking, sexual offending and mental disorders are usually related to various mental health conditions, including paraphilias, mood and anxiety disorders, learning disability, and personality disorders. According to previous publications, this group of offenders is more likely to receive the diagnosis of severe psychotic disorder, such as schizophrenia, and mood disorder, such as bipolar disorder, when compared to the general population (Fazel et al. 2008). In terms of disorder of sexual preferences or paraphilias, these include fetishistic transvestism, voyeurism, exhibitionism, paedophilia, sadomasochism, and other paraphilias including necrophilia, zoophilia, coprophilia, urophilia, frotteurism, etc. (see ICD-10 classification and Gunn and Tayler 2014).

20.11.1   Morbid Jealousy

There is a distinctive boundary between emotionally regulated jealousy in well-adjusted individuals and morbid or pathological jealousy associated with violence. Morbid jealousy could be associated with a psychotic disorder, and such cases could potentially be treated and managed more successfully than cases involving morbid jealousy associated with personality disorders or alcohol-substance misuse dependence (Gunn and Tayler 2014).

20.11.2   Erotomania

Perceived unrequited love and rejections certainly can trigger dangerous behaviours and violence driven by frustration and anger. Victims and family members can be put under a great deal of distress due to letters, messages, phone calls, etc.

---

[1] Intelligence quotient, or IQ, is a score derived from standardised tests. The most commonly used IQ test is the Wechsler Adult Intelligence Scale (WAIS).

20.12   Mental Health Legislation

Mental health legislation governs decisions about the compulsory detention and treatment of individuals who are affected with poor mental health. It applies in the circumstances in which a person with a mental disorder can be detained for treatment for that disorder without his or her consent (Mental Health Act 1983 (amended 2007)).

In practice, the specialty of psychiatry is different from other medical specialties when it comes to dealing with issues related to the individual's autonomy. In England and Wales the Mental Health Act 1983 (updated by the 2007 Act) and the Mental Capacity Act 2005, including the Deprivation of Liberty Safeguards, are the two elements of legislation that guide the way individuals suffering from mental health conditions receive appropriate health care and treatment (Fennell 2007). The Mental Capacity Act provides a legal framework to make decisions and act on behalf of those adults who lack mental capacity (for further information, see the Mental Capacity Act 2005). The Mental Health Act 1983 (amended 2007) provides mental health legislation that gives authority to mental health practitioners to force hospital admission or treatment for patients suffering from a mental disorder, without the individual's consent. The Mental Health Act 1983 (amended 2007) has a broad definition of mental disorder. According to this Act, mental disorder is 'any disorder or disability of the mind', but dependence on substance misuse is not considered a mental disorder, and learning disability is also excluded except for those individuals suffering from learning disability that is associated with 'abnormally aggressive or seriously irresponsible conduct'.

For detention, an individual has to be suffering from a mental disorder. The mental disorder has to be of a nature and/or degree to warrant detention in the best interest of the individual's health because without hospital admission and treatment the individual's health will deteriorate further. Additionally, detention provides safety for the individual and manages the risks associated with self-harming and/or committing suicide, along with providing protection from the risk of violence to others. Nature and degree are legal concepts. Degree refers to the severity of the disorder at the time of the assessment and nature refers to the previous course of the patient's disorder, for example a history of previous response to treatment, relapses of the disorder, and associated risks. Therefore, the Mental Health Act 1983 (amended 2007) legitimises detentions in hospitals whilst ensuring that the correct legal and ethical procedures are followed, and are according to the European Convention on Human Rights to safeguard against arbitrary deprivation of liberty and arbitrary interventions. The overall aim of mental health legislation is to ensure a balance between the individual's human rights to liberty and physical integrity, and society's privilege to ensure that an individual without ability to consent or refusal to consent can be lawfully assessed and treated fairly.

The Mental Health Act 1983 (amended 2007) takes care of people suffering from a mental disorder and protect them from being wrongly detained. Compulsory hospital admissions under the Mental Health Act 1983 (amended 2007) consist of Parts 2 and 3 of the Mental Health Act (see Table 20.1). Mental health assessments and decisions regarding the detention of an individual under the mental health law requires the input from various professionals who have well-defined legal roles. This include two medical practitioners (one doctor must be section 12 approved, a doctor who has special training in mental disorders), and an approved mental health practitioner.

Detained patients can appeal against hospital detention under the Mental Health Act 1983 (amended 2007). Patients detained under sections 2, 3, or 37 can apply to the Mental Health Act Managers (Manager's Hearing) or the Mental Health Tribunal (First-tier Tribunal) to be discharged from hospital detention or to review the detention status. These two panels have some similarities and differences. The Manager's Hearing involves a panel of three lay members of the community who act on behalf of the managers of the hospital where the patient is detained. The First-tier Tribunal is completely independent of the hospital and the three members of the panel are the chair, who is legally qualified, such as a judge, an independent doctor (psychiatrist), and a specialist lay member. For further information on First-tier Tribunals see https://www.gov.uk/mental-health-tribunal.

The field of forensic psychiatry in England and Wales includes assessment of an individual's mental health and the relationship between the individual's mental disorder and the index offence, and the treatment and rehabilitation of such individuals. Forensic psychiatry is also involved in the decision-making process needed to select the optimum placement for individuals to be treated and rehabilitated according to the level of security required. Individuals may be treated by local community forensic psychiatry services or admitted to low-, medium-, or high-security hospitals. Some treatment, particularly in the short term, may occur within prison. Individuals with mental disorders who are in prison can be transferred to a forensic mental health setting by court order under sections 35, 36, 37, 38, 41 of the Mental Health Act 1983 (amended 2007), and by the direction of the Home Secretary under sections 47, 48, 49 (see Table 20.1).

20.13   Section 48: transfer of unsentenced prisoners

20.13.1   Restriction orders and restriction directions

These apply to cases where a Crown court may add a restriction order to a hospital order as it appears to the court that a restriction order is necessary to protect the public from serious harm. The court requires oral evidence from one doctor who has recommended the hospital order. Restriction orders remove the doctor's authority to grant leave outside the hospital grounds, or to transfer or discharge the patient without the consent of the Secretary of State.

20.14   Section 41: restriction order

This restriction order may be added to a hospital order under section 37.

20.15   Section 49: restriction direction

This restriction order is the same as section 41 but it is attached to sections 47 or 48.

20.16   Specific psychiatric issues during criminal proceedings

20.16.1.1   Psychiatric Defences   In England and Wales two specific psychiatric defences are available to the defendant.

Table 20.1   Most commonly used sections.

Part 2 of the Act	Part 3 of the Act	Part 3 of the Act (Restricted Sections)
Applies to patients who are admitted to mental health hospitals detained under the Mental Health Act and are not subject to criminal proceedings.	Applies to patients who are involved in criminal proceedings against them. These admissions are directed by court orders.	Applies to patients who are usually detained in mental health secure units and are involved in criminal proceedings against them The restriction orders apply to individuals who are convicted of serious violence or sexual offence and are deemed to be dangerous. The restriction orders limit the decision-making powers of the treating clinician.
Section 2 Admission for *assessment* up to 28 days and cannot be extended. Two doctors must make this recommendation.	**Section 35** Remand to hospital for *assessment prior to trial* for a period of 28 days. The Crown court or the Magistrates' court, on the advice of <u>a</u> doctor, issues this court order. The court can renew the order for a period of 28 days at a time and for no more than *12 weeks* in total.	**Section 37/41** Hospital order 37 with a restriction order 41 because of concerns about public safety.
Section 3 Admission for *treatment* up to 6 months and can be extended. Two doctors must make this recommendation.	**Section 36** Remand to hospital for *treatment prior to trial* for a period of 28 days. The Crown court and *two* doctors are involved. The court can renew the order for a period of 28 days at a time and for no more than *12 weeks* in total.	**Section 41** This section applies to patients who were originally placed on section 37/41 to be discharged from hospital to the community but there are conditions imposed.
Section 4 Emergency admission for assessment up to 72 hours. Patients need to be assessed by a second doctor within 72 hours. One doctor is involved in the initial detention.	**Section 37** Hospital order. The Court and two doctors are involved. *After conviction* the court decided that instead of going to prison an individual should be in hospital for mental health treatment.	**Section 44** The magistrates may order that the patient be admitted to hospital rather than custody.
Section 5 (2) Detention of a patient who is already in hospital. One doctor is involved in the initial detention and it lasts for up to 72 hours.	**Section 38** Interim hospital order. This is a temporary hospital order to assess whether it may be appropriate to place the individual under hospital order 37. A court and two doctors are involved in the case of a person *convicted* of an imprisonable offence. It lasts a maximum period of 12 weeks and can be extended 28 days at a time and for no more than *12 months* in total.	**Section 45A. Hospital Direction and Limitation Direction** The sentenced prisoners could go straight from court to hospital to be treated. The individual (once treated) can be transferred back to prison to serve the remainder of the sentence. It authorises admission to hospital within 28 days and two doctors are required to provide evidence, one of whom would need to provide oral evidence to the court.

Table 20.1   (Continued)

Part 2 of the Act	Part 3 of the Act	Part 3 of the Act (Restricted Sections)
Section 5 (4) Nurse's powers to detain a patient who is already in hospital for up to 6 hours.	**Section 47 Transferred by Warrant of the Secretary of State** Transfer of *sentenced* prisoners to hospital. This section requires evidenced provided by two doctors that the individual suffers from a mental disorder that makes detention in hospital for medical treatment appropriate and appropriate medical treatment must be available.	**Section 47/49** Transfer of *sentenced* prisoners from prison to hospital with restrictions.
Section 136 Police take the individual to a place of safety from a public place up to 72 hours.	**Section 48 Transferred by Warrant of the Secretary of State** Removal to hospital of *unsentenced* prisoners. This section applies to prisoners on remand from Magistrates' or Crown courts, civil prisoners, and immigration detainees who are mentally disordered and who require urgent treatment in hospital. All conditions for detention as mentioned under section 47 apply.	**Section 48/49** Removal of prisoners *waiting to be sentenced* to hospital with restrictions.

Source: For further information, see Mental Health Act 1983 (as amended 2007).

The first is the defence of *not guilty by reason of insanity* (NGRI). This defence can apply to any crime. The legal test for this defence is based upon the McNaughton rules of 1843, following the case of an attempt to assassinate Queen Victoria's Prime Minister. Mr McNaughton fired a pistol at the Prime Minister's secretary, Edward Drummond, who subsequently died.

In order that a person could be found not guilty by reason of insanity, the jury must find that '... at the time of the committing of the act, the party accused was labouring under such a defect of reason, arising from a disease of the mind, as *not to know the nature and quality of the act* he was doing, or, if he did know it, that *he did not know what he was doing was wrong*'.

A person must be suffering from a mental disorder that results in him/her not being aware of what they were doing or not knowing that what they did was wrong. This is a very hard test to fulfil and it is only used rarely. A successful defence results in a special verdict of NGRI. At sentencing, options available to the judge include hospital treatment in a psychiatric hospital, supervision or a guardianship order, or an absolute discharge.

The second defence is manslaughter on the grounds of *diminished responsibility*. This defence is only available for a charge of murder. This was introduced in the 1957 Homicide Act to avoid sentencing mentally ill people who had committed murder to death. Murder carries only one sentence in courts in England and Wales, that of automatic life imprisonment. Section 52 of the Coroners and Justice Act 2009 replaces the definition of diminished responsibility as contained in the 1957 Homicide Act.

The test for this defence is three-fold:

- Is the defendant suffering from an abnormality of mental functioning?

- If so, has it arisen from a recognised medical condition?

- If so, has it substantially impaired his/her ability to understand the nature of his conduct or to form a rational judgement or to exercise self-control (or any combination)?

If convicted of manslaughter on the grounds of diminished responsibility, all sentencing options, including hospital treatment, are available to the judge.

20.16.1.2   Mens Rea and Actus Reus   A crime requires the combination of a mental and physical element. Mens rea means the 'guilty mind'. It refers to the individual's state of mind which makes the individual aware that his or her behaviour is a crime. Actus reus, the physical element, meaning the 'guilty act', requires some degree of mens rea in order to constitute a crime.

Mens rea could be absent in mental states of intoxication with alcohol and substance misuse. However, voluntary intoxication is not a defence to a crime. Other mental states in which mens rea may be absent is when the individual acts in a completely involuntarily manner, which is known as automatism. There are two types of automatism, 'non insane automatism', which is when an external factor has caused the individual to act in an involuntary manner, such as the use of substances, head trauma, etc., and 'insane automatism', which is related to an involuntary action as a result of an internal factor such as a physical health condition affecting the mind. These cases are very complex and there are difficulties in the way they are currently legislated (see the Law Commission UK website for further details, http://lawcommission.justice.gov.uk/areas/insanity.htm).

20.16.1.3   Fitness to Plead   The mental state of an individual at the time of the trial is crucial as a criminal trial can only go ahead if the individual is deemed 'fit to plead'. Forensic psychiatrists are often involved in assessing a defendant's fitness to plead.

In England and Wales, fitness to plead and be tried is based on the legal test known as the Pritchard criteria (from the case of R v Pritchard from 1836, Mr Pritchard was deaf and mute, and was accused of bestiality). This test assesses the mental state and abilities of the individual to ascertain whether the individual's mental state is affected by any mental health symptoms, including psychotic symptoms, learning disabilities, or neurological disorders. It involves demonstrating, on the balance of probabilities, whether the individual is capable of:

- understanding the charge or charges
- understanding and deciding whether or not to plead guilty
- following the court proceedings, which involves the individual being able to understand what the witness and the counsel are saying, and also being able to communicate with solicitors
- instructing solicitors and counsel, which means the individual being able to understand the questions put forward by lawyers, and being able to articulate an answer
- exercising the individual's right to challenge the jurors.

If the accused's defence team raise the issue of unfitness to plead, they must prove that the accused is unfit to plead on *the balance of probabilities*. However, if it is raised by the prosecution, they must prove that the accused is unfit to plead *beyond reasonable doubt*. If the judge finds that the defendant is unfit to plead, the jury will decide whether the defendant did the act or made the omission charged against him.

20.17   Serial Killers

There have been several definitions of what is a serial murder and they differ on specific details. The first thing to bear in mind is that serial killing is rare.

The Federal Bureau of Investigation (FBI) website has published a generic definition of what constitutes a serial murder: 'The unlawful killing of two or more victims by the same offender(s), in separate events'. The FBI has also identified three types of serial killers:

- *disorganised*, which includes individuals with a low level of intelligence. Usually these individuals are unable to interact adequately in social settings, and they tend to have an introverted personality. Their crimes are thought to be impulsive, there is no planning involved, and they tend to dispose of the victim's body at the scene of the crime.
- *organised*, which includes individuals with an average or above level of intelligence. They can observe balanced social interactions, they plan carefully the crimes, abduction of the victim could be involved, and they tend to dispose the victim's body at a different location.
- *mixed*, which involves a combination of both of the above.

Serial killers tend to be egocentric in character, expressing little consideration for others, tend to be dismissive of the rules of society, and show ritualistic behaviours. They tend to have unfulfilled fantasies, and the killing acts allow them to live out their fantasies.

The overall view about how an individual becomes a serial killer is that it involves complex social, biological, and psychological factors that are involved in expressing criminal behaviours. Broadly speaking, the psychological development of an individual is shaped by their exposure to bio-psycho-social experiences from birth to death. The behaviours expressed and the choices the individuals make are influenced by lifetime exposure to environmental stimulation (Gunn and Tayler 2014).

Violence is linked to early life disruptive psychosocial development such as when children have developed unhealthy early life coping strategies as a result of abuse and neglect. Children may learn through traumatic life experiences to focus on mental states of daydreaming and fantasy. Violent behaviours are linked to those individuals who are unable to utilise adequate coping strategies to relate to themselves and/or others because they never had the chance to learn them (Gunn and Tayler 2014).

20.18   Clinical Forensic Psychiatry

20.18.1   The role of the Forensic Psychiatrist

A psychiatrist is a medical doctor who has specialised in the assessment, diagnosis, and treatment of mental health disorders. Psychiatry is a medical specialty with a number of subspecialties, one of which is forensic psychiatry. Forensic psychiatrists have experience of working with individuals suffering from mental disorders who usually have a significant background history of violence and who also require long-term care. Rehabilitation programmes play a crucial part in the therapeutic service provided by forensic mental health settings and involve input from a range of disciplines, including psychiatry, clinical psychology, psychotherapy, occupational therapy, educational activities, art therapy, drama therapy, and nursing care.

In the UK, the majority of forensic psychiatrists work for the National Health Service (NHS) in specialised secure psychiatric hospitals. They may also provide in-reach into mental health services in prisons.

Broadly speaking the role of the forensic psychiatrist involves clinical assessment and diagnosis:

20.18.1.1   Clinical assessment and diagnosis

Mentally disordered offenders under the care of forensic mental health services usually have complex needs, which in turn require to be addressed in the formulation of the treatment and management plan. This process requires detailed assessment of background of the patient, the offending, other risk behaviours, and the clinical diagnosis. It is not uncommon for several diagnoses to be present in individuals, which is important to bear in mind as they could impact on the individual's offending behaviours, For example, an individual could just be suffering from a psychotic illness, or there could be a personality disorder diagnosis involved, or there could be a combination of both. In addition to this, substance misuse and dependence could also be added to the mix. Taking this into account, it is not surprising that clinical assessments and diagnosis can be a time-consuming process, requiring periods of ongoing clinical observations and input from a multidisciplinary team of professionals. This multidisciplinary approach facilitates an understanding of the nature of the offender's clinical diagnosis, and the degree to which the nature of the disorder has impacted on the individual's health and offending history.

20.18.1.2   Aspects of treatment and management

Treatment of mental health conditions involves the prescription of psychotropic medication, eg: antipsychotic medication to treat psychotic illness such as schizophrenia.

In addition to pharmacological treatment, the input from psychological therapies and a wide range of occupational therapies are crucial to the process of treatment and rehabilitation. It is paramount that both professionals and patients work together in achieving an understanding of issues related to risk of re-offending and relapsing into mental disorder.

This include enhancing the individual's awareness of the mental disorder, often patients struggle to understand the nature, significance, and severity of the mental disorder they suffer.

20.18.1.3   Addressing areas of risk

Forensic mental health services have strong focus on assessing risks and assisting patients to understand and reduce their risks. There are different tools to assess risks, but one of the most widely used structured tools is the historical, clinical, risk, management 20 (HCR-20) system, which assists professionals to structure decisions around the patient's risk of violence. Violence risk assessment and risk prediction are critical parts of the service delivery in a forensic mental health setting. Assessment of the level of risk that individuals pose to themselves, property, and others also involves input from a multidisciplinary team of professionals.

Overall, it is accepted that predicting oscillations in human behaviour and therefore predicting future risks is a challenging task (Gunn and Tayler 2014).

20.18.2 Providing a good-quality rehabilitation package

It is important to design a package of care that can offer a sustainable management plan to achieve a realistic level of care provided by forensic mental health teams, family members, and friends. This is crucial to a successful outcome regarding the individual's treatment, their rehabilitation, and their future discharge from hospital care. An effective relapse prevention plan is also crucial in order to prevent frequent readmissions to secure hospitals.

The Care Quality commission (CQC) is an independent regulator that carried out inspections to registered health care providers to ensure that the standards of quality of health care are being met (Care Quality Commission, 2014).

20.19   Secure Forensic Mental Health Services

In England and Wales, the NHS or the private sector may manage secure units. Usually, forensic mental health services care is for individuals who suffer from a mental disorder and have been arrested, those who are in prison but have not been tried or convicted, and individuals who have been to court and have been found guilty of a crime. However, there can be circumstances when individuals suffering from a mental disorder are admitted to secure psychiatric hospitals without having to go through the criminal justice system if they are deemed to be at high risk to members of the public and property. There are also circumstances when someone suffering from a mental disorder comes into contact with the police or the courts, but will not necessarily require a referral to a forensic psychiatric service. This would depend on the nature and the degree of the mental disorder and how this is linked to the type of criminal offence committed, background history of non-violent and violent offending profile, and the level of risk individuals could pose to themselves and/or others.

Forensic secure units in England and Wales are classified as low, medium, or high, related to the level of risk involved in each individual case, and aim to provide the most appropriate therapeutic milieu and treatment and to manage the patient safely. There are also specialised units providing care for particular groups of offenders, such as those with learning disabilities, severe personality disorders or other specific conditions such as autistic spectrum disorders or brain injury.

Sometimes, forensic mental health units also care for patients whose very high-risk behaviour towards both themselves and others has made it impossible for them to be managed safely in general psychiatry hospitals.

Patients can be referred to forensic mental health services at any stage throughout the criminal justice system from police stations, prisons, courts, general psychiatry hospitals, or community mental health services.

The admission criteria to a secure hospital varies according to the level of security required. In general, it depends on the assessment of the level of risk to others, the severity of the offence committed, the type of clinical diagnosis, and offending background history.

The admission criteria to the different levels of secure services are summarised in the following sections.

20.19.1 Admission Criteria to High Security Services

This level of physical security is similar to category B prisons, and caters for patients who pose grave and immediate danger to others and those who cannot be safely managed in a less secure environment. Mentally disordered offenders fitting this criteria include those who have used weapons and have committed serious and random unprovoked assaults.

20.19.2 Admission Criteria to Medium Secure Services

Patients admitted to this level of security include mentally disordered people who are a serious risk to the public, present a significant risk of escape or abscond, but do not present grave and immediate danger to others.

20.19.3 Admission Criteria to Low Secure Services

Patients admitted to this level of security include individuals suffering from a mental disorder who are a high risk to themselves and those who are at risk of low-level violence such as common assault (Rethink.org).

20.19.4 Specific provision

It is recognised that there is a gender difference when it comes to meeting the mental health needs of the mental health service users, therefore single-sex accommodation is available.

Within the secure forensic mental health service settings there are three types of security: physical, procedural, and relational.

20.19.4.1 Physical Security Physical security measures put in place in mental health settings include robust windows, locked doors, high fences, etc.

20.19.4.2 Procedural Security This relates to procedures or guidelines based on policies, which would address security controls to mitigate the identified risks. For example, security controls to avoid access to weapons, illicit substances, social media, and escape from a secure setting (Kennedy 2002). In Practice, procedural security may involve compulsory searches or inspections, substance misuse testing, investigation of incidents, and specific risk management procedures.

20.19.4.3 Relational Security Systems and processes are provided that ensure good-quality multidisciplinary assessment and treatment of patients. Its aim is to encourage productive therapeutic relationships between patients and members of the clinical team. An overall aim is to stabilise the individual's mental state and reduced recurrence of disturbed behaviours in the least restrictive setting.

20.20 Conclusions and final thoughts

The relationship between mental disorder, violence, and criminal behaviour is not straightforward despite the extensive research that has been carried out to establish links (Appelbaum et al. 2000). In other words not all criminals suffer from mental disorder and not all psychiatry patients are offenders. A recent study suggests that offenders with mental disorders are more likely to reoffend if untreated (Mela and Depiang 2016).

Forensic mental health services have an ethical duty to protect the patient's human rights, a duty to encourage the patient's autonomy, and are ethically and legally responsible for the patient's treatment and the provision of an appropriate rehabilitation programme. Individuals have different therapeutic needs, therefore therapeutic decisions need to be tailored to meet the individual's needs. This personalised care management approach also involves relevant consideration of matters related to public safety. A forensic psychiatrist aims to treat and stabilise the individual's mental state and behaviours in order to maximise as much as possible the individual's quality of life and reduce the patient's risk of harming themselves and/or harming others.

Detaining someone under mental health legislation involves restriction of the individual's autonomy. It is therefore not surprising that the practice of forensic psychiatry is not free of potential moral, ethical, and philosophical dilemmas or debate. German philosophy, and in particular the work initially carried out by Friedrich Nietzche (Nietzsche 2003), which was later taken forward by the French philosopher Michel Foucault, contributed to the development of a genealogical model to analyse society (Foucault 1995; Faubion 1998). This model argues that history has shaped society and also argues that history has intrinsically influenced the link between knowledge, institutional power, and the human subject in modern society. It also facilitates conceptual tools to understand how historical influences have shaped humans as 'subjects'. This seems to be reflected throughout the historical development and current perspectives pertinent to forensic mental health services and the law, in many respects both of these take the individual's autonomy away when an individual is detained.

References

American Psychiatry Association (2013). *Diagnostic and Statistical Manual of Mental Disorders (DSM-5)*, 5e. America Psychiatry Publishing.

Amos, J.J. and Robertson, R.G. (2010). *Psychosomatic Medicine: An Introduction to Consultation-Liaison Psychiatry*. Cambridge University Press.

Appelbaum, P.S., Robbins, P.C., and Monahan, J. (2000). Violence and delusions: Data from the MacArthur violence risk assessment study. *American Journal of Psychiatry* 157 (4): 566–572.

Bluglass, R. and Bowden, P. (1990). *Principles and Practice of Forensic Psychiatry*. Churchill Livingstone: Edinburgh.

Care Quality Commission (2014). www.cqc.org.uk.

Carr, A. (2005). Contributions to the study of violence and trauma: Multisystemic therapy, exposure therapy, attachment styles, and therapy process research. *Journal of Interpersonal Violence* 20 (4): 426–435.

David, A.S., Fleminger, S., Kopelman, M.D. et al. (2012). *Lishman's Organic Psychiatry A Textbook of Neuropsychiatry*. Wiley-Blackwell.

De Coster, S. and Heimer, K. (2001). The relationship between law violation and depression: an interactions analysis. *Criminology* 39 (4): 799–836.

Faubion, J.D. (1998). *The Essential Works of Foucault: Aesthetics, Method, and Epistemology*, vol. 2. New York: The New York Press.

Fazel, M., Långström, N., Grann, M., and Fazel, S. (2008). Psychopathology in adolescent and young adult criminal offenders (15–21 years) in Sweden. *Social Psychiatry and Psychiatric Epidemiology* 319–24 (512): 43.

Fazel, S., Gulati, G., Linsell, L. et al. (2009). Schizophrenia and Violence: Systematic review and meta-analysis. *PLoS Medicine* 6 (8): e1000120. doi:10.1371/journal.

Fazel, S., Wolf, A., Chang, Z. et al. (2015). Depression and violence: a Swedish population study. *The Lancet Psychiatry* 2 (3): 224–232.

Fennell, P. (2007). *Mental Health, The New Law*. Jordan Publishing.

Foucault, M. (1995). *Genealogy as Critique*. Verso Publications.

Gelder, M., Andreasen, N., Lopez-Ibor, J., and Geddes, J. (2012). *New Oxford Textbook of Psychiatry*, vol. 1 and 2. Oxford University Press.

Gunn, J. and Tayler, P.J. (2014). *Forensic Psychiatry*, 211–242. CRC Press. Chapter 9.

Hall, K.A. and O'Connor, D.W. (2004). Correlates of aggressive behaviour in dementia. *International Psychogeriatrics* 16 (2): 141–158.

Hughes, K., Bellis, M.A., Jones, L. et al. (2012). Prevalence and risk of violence against adults with disabilities: a systematic review and meta analysis of observational studies. *Lancet* 379: 1621–1629.

Kennedy, H.G. (2002). Therapeutic uses of security: mapping forensic mental health services by stratifying risk. *Advances in Psychiatry Treatment* 8: 433–443.

Mahowald, M.W., Bundlie, S.R., Hurwitz, T.D., and Schenck, C.H. (1990). Sleep violence – forensic science implications: polygraphic and video documentation. *Journal of Forensic Sciences* 35: 413–432.

Mela, M. and Depiang, G. (2016). Clozapine's effect on recidivism among offenders with mental disorders. *Journal of the American Academy of Psychiatry and the Law* 44 (1): 82–90.

Nielssen, O.B., Malhi, G.S., and Large, M.M. (2012). Mania, homicide and serious violence. *Australian and New Zealand Journal of Psychiatry* 46 (4): 357–363.

Nietzsche, F. (2003). *The Genealogy of Morals*. Dover Thrift Editions.

Oakley, C., Hynes, F., and Clark, T. (2009). Mood disorders and violence: a new focus. *Advances in Psychiatric Treatment* 15 (4): 263–270.

Reed, J. (1992). *Reed Report: Review of Mental Health and Social Services for Mentally Disordered Offenders and others Requiring Similar Services*. London: HMSO.

Scull, A. (1979). *Museums of Madness*, 64–66. London: Allen Lane.

Senior, J., Lennox, C., Noga, H., and Shaw, J. (2011). *Liaison and Diversion Services: Current Practices and Future Directions*. The Offender Health Research Network.

Siclari, F., Khatami, R., Urbaniok, F. et al. (2010). Violence in sleep. *Brain* 133 (12): 3494–3509.

Sirotich, F. (2008). Correlates of crime and violence among persons with mental disorder: an evidence-based review. *Brief Treatment Crisis Intervention* 8 (2): 171–194.

Skultans, V. and Cox, J. (2000). *Anthropological Approaches to Psychological Medicine: Crossing Bridges*. Jessica Kingsley Publishers.

Soyka, M. (2000). Substance misuse, psychiatric disorder and violent and disturbed behaviour. *British Journal of Psychiatry* 176: 345–350.

Stuart, H. (2003). Violence and mental illness: an overview. *World Psychiatry* 2 (2): 121–124.

Swanson, J.W., Holzer, C.E. 3rd, Ganju, V.K., and Jono, R.T. (1990). Violence and psychiatry disorder in the community: evidence from the Epidemiologic Catchment Area surveys. *Hosp Community Psychiatry* 41 (7): 761–770.

Walsh, E., Moran, P., Scott, C. et al. (2003). Prevalence of violent victimisation in severe mental illness. *British Journal of Psychiatry* 183: 233–238.

Waterhouse R & Williams R (1993) The Clunis Case: Passing the buck carried on until an innocent man died: *The Independent*'s own investigation of events that led to a ramdon killing. *The Independent* [Online] 19 July.

World Health Organization (1992) Pocket Guide to ICD-10 Classification of Mental and Behavioural Disorders: with glossary and diagnostic criteria DCR-10. Churchill Livingstone.

World Health Organizaion (2009). *Interpersonal Violence and Illicit Drugs*. Liverpool: Centre for Public Health John Moores Uiversity.

World Heath Organization and United Nations Office on Drugs & Crime (2014). Global Status Report on Violence Prevention. WHO publications.

21
Maternal Deaths

Mahomed Dada
Histopathology Department, Cheltenham General Hospital, Cheltenham, UK

21.1   Introduction and definitions

The 10th International Classification of Diseases (ICD-10) (WHO 1994) defines maternal death as 'the death of a woman while pregnant or within 42 days of the termination of pregnancy (includes delivery, ectopic pregnancy, miscarriage or termination of pregnancy), irrespective of the duration and site of the pregnancy, from any cause related to or aggravated by the pregnancy or its management but not from accidental or incidental causes.'

Maternal deaths can be further categorised into direct, indirect, and coincidental (fortuitous) deaths (Confidential Enquiries into Maternal Deaths in the United Kingdom 2011):

a.   Direct deaths result from obstetric complications of the pregnant state (pregnancy, labour, and puerperium) from interventions, omissions, incorrect treatment or from a chain of events resulting in any of the above (Table 21.1).

b.   Indirect deaths are defined as those resulting from previous existing disease or disease that develops during pregnancy and which was not the result of direct obstetric causes, but which was aggravated by the physiological effects of pregnancy. Examples of indirect death are epilepsy, diabetes, and cardiac disease. In the UK, deaths from hormone-dependent malignancies are included (Table 21.2).

c.   Coincidental (or fortuitous) deaths result from unrelated causes which happen to occur in pregnancy or the puerperium (Table 21.3).

Essential Forensic Medicine, First Edition. Edited by Peter Vanezis.
© 2020 John Wiley & Sons Ltd. Published 2020 by John Wiley & Sons Ltd.

Table 21.1 Direct causes of maternal death.

- Venous thrombosis and pulmonary embolism
- Hypertensive disease of pregnancy [pre-eclampsia (PET), eclampsia]
  a. Subtype of PET: HELLP syndrome in PET (haemolysis, elevated liver enzymes, low platelets)
- Peripartum haemorrhage
  a. Uterine atony
  b. Abruption of the placenta
  c. Placenta praevia
  d. Abnormally adherent placenta (placenta accreta, increta, percreta)
  e. Retained placenta
  f. Tear or rupture of genital tract
     i. Spontaneous
     ii. Iatrogenic
- Life support for peripartum haemorrhage
  a. TRALI (transfusion-associated lung injury)
  b. Fluid overload
- Peripartum dilated cardiomyopathy (defined as cardiac failure from last month of pregnancy up to 5 months postpartum; other causes excluded)
- Amniotic fluid embolism
- Early pregnancy deaths
  a. Ectopic pregnancy and haemorrhage
  b. Spontaneous miscarriage
  c. Legal termination
- Genital tract sepsis – puerperal sepsis
- Anaesthetic (general and regional anaesthesia)
- Air embolism
- Ogilvie's syndrome (pseudo-obstruction of the large bowel)
- Choriocarcinoma and hydatidiform mole
- Ovarian hyperstimulation syndrome (OHSS)
- Acute fatty liver of pregnancy

Source: Moodley et al. (2001).

Late maternal deaths refer to deaths occurring between 42 days and 1 year after abortion, miscarriage or delivery that are the result of *direct* or *indirect* maternal causes. Some deaths are multifactorial, e.g. suicide due to postpartum depression (which affects up to 15% of mothers) (Pearlstein et al. 2009). Psychiatric causes (Oates 2003) of maternal deaths are deaths that would not have occurred in the absence of the psychiatric disorder. The death may be due to suicide (most common cause), substance abuse, adverse drug reaction or homicide.

WHO (2013) estimates that in 2010 there were approximately 287 000 maternal deaths, 99% of which occurred in developing countries. Most of these maternal deaths were preventable if appropriate life-saving preventative and therapeutic interventions had taken place. The report identifies three components associated with maternal morbidity and mortality: delays in seeking care, delays in reaching care, and delays in receiving care at the facility (the three delays). Recognition of the links between development and women's health is incorporated in one of the United Nations' Millennium Development Goals (MDG5) (United Nations General Assembly 2000). The aim of this goal is to reduce the maternal mortality ratio (MMR) by three quarters. The MMR is the number of direct and indirect deaths per 100 000 live births and represents the risk associated with each pregnancy, i.e. the obstetric risk. In the UK, the maternal mortality rate is used and is based on the

Table 21.2 Indirect causes of maternal death.

- Cardiac
  a. Congenital heart lesion with pulmonary hypertension
  b. Inheritable cardiomyopathy, e.g. hypertrophic cardiomyopathy (HOCM)
  c. Arrhythmogenic right ventricular cardiomhopathy (ARVCM)
  d. Acquired cardiac muscle disease, e.g. ischaemic heart disease, endocardial fibroelastosis
  e. Obesity and sudden cardiac death
  f. Valvular disease, e.g. in IV drug users, rheumatic mitral stenosis
- Systemic hypertension
- Idiopathic arterial (primary) pulmonary hypertension
- Pre-existing thrombophilia states, including antiphospholipid syndrome
- Thrombotic thrombocytopaenic purpura (TTP)
- Stroke
  a. Subarachnoid haemorrhage
  b. Cerebral infarction
  c. Cerebral venous sinus thrombosis
- Other cardiovascular diseases
  a. Dissection of aorta
  b. Dissection of coronary artery
  c. Dissection of splenic artery
- Psychiatric, including suicide related to pregnancy and delivery
- Epilepsy [sudden unexplained death in epilepsy (SUDEP)]
- Malignant disease worsened by pregnancy (breast, cervix)
- Community-acquired sepsis
- Acute anaphylaxis from drug treatment, e.g. antibiotics
- Other diseases:
  a. HIV/AIDS and tuberculosis
  b. Sickle cell disease (HbSS and HbSC)
  c. Connective tissue disease – systemic lupus erythematosus (SLE)
  d. Diabetes mellitus – gestational and pre-existing diabetes; this includes the hypoglycaemic 'dead in bed' syndrome
  e. Influenza (e.g. epidemic type A–H1N1)
  f. Cirrhosis
  g. Any other clinico-pathological condition that the pregnant state makes worse; these include inherited and acquired conditions, and the patient may have been specifically warned of the hazards of becoming pregnant

Source: Moodley et al. (2001).

Table 21.3 Coincidental causes of maternal death.

- Death by own hands (suicide – some cases are unrelated to pregnancy, reflecting underlying mental health issues; note that only coroners/procurator fiscals can make the verdict of 'suicide'
- Other malignant disease
- Stroke (early in pregnancy)
- Transportation death (mostly road traffic collision)
- Homicide
- Toxic/illicit drug overdose
- Any other significant clinico-pathological condition

Source: Moodley et al. (2001).

Table 21.4   Causes of maternal death.

Cause	Frequency (%)
Haemorrhage	24
Infection	15
Unsafe abortion	13
Eclampsia	12
Obstructed labour	8
Other direct	8
Indirect	20

Source: WHO (2013).

number of direct and indirect deaths per 100 000 maternities. Maternities are defined as the number of pregnancies that result in a live birth at any gestation or stillbirths occurring at or after 24 completed weeks of gestation, and they are required to be notified by law (Pearlstein et al. 2009).

Despite a decline in maternal mortality, there are still significant differences in the MMR between developed and developing countries, and between urban and rural areas in some countries. Education of girls, provision of contraceptive services, and the presence of skilled birth attendants have been associated with lower maternal mortality (United Nations 2013).

21.2   Causes of maternal deaths

Leading medical causes of maternal death include haemorrhage, infection, eclampsia, obstructed labour, unsafe abortion, indirect causes, and other direct causes (Table 21.4).

During the period 2006–2008 (Pearlstein et al. 2009) the MMR in the UK was 11.39 per 100 000 maternities. Deaths from thrombo-embolism and haemorrhage had declined but deaths due to genital tract sepsis had increased. Cardiac disease was found to be the most common cause of indirect deaths. Substandard care was identified in 70% of direct deaths and 55% of indirect deaths.

21.3   The autopsy in maternal death

To improve the quality and standard of data obtained from maternal autopsies, the autopsies should be done in regional centres by pathologists with special interest and experience in the field.

Prior to the autopsy, the pathologist must know the full history of the patient and should have access to the clinical notes and, if necessary, consult with clinical colleagues (obstetricians, midwives, and anaesthetists) and others involved in the care of the patient. The presence of clinicians at the autopsy is helpful in correlating the clinical events to the findings at autopsy.

According to the Royal College of Pathologist Guidelines (RCPath 2010), relevant clinical information includes:

- all clinical information on past and present pregnancy history

- where the delivery took place (at home or in hospital) and whether a patient transfer was involved

- the delivery process, e.g. Caesarean, forceps, transfusions

- clinical and drug information on pre-existing medical conditions, including pre- eclampsia, renal disease, cardiac disease, and haematological conditions such as sickle cell disease

- family history of thrombosis and thromboembolism

- foetal/neonatal information, e.g. infected peri-partum, small-for-dates, traumatised

- pre-mortem laboratory data, e.g. blood cultures, blood clotting and platelet counts, liver and renal function tests.

The standard autopsy procedure should be followed but it must be remembered that certain complications of pregnancy are either unique or unusual, such as air embolism, amniotic fluid (AF) embolism, dissecting aneurysms of the aorta or coronary arteries, local aneurysms of mesenteric, splenic, hepatic, uterine or ovarian arteries, aspiration of gastric contents, perforations of the intestines in cases of abortion, trauma to the bladder and urethra, and trauma and tears to the external and internal genitalia. Routine sections should be taken for histological assessment. In addition, blocks from any abnormal tissue found at autopsy, the pituitary, right and left ovaries, right and left fallopian tubes, placental site of uterus, cervix, and placental tissue should be taken (Moodley et al. 2001).

A procedure which involves retention of samples and laboratory tests will be necessary. Prior discussions with a microbiologist and a toxicologist may be helpful. It is also prudent to retain samples of peripheral blood, gastric and intestinal contents, vitreous humour, and urine as well as samples for microbiological analysis at the start of an autopsy; these can be discarded later if they are not required.

External examination may reveal petechial haemorrhages as a sign of disseminated intravascular coagulopathy due to sepsis. The external genitalia should be examined for sepsis, trauma or excessive haemorrhage. Tests for pneumothorax and air embolism should be undertaken. Air embolism can occur in the event of placental disruption, during delivery of the placenta, or during intercourse or acts resulting in vaginal insufflation (Christiansen and Collins 2006). The pulmonary artery should be examined for thrombo-emboli and the source of emboli should be noted.

The pathologist undertaking a maternal post mortem should also examine or review any recent surgical resection specimen, such as a caesarean or postpartum hysterectomy or products of conception (Moodley et al. 2001).

In arriving at the cause of death, the pathologist should take into account the history, the autopsy findings, and the results of the special investigations undertaken at autopsy. The clinco-pathological summary should be comprehensive to assist the clinical team, the coroner or other judicial officer (if a medico-legal autopsy), National Confidential Enquiries into Maternal Deaths, and local audit. The cause of death may sometimes only be formulated after a multidisciplinary meeting with other clinical role players (Moodley et al. 2001).

Decide whether the death is direct, indirect or coincidental in relation to the pregnancy. Audit committees may also want to determine if the death was preventable so that recommendations could be made to reduce deaths from similar causes or circumstances (Moodley et al. 2001).

Rushton and Dawson identified the following pitfalls in autopsies performed on patients with maternal deaths:

d. lack of details in the autopsy report

e. inadequate post-mortem examination

f. sources of pulmonary emboli not determined

g. histology of lungs not performed for suspected amniotic fluid examination

21.4   Specialised pathology in pregnancy

21.4.1   Amniotic fluid embolism

Amniotic fluid (AF) embolism is a rare and severe complication during pregnancy or shortly after delivery. In a UK study (Knight et al. 2010) AF embolism was significantly associated with induction of labour, multiple pregnancy, and older, ethnic minority women.

The clinical features are similar to pulmonary embolism, septic shock, anaphylaxis, and eclampsia, and the clinical diagnosis is based on one or more of the four key clinical signs and symptoms: cardiovascular collapse, respiratory distress, coagulopathy, and/or coma/seizures. The incidence varies from 1 in 8000 to 1 in 80000 deliveries. The mortality rate is between 61 and 86% (Rushton and Dawson 1982). AF embolism occurs in the third trimester of pregnancy, in labour, or during traumatic or rapid deliveries.

The most reliable diagnosis is the finding of foetal material in the maternal pulmonary circulation at autopsy (Benson 2012). AF contains foetal squames, mucous (from the foetal meconium) and lanugo, which consists of fatty material with some hair derived from the foetal skin vernix), meconium, cells from the chorion and amnion, and other cellular debris. The particulate elements are usually impacted in the lung capillaries, but rarely found in the systemic circulation (kidney, liver, and brain). The actual fluid is undetectable histologically.

To diagnose AF embolism one has to identify one or more of the above particulate materials. Fat may be seen in frozen sections of the lung using the Oil Red O or Sudan stains. The other elements may be demonstrated using Attwood's stain (alcian blue or green-phloxine tartrazine technique). Foetal squames may also be demonstrated using immunohistochemical markers.

21.4.2   Pre-eclampsia, eclampsia, and hypertension

Hypertensive disease in pregnancy is common and is an important contributory cause to maternal deaths (Knight et al. 2010). Clinically the hypertension may be evident prior to conception or may become manifest during pregnancy. Furthermore, essential hypertension may be complicated by pre-eclampsia or eclampsia. Hypertensive disorders of pregnancy (HDP) represent a group of conditions associated with high blood pressure during pregnancy, proteinuria, and in some cases convulsions. Pre-eclampsia and eclampsia are associated with vasospasm, vascular lesions in multiple organ systems, increased platelet activation, and subsequent activation of the coagulation system in the micro-vasculature. Eclampsia is pre-eclampsia with central nervous system seizures. The patient is often left unconscious and death may occur if untreated. The incidence of pre-eclampsia is estimated at 3.2% of live births (approximately over 4 million cases each year), resulting in over 72 000 deaths (AbouZahr 2003).

The morphological changes of hypertension in pregnancy may be seen in the kidney, brain, heart, pituitary, and placenta (Christiansen and Collins 2006). The placental changes include:

h. placental infarcts

i. retroplacental haematomas

j. features of villus ischaemia such as prominent syncytial knots, thickening of the trophoblastic basement membrane, and villus hypovascularity

k. fibrinoid necrosis associated with large numbers of lipophages in the vessel wall (acute atherosis).

21.4.3 Haemorrhage

Obstetric haemorrhage may occur antenatally, postnatally, and intrapartum. Examples include placenta praevia and accreta, placental abruption, and postpartum haemorrhage. Please refer to textbooks of obstetrics for diagnostic criteria and guidelines.

References

AbouZahr, C. (2003). Global burden of maternal death and disability. *Br. Med. Bull.* 67: 1–11.

Benson, M.D. (2012). Current concepts of immunology and diagnosis in amniotic fluid embolism. *Clin. Dev. Immunol.* 2012: 1–7.

Centre for Maternal and Child Enquiries (CMACE) (2011). Saving Mothers' Lives: reviewing maternal deaths to make motherhood safer: 2006–08. The Eighth Report on Confidential Enquiries into Maternal Deaths in the United Kingdom. *BJOG* 118(Suppl. 1: 1–203.

Christiansen, L.R. and Collins, K.A. (2006). Pregnancy-associated deaths: a 15-year retrospective study and overall review of maternal pathophysiology *Am. J. Forensic Med. Pathol.* 27: 11–19.

Knight, M., Tuffnell, D., Brocklehurst, P. et al. (2010). UK obstetric surveillance system. Incidence and risk factors for amniotic fluid embolism. *Obstet. Gynecol.* 115: 910–917.

Moodley, J., Moorad Nielsen, R.G.R., McQuoid-Mason, D.J. (2001). Obstetrics and Gynaecology. In: *Introduction to Medico-Legal Practice* (ed. Dada M.A and McQuoid-Mason D.J.), 74–76. Durban: Butterworths.

Oates, M. (2003). Suicide: the leading cause of maternal death. *Br. J. Psychiatry* 183: 279–281.

Pearlstein, T., Howard, M., Salisbury, A., and Zlotnick, C. (2009). Postpartum depression. *Am. J. Obstet. Gynecol.* 200: 357–364.

Royal College of Pathologists Guidelines on Autopsy (2010). *Practice Scenario 5: Maternal Death.* London: Royal College of Pathologists Available from https://www.rcpath.org/uploads/assets/827a1a8c-5ed4-4203-9eb336e0 de0f7d2d/g100autopsypracticesection5maternaldeathfinaloct2010.pdf

Rushton, D.I. and Dawson, I.M.P. (1982). The maternal autopsy. *J. Clin. Pathol.* 35: 909–921.

United Nations The Millennium Development Goals Report 2013, United Nations, 2013; UNDP, UNFPA; UNICEF; UN Women; WHO.

United Nations General Assembly. United Nations Millennium Declaration. A/RES/55/2. 1–9-2000. UN General Assembly, 55th session, agenda item 60(b).

World Health Organization (1994). *International Classification of Diseases (ICD) 10.* Geneva: World Health Organization. Available from: http://www.who.int/classifications/icd/en.

World Health Organization (2013). *Maternal Death Surveillance and Response: Technical Guidance. Information for Action to Prevent Maternal Death.* Geneva: World Health Organization. Available from: http://apps.who.int/iris/ bitstream/10665/87340/1/9789241506083_eng.pdf?ua=1.

22

The Examination of Detainees and Death in Custody

Peter Vanezis
Queen Mary University of London, London, UK

It has been said that the appropriate treatment of detainees is a measure of the value and respect that a society has for the rights of its citizens. This chapter discusses the various aspects of the requirements of detainees and the investigation of deaths that occur in a custodial environment or in contact with authority.

22.1 Defining death in custody

It is practical to deal with the investigation of deaths that occur in custody together with those that come into contact with the police although not necessarily in a custodial environment. Indeed, the Crown Prosecution Service (CPS) (cps.gov.uk (2017) www.cps.gov.uk/legal/d_to_g/deaths_in_custody/#a01) describe 'death in custody' as being a generic term which refers to deaths of those in the custody of the state and lists the following circumstances that may apply to this definition:

- whilst under arrest in a police station

- whilst held as a prisoner in a prison or police station

- whilst under arrest by a police officer

- whilst being detained for the purposes of a search

Essential Forensic Medicine, First Edition. Edited by Peter Vanezis.
© 2020 John Wiley & Sons Ltd. Published 2020 by John Wiley & Sons Ltd.

- whilst in other lawful detention, e.g. immigration detention (but not where the victim is compulsorily detained under the Mental Health Act 1983 except where the person is still in police custody before being transferred to a medical facility)

- whilst a child or young person is in custody for their own protection

- as a result of being shot by a police officer

- following any other contact with the police where there may be a link between the contact and the death.

The guidelines produced by the CPS are useful in many respects but it is recognised that the scope for such deaths is more complex and requires the concept of custody to be flexible. Ruiz et al. (2014) argue that the lack of an internationally recognised standard definition of death in custody is of major concern. They maintain that defining death in custody based on the place where death occurs has shortcomings, as it provides authorities with the opportunity to reduce the overall number of such deaths. This is mostly done by transferring or releasing detainees to hospitals or any other place immediately prior to their death to reduce custody death numbers. Since these transfers or releases may take place for imprisoned persons attempting to commit suicide or those who may become victims of drug overdose and violent injuries, these deaths would not be included in the definition of death in custody, as they occurred outside the prison environment.

For the purposes of investigation and monitoring, custody deaths include those that occur in prison, police custody or detention as a juvenile, and where there is a concern that death was caused or contributed to by:

- traumatic injuries

- lack of proper care whilst in custody or detention

- the deceased escaping or attempting to escape from police custody or juvenile detention.

22.2   Ministerial Council on Deaths in Custody

As a result of concerns of the increasing numbers of deaths in custody, the Ministry of Justice announced the creation of a three-tier Ministerial Council on Deaths in Custody in 2008, following publication earlier that year of the Fulton Report (Fulton 2008). The Fulton Report recommended the creation of a new structure to replace the Ministerial Roundtable on Suicide and the Forum for Preventing Deaths in Custody. The shared purpose of the Ministerial Council is to bring about a continuing and sustained reduction in the number and rate of deaths in all forms of state custody in England and Wales. It is jointly funded by the Ministry of Justice, Department of Health, and the Home Office and incorporates senior decision-makers, experts, and practitioners in the field. This extended, cross-sector approach to deaths in custody is intended to allow for better learning and sharing of lessons across the custodial sectors. The Ministerial Council consists of three tiers: the Ministerial Board on Deaths in Custody, an independent advisory panel (IAP), and a practitioner and stakeholder group.

The fifth statistical report by the IAP into deaths in custody, published in December 2015, which covered the period between 2000 and 2014, includes all deaths which occurred in the following locations:

- prisons

- in or following police custody

- secure training centres/secure children's homes

- immigration removal centres

- Approved Premises

- hospitals, when detained under the Mental Health Act 1983.

22.3 Deaths in custody in England and Wales

There were 8129 deaths in custody recorded in England and Wales for the 15 years from 2000 to 2014: 73% men ($N = 5918$) and 27% women ($N = 2211$). There were 21% fewer total deaths in 2014 ($N = 479$) compared to 2000 ($N = 607$) (Independent Advisory Panel 2017) (Figure 22.1). The majority (59%) of these 8129 deaths were patients detained under the Mental Health Act. The second highest number were within prison settings, at 34% of all deaths. Overall, the numbers of deaths amongst detained patients appears to be decreasing year on year whilst the prison sector has had a continued increase from 2006 onwards.

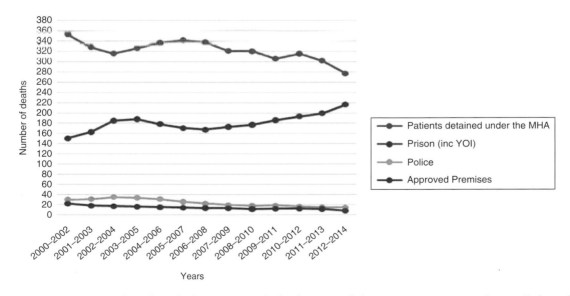

Figure 22.1 Average number of deaths in state custody for four custodial sectors 2000 to 2014. Source: Independent Advisory Panel Report, www.iapdeathsincustody.independent.gov.uk.

In 2014, there were 479 recorded deaths in state custody (a decrease of 15% from 2013). The largest cause of recorded death in that year was related to natural causes (67%), followed by self-inflicted deaths (23%). White males accounted for the majority of deaths. The largest age band was in those aged 61 and over who were patients detained under the Mental Health Act 1983 ($N = 121$); all but one of the deaths were from natural causes.

The latest figures reveal that there were 310 deaths in prison custody in the 12 months to June 2018, down 2% from the previous year. Of these, five were homicides, up from two incidents in the previous year. There were 77 self-inflicted deaths, down from 99 in the previous year, three of which occurred in females, compared to six incidents in the previous 12 months (Ministry of Justice, National Statistics 2018).

22.4   Management of detainees in police custody

Managing persons brought into police custody requires the understanding of healthcare needs and the various risks which impact on the outcome of the well-being of the detainee. Both healthcare staff and police have important roles to play.

22.4.1   Risk assessment

It is essential to assess the risk and potential risk that each detainee presents to themselves, staff, other detainees, and other people coming into the custody suite. An officer making an arrest is personally responsible for the risk assessment and welfare of the detained person until the suspect is handed over to the custody officer for a decision regarding detention. The dynamic nature of the incident and the process of arrest may have a bearing on the assessment which, by its very nature, is likely to be continuous and needs to respond to any changing circumstances. The assessment needs to be documented at the earliest opportunity (College of Policing 2017).

The custody officer is responsible for documenting and recording the risk assessment for every detainee in the custody record in accordance with paragraphs 3.6–3.10 of the Police and Criminal Evidence Act 1984, Code C (1984)(the code is revised on a regular basis).

The custody officer must ensure that all those responsible for the detainee's custody are briefed about the risks. They should ensure their responses to risk are dynamic, reviewed, and communicated to all people involved in the care of the detainee, including relevant healthcare staff.

The arresting or escorting officer should check any immediately available sources of information relevant to the welfare of the arrested person. This may include:

- the detainee

- the detainee's friends or relatives

- witnesses

- all staff involved in the person's arrest and detention

- the Police National Computer (PNC), Police National Database (PND), and other local IT systems

- healthcare professionals (HCPs), including general practitioners (GPs)

- legal representatives

- an appropriate adult

- other detainees

- other relevant bodies and organisations, e.g. the youth offending team.

22.4.1.1 Role of the doctor Healthcare needs in custody include management of chronic medical conditions, initial management and referral as emergencies if appropriate, in cases of drug and alcohol misuse, mental health disorders, and trauma management. In addition there may be health needs related to the concealment of drugs, for example body packing or stuffing. Healthcare may also be required arising from police procedures leading to detention, for example the use of various restraining agents, including the use of Taser, irritant sprays, handcuffs manual restraint, and the use of batons.

The healthcare professional, from management and assessment of the detainee, will advise the police whether the detainee is fit to be detained, interviewed, charged or released.

22.5 Role of the Independent Office for Police Conduct

The Independent Police Complaints Commission (IPCC) came into force on 1 April 2004 and replaced the Police Complaints Authority as the guardian of the complaints procedure. The legal framework for the investigation of complaints arises from the Police Reform Act 2002. The IPCC was replaced by the Independent Office for Police Conduct (IOPC) in January 2018 (see the end of this chapter).

The circumstances of all deaths referred to the IPCC between 2000 and 2014 were evaluated (Figure 22.2) to determine whether or not they met the criteria for inclusion in one of the following categories:

- fatal road traffic incidents

- fatal shooting incidents

- deaths in or following police custody

- deaths during or following other types of police contact.

22.5.1 Investigation types

Independent investigations: conducted solely by IOPC investigators who have the powers of a police constable and are able to enter police premises and seize and retain documentation or other evidence where necessary.

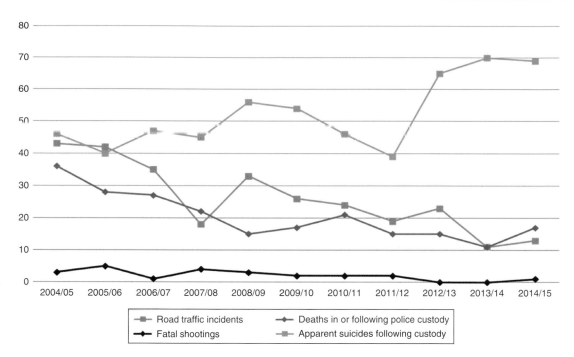

Figure 22.2 Incidents by type of death and financial year, 2004/05 to 2014/15, investigated by the IPCC. Source: Independent Police Complaints Commission (now the Independent Office for Police Conduct).

Managed investigations: conducted by police officers under the direction and control of the IOPC, which is responsible for setting the terms of reference, approving the investigating officer, and monitoring the progress of the investigation to ensure it is conducted in an accurate and timely manner.

Supervised investigations: conducted by police officers but the IOPC agrees the choice of investigating officer and terms of reference. The responsibility for maintaining the record of decisions and for conducting a timely investigation rests with the police officers undertaking the investigation.

Local investigations: conducted by police officers when the IOPC decides that the force has the necessary resources and experience to carry out an investigation without external assistance.

22.6   Deaths related to restraint

Restraining someone in certain circumstances is essential when dealing with a non-compliant or violent individual behaving in a threatening manner to the restrainers. The problem arises when the subject is an unwilling party to the restraint and contributes to its potential danger by reacting violently. There are a number of questions which need to be carefully considered when restraint is employed. One of these is whether the type and amount of force used is appropriate and safe. It is therefore incumbent on the restrainers to minimise the potential risks and use physical restraint only as a last resort. Nevertheless, whatever type of restraint might be used, if the subject dies during this process the method will be questioned, no matter how safe it was thought to be.

The risk of fatalities could be viewed as present in any restraint position, with forceful restraint being the highest risk factor, and de-escalation being the intervention of choice in managing violence and aggression. However, de-escalation may not always be effective and, in order to prevent harm to others, restraint or seclusion may be necessary.

In deaths in custody there will always be the additional difficulty of separating any potential contribution of control measures from the underlying pathology. For example, was death due to the police control method, or to positional asphyxia, or from excited delirium syndrome/acute behavioural disturbance (ABD) or from the interplay of all these factors?

22.7 Excited Delirium Syndrome/Acute Behavioural Disturbance

Restraint may be required in cases where the subject is agitated and aggressive, and is likely to have taken stimulant drugs such as cocaine, with which excited delirium syndrome/acute behavioural disturbance (EDS/ABD) is frequently associated. In relation to such a situation, the term EDS or ABD is applied, yet there are difficulties around identifying and studying this condition because of the lack of a well-defined, consistent epidemiological case definition and overlap with other established diseases (deBard 2009; Adler et al. 2012; Vilke et al. 2012) such as neuroleptic malignant syndrome. Stress-related cardiomyopathy may be a factor in restraint-related deaths but more analysis is needed of timelines before and during the restraint to confirm this.

The syndrome comprises the following sequence of events: hyperthermia, delirium with agitation, respiratory arrest, and death. Initially the person is hyperthermic, grossly psychotic, and displays a great deal of physical agitation and a marked increase in physical strength. After a relatively short interval, the individual becomes quiet and deaths follows shortly thereafter in nearly all cases. Some may well have been hog-tied with their wrists and ankles bound together behind their back. It should also be appreciated that 'agitated delirium' may be the result of medical conditions other than cocaine or the effect of stimulant drug toxicity. It has been suggested that it is a variant of neuroleptic malignant syndrome (Kosten and Kleber 1988). There is growing evidence that the stress associated with restraint makes death more likely. Particularly in chronic cocaine users, death is thought to be due to the effect of a surge of catecholamines on a sensitised myocardium.

Such deaths can be seen to be multifactorial and consideration should be given not only to biophysiological mechanisms but should include the circumstances, which may be complex, surrounding each death (Aiken et al 2011) (Figure 22.3).

22.8 Conflict resolution (De-escalation)

Police forces in the UK have devised models for conflict resolution to achieve control over a subject. The guidelines produced are designed to take into account the interaction of offender behaviour, impact factors, and reasonable officer responses. As offender behaviour becomes increasingly more hostile, the officer will consider a number of impact factors, such as possible imminent danger and size of the offender, when deciding on the level of response. Such a response will be correspondingly more robust to affect compliance and neutralise any perceived or real threat to the members of the general public or police officers.

▶ Pre-existing lung disease such as chronic obstructive pulmonary disease
▶ Various types of heart conditions, particularly cardiomyopathy.
▶ Postural (positional) asphyxia with the individual and restrained in a prone, supine or basket hold position
▶ Catecholamine release resulting from stress
▶ Alcohol and/or drug intoxication particularly cocaine coupled with violent/erratic behaviour
▶ Excited delirium/acute behavioural disturbance
▶ Metabolic acidosis from exertion.
▶ Thrombo-embolic disease.

Figure 22.3   Multifactorial causes of restraint-related death. Source: Adapted from Aitken 2011.

Conflict resolution training has attempted to provide a more standardised approach to the issue of de-escalation (Miller 2003). Although there appears to be a lack of high-level evidence for the process of de-escalation, it is clear that the concept and process of de-escalation is part of many interventions available for the prevention, management, and reduction of violence and aggression that sit within an overall organisational framework of violence reduction (Colton 2010).

22.9   Methods of restraint

A number of restraint methods have been used in the past or are currently in use.

22.9.1   Physical contact involving pressure to the body

The danger of any form of restraint where there is the potential of depriving the restrained person of oxygen is particularly prevalent where pressure is applied either directly or indirectly to certain parts of the body using the following techniques:

- neck holds: bar or 'choke' hold, carotid sleeper

- other forms of neck pressure to cause immobilisation

- mouth obstruction by taping

- hand cuffing (anterior or posterior), arm restraint, feet tying, tying the hands and feet together at the back ('hog tying'), and trunk immobilisation, particularly in the prone position.
    Pressure on the chest, abdomen, and/or body position is the most common cause of death related to hypoxia. When an individual is restrained or in a prone position, three things happen that compromise the body's ability to breathe:
    – there is direct occlusion of the upper airways (Belviso et al. 2003)
    – compression by weight or restriction in the movement of the ribs limits their ability to expand the chest cavity and breathe (Stratton et al. 2001; Parkes 2008)
    – pushing of abdominal organs upwards, restricting movement of the diaphragm and further limiting breathing (Reay et al. 1992; Parkes 2008).

Nowadays, following a number of tragic deaths in such circumstances, forms of restraint which might compromise the ability to breath or in some other way deprive the body of oxygen by mechanical means are avoided as far as possible, in preference to other techniques thought to be safer.

22.9.2 Use of baton guns (previously 'rubber bullets')

The plastic baton gun was approved by the Home Office in the UK in 2001 as 'a less lethal option' for use by the police. It replaced rubber bullets, which had been used in civil disturbances in Northern Ireland since 1970. Hughes et al. (2005) in their series of 28 patients found 30 injuries, all of which were non-fatal. Injuries were to the upper limbs, lower limbs, and chest. No head injuries were found in their series. Of the 14 deaths attributable to plastic baton rounds in Northern Ireland, all have been the result of head or chest trauma (Rocke 1983).

22.9.3 Conducted electrical device CED (Taser gun)

The Taser is a development of the stun gun is used by British police forces as a 'less lethal' weapon. The barbs attach to the subject's skin or clothing and deliver up to 50 000 V of electricity in rapid pulses over five seconds. The electric current causes uncontrollable muscle contraction and overwhelming pain that incapacitates the subject. The weapon can be turned off before the end of the five seconds default period. The barbs remain attached until removed, thus allowing further electrical discharges to be delivered via the copper wires should the subject resume non-compliant and threatening behaviour. The cartridge can be detached from the weapon, allowing it to be used as a stun gun in close quarters.

The UK Government has recently approved controversial plans to issue police officers in England and Wales with a new and more powerful X2 Taser gun, which has a second shot in case the first should fail (Lewis 2017). The weapon also has an electric crackle warning noise and pulsating light to try to encourage a suspect to surrender before being fired upon. Both the new and old X26 model give a 50 000-V electric shock.

At least 11 deaths in the UK have been linked to the use of Tasers over the 13 years since they were first introduced, but experts have been unable to say whether the stun gun was directly responsible for any of those deaths. The overall conclusion from experience in the use of the Taser over many years is that they are generally safe when used according to manufacturer's instructions and police guidelines on healthy subjects who are not under the influence of drugs or alcohol, and are not suffering from pre-existing cardiac or respiratory conditions. Clinical studies (Cevik et al. 2009) indicate that high-voltage electrical pulses do not cause cardiac arrhythmia but instead acute stress cardiomyopathy may be an explanation for deaths associated with electronic weapons. Patients with acute stress cardiomyopathy usually have had an emotional or physical stress, have high circulating levels of catecholamines, and present with an acute coronary syndrome but have normal coronary vessels without significant thrombus formation.

Tasers also have the potential to cause severe injuries and other adverse effects resulting from the unique penetrating action of Taser barbs, from muscular contractions, or, indirectly, from falls (Bleetman et al. 2004; SACMILL 2017).

22.9.4 Chemical sprays/gas

Substances used for immobilisation of individuals or crowds include CS gas (tear gas), the active component of which is 2-chlorobenzalmalononitrile, a cyanocarbon; the chemical agent 2-chloroacetophenone, (CN gas or mace), is an aerosol spray and OC oleoresin capsicum (pepper spray) (Schep et al. 2015). These are all are highly irritant incapacitating agents. They cause severe irritation and watering of the eyes, as well as stinging or burning to the nose, tight chest, sore throat, coughing, difficulty breathing, and skin irritation. Payne-James et al. (2014) in their study of the use of such sprays by the Metropolitan Police (London) found that symptoms and signs of exposure to incapacitant sprays lasted longer than was expected (a mean of 2.8 hours). Approximately 30% of those exposed had ocular effects and 20% had skin effects.

22.9.5 Drug administration

Drugs may be used to sedate an individual to restrict their movement. They are used in an emergency situation and/or within a psychiatric environment to control agitated or aggressive patients who may be threatening or causing harm to themselves or others (Hopper et al. 2015). Such drugs often used include include benzodiazepines, antipsychotics, and dissociative anaesthetics such as ketamine.

22.10 Addendum

22.10.1 Recent developments in the UK

A recent independent report into deaths and serious incidents in police custody was chaired by Dame Elish Angiolini and published in October 2017 (Angiolini 2017). The report is comprehensive and outlines the concerns of both families and other professionals and organisations. It makes many recommendations and the reader is directed to the report for further information.

The Independent Office for Police Conduct (IOPC) replaced the IPCC on 8 January 2018, taking over the same role. Further information can be accessed at www.policeconduct.gov.uk.

References

Adler, J., Czarnecki, F., Heck, J., and Bozeman, W.P. (2012). Excited delirium syndrome (ExDS): defining based on a review of the literature. *J. Emerg. Med.* 43: 897–905.

Aiken F, Duxbury J, Dale C, Harbison I. Review of the Medical Theories and Research Relating to Restraint Related Deaths (2011). University of Central Lancashire and Caring Solutions (UK).

Angiolini E. (2017). Independent report. Deaths and serious incidents in police custody. http://www.gov.uk/government/publications/deaths-and-serious-incidents-in-police-custody. Accessed August 2018.

Belviso, M., De Donno, A., Vitale, L., and Introna, F. Jr. (2003). Positional asphyxia: reflection on 2 cases. *Am. J. Forensic Med. Pathol.* 24: 292–297.

Bleetman, A., Steyn, R., and Lee, C. (2004). Introduction of the Taser into British policing. Implications for UK emergency departments: an overview of electronic weaponry. *Emerg. Med. J.* 21: 136–140.

Cevik, C., Otahbachi, M., Miller, E. et al. (2009). Acute stress cardiomyopathy and deaths associated with electronic weapons. *Int. J. Cardiol.* 132: 312–317.

Code C. Revised code of practice for the detention, treatment and questioning of persons by police officers. Police and criminal evidence act 1984 (PACE) – Code C. Presented to Parliament pursuant to Section 67(7B) of the Police and Criminal Evidence Act 1984.

College of Policing (2017). Detention and custody. www.app.college.police.uk/app-content/detention-and-custody-2/risk-assessment. Accessed August 2017.

Colton, D (2010) Checklist for Assessing your Organisations Readiness for Reducing Seclusion and Restraint. Staunton, Staunton, Virginia.

Crown Prosecution Service. Deaths in custody. www.cps.gov.uk/legal/d_to_g/deaths_in_custody/#a01. Accessed August 2017.

DeBard (Chair), 2009. White Paper Report on Excited Delirium Syndrome. American College of Emergency Physicians. American College of Emergency Physicians Excited Delirium Task Force.

Fulton R (2008). Review of the forum for preventing deaths in custody. Report of the Independent Reviewer, Ministry of Justice. www.iapdeathsincustody.independent.gov.uk/about/ministerial-council-on-deaths-in-custody. Accessed August 2017.

Hopper, A.B., Vilke, G.M., Castillo, E.M. et al. (2015). Ketamine use for acute agitation in the emergency department. *J. Emerg. Med.* 48: 712–719.

Hughes, D., Maguire, K., Dunn, F. et al. (2005). Plastic baton round injuries. *Emerg. Med. J.* 22: 111–112.

Independent Advisory Panel on Deaths in Custody (2014). http//iapdeathsincustody.independent.gov.uk. Accessed August 2017.

Kosten, T.R. and Kleber, H.D. (1988). Rapid death during cocaine abuse: a variant of the neuroleptic malignant syndrome? *Am. J. Drug Alcohol Abuse* 14: 335–346.

Lewis B. (2017) Policing: Written statement HCWS517. http://www.parliament.uk/business/publications/written-questions-answers-statements/written-statement/Commons, 2 March 2017. Accessed December 2017.

Miller, G. (2003). *Safer Services, Promoting Safer Therapeutic Services*. London: Security Management Service NHS Trust.

Ministry of Justice. (2018). Safety in Custody Statistics, England and Wales: Deaths in Prison Custody to March 2018 Assaults and Self- harm to December 2017.

Parkes, J. (2008). Sudden death during restraint: do some positions affect lung function? *Med. Sci. Law* 48: 137–141.

Payne James, J., Smith, G., Rivers, E. et al. (2014). Effects of incapacitant spray deployed in the restraint and arrest of detainees in the metropolitan police service area, London, UK: a prospective study. *Forensic Sci. Med. Pathol.* 10: 62–68.

Code C. Revised code of practice for the detention, treatment and questioning of persons by police officers. Police and criminal evidence act 1984 (PACE) – Code C. Presented to Parliament pursuant to Section 67(7B) of the Police and Criminal Evidence Act 1984.

Police Reform Act 2002.

Reay, D.I., Fligner, C.I., Stilwell, A.D., and Arnold, J (1992) Positional asphyxia during law enforcement transport. *Am. J. Forensic Med. Pathol.* 13: 90–97.

Rocke, L. (1983). Injuries caused by plastic bullets compared with those caused by rubber bullets *Lancet* 1 (8330): 919–920.

Ruiz, G., Tenzin Wangmo, T., Mutzenberg, P. et al. (2014). Understanding death in custody: a case for a comprehensive definition. *J. Bioeth. Inq.* 11: 387–398.

SACMILL Statement on the Medical Implications of Use of the TASER X2 Conducted Energy Device System. Scientific Advisory Committee on the Medical Implications of Less Lethal Weapons. http://www.gov.uk/government/publications/medical-implications-of-the-taser-x2. Accessed December 2017.

Schep, L.J., Slaughter, R.J., and McBride, D. (2015). Riot control agents: the tear gases CN, CS and OC – a medical review. *J. R. Army Med. Corps* 161: 94–99.

Stratton, S.J., Rogers, C., Brickett, K., and Gruzinski, G. (2001). Factors associated with sudden death of individuals requiring restraint for excited delirium. *Am. J. Emerg. Med.* 19: 187–191.

Vilke, G.M., DeBard, M.L., Chan, T.C. et al. (2012). Excited delirium syndrome (ExDS): defining based on a review of the literature. *J. Emerg. Med.* 43: 897–905.

23
Forensic Toxicology: Clinico-pathological Aspects and Medico-legal Issues

Nadia Porpiglia, Chiara Laposata, and Franco Tagliaro
Department of Diagnostics and Public Health, University of Verona Italy, Verona, Italy

23.1 Introduction

In a large proportion of deaths there is a need to examine samples taken from the deceased for the presence of substances in order to ascertain the contribution, if any, that they have made to the cause of death or if they might be in any other way relevant to the circumstances leading to death.

In this chapter, an account will be given of the clinico-pathological effects of substances that are most commonly encountered in forensic practice, which are subject to toxicological analysis.

The vast majority of deaths related to poisoning or other adverse effects are either related to intentional self-harm or are events in which the substances are taken or encountered accidentally, without the intention of causing death, but which may put the individual at risk. Differently from the past centuries, in modern times substances are used with homicidal intent less frequently, although with some notable exceptions.

23.2 Biological samples collected for toxicological analysis

In the living individual, typical biological samples for toxicological analysis include blood, urine, hair, saliva, breath, and gastric contents (from vomitus or after stomach wash). In the deceased, it is not only important to collect similar samples as above, but also to access other body fluids such as vitreous humour, bile, cerebrospinal fluid, as well as the organs and muscle tissue (Table 23.1).

Table 23.1   Recommended specimens collected in post-mortem cases.

Type of death	Recommended specimens
Suicides, motor vehicle crashes, industrial accidents	Blood, urine, vitreous humour, liver, stomach contents, hair
Homicides, suspicious	Blood, urine, vitreous humour, stomach contents, bile, liver, hair, nails
Drug-related	Blood, urine, vitreous humour, stomach contents, bile, liver, hair, nails
Volatile substance abuse	Blood, urine, vitreous humour, lung fluid or tied-off lung, liver
Heavy metal poisoning, exposure to other poisons	Blood, urine, vitreous humour, liver, hair, kidney, bone

23.2.1   Blood

Blood is often the specimen of choice for detecting, quantifying, and interpreting drugs and other toxic substances. Their concentrations (including the concentrations of their metabolites) may be useful for establishing when the substance was ingested and its effect on the deceased at the time of death. Blood taken after death presents problems due to post-mortem redistribution, decomposition, and changes of concentrations at different sites. In the decomposing body it may be difficult to obtain uncontaminated blood and one frequently relies on vitreous humour, if available.

23.2.2   Urine

Urine testing results do not directly correlate to drug effects at the time of sample collection because of the time it takes the body to eliminate these drugs or their metabolites in the urine. Often drug metabolites detected in urine are pharmacologically inactive. Urine testing is useful for demonstrating that a substance found in the urine had been in the blood at an earlier time. It is also important to know that the concentration of urine is highly influenced by the hydration condition of the subject and therefore the quantitative interpretation of the results is questionable. Also, it should be emphasised that the urinary elimination time of different drugs is extremely variable, ranging from hours up to weeks.

23.2.3   Liver

The liver is only occasionally retained for analysis. Many drugs become concentrated in the liver and can be found even when there are no levels in the blood. In this latter situation, however, interpretation of findings is complex. Being a fluid, bile is in general preferred to liver tissue.

23.2.4   Vitreous humour

The vitreous humour can be a useful fluid to screen for a range of drugs, and it is most commonly analysed for alcohol concentrations. Since the alcohol content in fluids and tissues is proportional to their content of water, its concentration in the vitreous humour is higher than in blood because of its higher content of water. Interpretation of other toxicological findings in the vitreous humour is more complex because for proper use of the data the diffusion rate of each molecule from blood into the vitreous humour needs to be known.

23.2.5 Stomach contents

Because drugs and poisons can often be ingested, stomach contents can provide important investigative clues. In a case of potential overdose or acute poisoning, high concentrations of drugs or toxins may be detected, depending on how much time elapsed between ingestion and death. In many cases of acute poisoning, undissolved capsules or tablets may be discovered, allowing relatively simple drug or poison identification. The total amount of a drug or poison present in the stomach is more important than its concentration; moreover, it should be taken into consideration that the drugs present in the stomach (particularly if not dissolved) have not been absorbed and consequently have not acted.

23.2.6 Hair and nails

Hair specimens, usually taken from the vertex posterior of the head, can be used to test for exposure to heavy metals and drugs over a period of weeks to months. Hair is predominantly used to test for controlled drugs and psychoactive compounds, such as amphetamines, cocaine, marijuana (THC), and heroin; more recently, assays have been created to determine if the deceased had been drinking heavily in the last few months before death. Drug analysis can also be done on fingernails and toenails in order to provide an even longer potential window of exposure than hair. However, relatively little is known about how the nails interact with drugs, thus interpretation of results is quite difficult. Hair content is affected by external contamination issues that can mitigate its value as forensic evidence, so special sample preparations in the laboratory may be needed for a given case.

23.3 Interpretation of toxicology results

One of the key questions in post-mortem toxicology is always 'Did a drug (and what drug) cause or contribute to the death?' (Ferner 2008).

The answer can be found by taking into account the following:

- the medical history

- the reported circumstances and manner of death

- the quantitative determination of the concentration of drugs and toxicants and their active metabolites in the biological samples of the deceased

- the knowledge of the effects of the compounds detected in the post-mortem samples

- the knowledge of the interactions between drugs and their role

- the exclusion of other potential causes of death or illness.

Modern forensic toxicology is based on the integrated interpretation of the results (both qualitative and quantitative) derived by the application of up-to-date analytical methods (in general,

GC/MS and/or HPLC/MS) to the post-mortem (and pre-mortem, if available) biological samples (blood, urine, bile, gastric content etc.)

Qualitative analysis indicates/excludes the presence of a substance in the sample, without providing accurate information with regards to the concentrations. A 'positive' result, indicating the presence of a drug or its metabolites in post-mortem samples at concentrations above the limit of detection of the used method, can lead to the reinforcement of suspicions of the linkage between the drug and the death. However, it is not possible to assess that the substance caused death, or that it did not, only by the mere positive/negative result of a qualitative test. Quantitative analysis, on the other hand, could help in assessing whether the concentration of a substance was potentially poisonous enough to cause death. This approach, however, must be adopted with great caution, taking into account the issues discussed below.

First of all, the analytical methods, and particularly immunometric assays (still used in clinical contexts), can erroneously give false-positive or false-negative results due to several conditions:

- lack of analytical specificity (interference from congeners of the analyte)

- lack of analytical sensitivity

- interference from compounds generated post mortem

Other possible causes of inaccuracy are: i. contamination of the sample, ii. post mortem degradation of the compound, iii. post-mortem redistribution (PMR) of substances. In particular, PMR is a complex process that starts immediately after death and includes the passive release of drugs from their reservoir sites (gastrointestinal tract, lungs, liver, kidney etc.) because of the autolysis of cells and the putrefactive process (Launiainen and Ojanperä 2014).

It is, therefore, extremely important to emphasise that for many drugs there are marked differences between post-mortem concentrations obtained from peripheral and central sites samples. Moreover, most drug assays in samples from living patients are made on plasma or serum, whereas whole blood is preferred during autopsies. In the most favourable circumstances, it is possible to withdraw whole blood flowing from femoral veins (because it is thought to be least susceptible to post-mortem change and redistribution).

Even in life, the concentration ratio between whole blood and plasma varies from drug to drug because of the different water content of the two fluids and the different water solubility of the compounds.

On the side of interpretation, quantitative analysis used to compare concentrations in suspected cases with concentrations previously attributed to poisoning is potentially misleading. The designation of 'lethal dose' in humans is, in fact, not straightforward and has not been defined for all known substances. In such cases, lethal doses determined in animal studies are instead considered, but relevant limitations arise from this approach because of major inter-species differences of the drug potency.

In conclusion, the answer to the question 'Does the post-mortem concentration indicate that the deceased died from the action of the drug or was the drug present incidentally?' can be given more easily when only one drug is involved and its PMR is negligible. In the other circumstances, a correct reply needs an accurate study of the particular case, including clinical history and autopsy

Table 23.2 Fatal concentrations (expressed in mg L^{-1} or kg) reported for most common substances of abuse.

Substance	Range	Mean
Morphine		
Blood	0.2–2.3	0.7
Urine	14–18	3.0
Liver	0.4–18	52
Cocaine		
Blood	0.9–21	5.2
Urine	1.4–215	47
Liver	0.1–20	4.3
Amphetamine		
Blood	0.5–41	8.6
Urine	25–700	237
Liver	4.3–74	30
Phencyclidine		
Blood	0.3–25	4.8
Urine	0.4–120	35
Liver	0.9–170	23

findings, the knowledge of the reliability of the analytical methods used, and, last but not least, a sound knowledge of the pharmacology and toxicology of all the compounds quantitatively identified in the samples.

As mentioned above, it is extremely difficult to define the fatal concentrations of a drug/poison in the bodily fluids. However, based on literature, data concentration ranges associated with the death of the subject have been published. Table 23.2 illustrates, as examples, the concentrations that have been reported for common abuse substances (Baselt and Cravey 1995)

23.4 Interactions between drugs

In the vast majority of clinical or forensic toxicology cases more than one drug is potentially involved because of multidrug therapy or abuse of more than one drug, including, potentially, alcohol.

Interactions between drugs can occur in the same way as interactions amongst chemicals that an individual may come into contact with at any given time before death. Compounds of a various nature administered by an individual, accidentally or not, may interact amongst themselves in a variety of ways, making the interpretation of data even more complicated. It is said that two chemicals ingested simultaneously produce an *additive* response when their effects are simply combined and equal to the sum of the effects of each agent given alone. The additive effects of two drugs with the same pharmacological action may prove fatal even though the individual drug concentrations are not per se toxic. When the combined effects of two compounds are greater than the sum of each agent given alone, a *synergistic* effect occurs. *Potentiation* occurs when a substance does not generally have a toxic effect on humans but, when added to another compound, it is toxic. Finally, when two substances interfere with each other's actions or one of the two interferes with the action of the other, the result is defined as *antagonism* (Klaassen and Watkins III 2010).

23.5 Assessing the cause of death

The difference between assessing the 'cause of death' and the 'mode (manner) of death' implies a difference in the actions to be taken following the discovery of a dead body. The cause of death is strictly related to a medical perspective, e.g. lung emboli, sepsis, hypertensive intracerebral haemorrhage, intoxication by cyanide etc. The circumstances surrounding death and their legal relevance refer to the mode or manner of death. Assigning a single, unique, and nameable cause of death is not always possible. Information on the cause of death can be gained from a number of clinical chemical parameters, symptoms, and syndromes in terms of particular poisons or groups of active substances. For example, when insulin, oral antidiabetic agent, and salicylate poisoning is suspected, hypoglycaemia may be present, whereas acidosis is indicative of ethyl glycol, methanol, salicylate, and cyanide poisoning. Agents such as carbon monoxide, cyanide, nitrate, nitrite, and aniline derivatives cause haemoglobin changes.

In addition to these primarily clinical aspects, a list of noticeable circumstances should indicate warning signals and the possibility of poisoning should be considered, for example:

- unexpected death of a young, otherwise healthy, person

- unconsciousness of a patient

- sudden illness in a child with no previously diagnosed disease

- known or suspected drug addiction

- easy access to toxic substances

- medication packaging found near the corpse

- injection sites or needle tracks (i.e. a line of needle-entry wounds).

Although variable approaches of dissection at autopsy exist, all autopsies generally include recording basic data (such as height and weight of the corpse, descriptions and weight of the organs) and taking specimens for further forensic toxicology and histopathology investigations.

The collection of specimens at autopsy for chemical-toxicological and histological or immuno-histo-chemical analysis commonly includes brain, liver, peripheral vein blood, bile fluid, vitreous humour, cerebrospinal fluid, urine, muscles, hair, and gastric content. However, depending on the line of inquiry, it is often necessary to take additional specimens for chemical-toxicological analysis, for example lungs (in headspace vials to detect, e.g. volatile gases).

Although most of the morphological features found during the autopsy do not provide information on the medicinal poison/s that caused the death, some distinctive features may suggest which toxic substance or class of substances caused the death. For example, corrosive poisons have the propensity to cause burns to the skin near and inside the mouth, on the mucosa of the oesophagus, and the stomach. The appearance of bright red colour to lividity, blood, and muscles suggests intoxication with carbon monoxide; a brownish colour suggests intoxication with methaemoglobin-forming substances (e.g. nitrites). Pulmonary oedema is commonly seen in opiate overdosing and hypertrophic cardiomyopathy associated with chronic abuse of cocaine.

23.6 Alcohol

In different forms, alcohol use and abuse is a phenomenon characterising almost the whole of humankind. In general, the term alcohol most often indicates ethanol (ethyl alcohol) present in beverages and food, but more properly this term includes also other alcohols, such as methanol (methyl alcohol) and isopropanol (isopropylic alcohol), which occasionally are consumed and may cause severe intoxication.

Morbidity and mortality related to the effects of alcohol are ubiquitous in forensic medical practice and regularly encountered by both the forensic medical examiner and the pathologist. Deaths involving alcohol consumption may be either directly or indirectly related to its use in a number of ways. Deaths resulting from the direct effects of alcohol that has been consumed within a short time before death include alcohol poisoning, when alcohol is mixed with drugs, complications from alcohol intoxication, and sudden death following bingeing. Death in heavily inebriated individuals may be due either directly or indirectly to intoxication. In any case, the excessive consumption of alcohol may impair judgement, psychomotor performance, and the ability to protect themselves from traumatic agents, and, consequently, increase the risk of the occurrence of accidents. Alcohol-related deaths may result from accidental events such as fires, road traffic accidents, falls, hypothermia, and drowning or from intentional events such as suicides and homicides.

As mentioned above, drunken individuals are often involved in fatal traumas, such as traffic fatalities, which may be caused by either drunken drivers or drunken pedestrians, or workplace accidents. According to the literature, these lethal fatalities involve drunken individual in 22–41% of cases (Sjögren et al. 2000). Moreover, there is substantial evidence that alcohol increases the risk of falls, which are not only extremely frequent but sometimes fatal. In fact, alcohol has been reported to be involved in 19–77% of fatal falls (and in 17–53% of non-fatal falls) (Hingson and Howland 1987). Drunken individuals may often fall down the stairs and subsequently suffer from head injuries. Carelessness or unsteady gait can cause falls from high places but this is less common (Saukko and Knight 2004). Alcohol-related falls differ from other types of falls because of a greater incidence of craniofacial injury and a greater severity of injury. This may be caused by the inhibition of protective reflexes in intoxicated patients and by the inability to outstretch their hands to break the fall, resulting in a greater incidence of head injuries.

Additionally, alcohol consumption may increase the occurrence of hazardous situations involving burn-causing agents. Frequently, drunken individuals fall asleep whilst smoking and the cigarette may start a fire. A different scenario involves the accidental spill of alcohol over a gas or kerosene heater, provoking a fatal fire (Saukko and Knight 2004). Consequently, the individual can be either intoxicated by carbon monoxide or affected by a burn injury.

With regards to alcohol-related drowning, it is common that drunken persons walk by a river or other waterways and fall into the water. However, death is not always caused by drowning but can occur by sudden vagal cardiac arrest as a consequence of the impact with cold water or by its sudden flood into the pharynx and larynx. The marked cutaneous vasodilatation favoured by alcohol is thought to arouse vasovagal shock (Saukko and Knight 2004).

A general exposure of the organism to cold and consequent hypothermia is worsened by alcohol. Although it has been suggested that alcohol can antagonise the arrhythmogenic effects of hypothermia and thus may be a protective factor against lethal hypothermia, alcohol intoxication must be regarded as a risk factor for hypothermia through a great variety of mechanisms. First, the effect of alcohol increases heat loss through peripheral vasodilation and increased sweat production but it decreases the perception of cold temperatures. Furthermore, alcohol impairs the ability to produce heat by causing muscle relaxation and, in high concentrations, it affects directly the hypothalamus centre for temperature regulation, whereas in chronic alcohol abusers the hypothalamic dysfunction is permanent because it is affected by Wernicke's encephalopathy.

By impairing psychomotor functions, alcohol intoxication also increases the risks of trauma and, subsequently, the risks of hypothermia. It, directly and indirectly, hampers an individual's ability to move away from an area of cold exposure (i.e. unconsciousness after head injury or severe injuries, such as fractured extremities which limit walking) (Turk 2010).

Alcohol intake is extremely common also in intentional events, as suggested by its involvement in 31–42% of suicides (Sjögren et al. 2000). For example, it is widely known that acute alcohol intoxication plays a causal role in suicidal behaviour because it affects the mood and cognitive states. In addition, chronic abuse of alcohol can have negative effects on mental health, causing psychiatric disorders such as depression, thus increasing the risk of suicide. Furthermore, current thinking indicates an association between alcohol dependence and impulsive suicide attempts (Smith et al. 1999).

Similarly, the majority of homicides are triggered by the aggressive behaviour stimulated by alcohol. Studies suggest that a moderate alcohol concentration in blood was found in a significant percentage of the victims of homicides (46–62.8%). Alcohol impairment reduces the reaction of victims, making them more vulnerable (Smith et al. 1999).

23.6.1   Physiological effects of alcohol with a forensic interest

Alcohol is a sedative drug which depresses the central nervous system in a dose-related manner. Amongst the first parts of the brain to be affected are those relating to acquired behaviour patterns and which provide for self-restraint.

Acute effects on the respiratory and cardiovascular systems are not usually important except at high concentrations of alcohol in blood, when potentially life-threatening depression of these systems occurs. However, alcohol also causes dilatation of the skin capillary blood vessels, giving rise to flushing of the face, but also the danger of death due to hypothermia in exposed conditions, as previously stated.

23.6.2   Effects on performance and behaviour

23.6.2.1 General effects and symptoms   The sedative effects of alcohol have, although with a high inter-individual variability, a dose-related manner of expression. Its apparent action as a stimulant, at low doses, is also due to depression of the inhibitory control mechanisms in the brain.

23.6.2.2 Schematic summary of alcohol-related effects

Blood alcohol level 0–50 mg dL^{-1}: No pronounced effects. There may be a slight flushing of the face, elevation of mood in company and tendency to talkativeness, feeling of well-being, beginning of loss of inhibition.

- 50–100 mg dL^{-1}: First obvious signs can be seen: flushed face, loss of inhibition and self-control, bravado in company; loss of some physical and mental coordination, including possible slurred speech and deterioration of sensory perception (sight, touch etc.); beginnings of the loss of judgement and self-critical faculty.
- 100–200 mg dL^{-1}: More pronounced effects: increasing physical and mental discoordination, impairment of concentration, slurred speech, staggering, sometimes nausea and sleepiness, nystagmus (involuntary side-to-side movement of the eyes); poor judgement and self-critical faculty, subjective feeling of being unwell.
- 200–300 mg dL^{-1}: Deterioration into unconsciousness, loss of pain sense, vision severely impaired.
- >300 mg dL^{-1}: Stupor and often coma.
- >450 mg dL^{-1}: Usually fatal, due to respiratory depression.

It is well established, however, that the above effects caused by alcohol ingestion strictly depend on previous exposure and habituation of the individual to alcohol, Moreover, effects also depend on the mood of the individual, on the environment in which alcohol is consumed, and, last but not least, on the co-administration of other substances (e.g. cannabis). Finally, alcohol-related effects on performance and behaviour depend significantly on the absorption status of alcohol: greater effects are observed during the absorption phase (when the alcohol level is rising), than in the elimination phase (when it is falling). As a result, it is not possible to predict exactly the effects of alcohol on an individual or to say with any certainty how a person would have behaved at a specific blood alcohol level.

Retrograde amnesia (i.e. the inability to recall an event which took place) due to alcohol intoxication is an established effect. However, in many jurisdictions, alcohol intoxication, intentional or negligent, cannot be pled as a defence, claiming that the defendant was 'unaware of what they were doing'. However, in case of alcohol intoxication due to 'force majeure', the responsibility of the subject can be abolished or diminished.

'Binge drinking' is a common pattern of alcohol consumption, particularly amongst youth. It has been defined as the consumption of five or more alcoholic drinks in one episode for men and four or more for women. It generally results in acute impairment and may have numerous adverse health consequences, including being the victim of a drunken attack, cases of liver cirrhosis or alcohol poisoning, and injuries in alcohol-related accidents, including car crashes.

The Director of the Centre for Public Health at Liverpool John Moores University has stated 'A lot of attention is paid towards binge drinking in younger people, but large numbers of people of all ages are simply drinking too much. High levels of excessive drinking are contributing to significant ill-health, which has immediate consequences for individuals and also puts pressure on the NHS, the police and the courts' (Hickley 2007). Concerning the effects on society of binge drinking, serious violence near pubs and clubs should be mentioned, as well as the most serious types of crimes, including murder and manslaughter.

23.6.3 Alcohol and driving

Basic skills, such as sensory, perceptual, cognitive, and motor control skills, which are strictly interconnected to perform complex activities, such as operating a motor vehicle in traffic, are affected by alcohol. The evidence that driving under the influence of alcohol increases traffic accidents is supported by unquestionable observational and experimental studies, the most famous of which was the Grand Rapids Study first published by Borkenstein et al. in 1964. Many other studies have followed up to the present time, leading to consistent data on an increase of crash risk when driving under alcohol influence (see also Canfield 2014, pp. 10–19). In particular, 'man–machine interaction' studies can be performed in the form of laboratory tests and simulation or actual driving in order to evaluate the complex abilities and actions required to drive motor vehicles and complex machinery (e.g. in the industrial field), such as attention, alertness, accommodation reflex, response to visual and auditory stimuli, deviation from the standard lateral position (SDLP), judgement of speed and safety distances. Laboratory tests include visual reaction time tests, attention, hand-eye coordination, and information processing tasks, state or dynamic body sway, and divided attention, which includes response competition and short memory.

In short, the effects of alcohol depend on the blood alcohol concentration (BAC), traditionally expressed as *mg* of ethanol per *dL* = 100 mL of blood, and more recently as *mg* of ethanol per *mL* of blood or *g* of ethanol per *L* of blood, but also on genetic and acquired individual variables, which cause changes of almost all the above-mentioned functions, primarily the reaction time to stimuli, in terms of perception as well as motor reaction, which is critical for fitness to drive vehicles. It is generally accepted that the traffic injury risk nearly doubles at BAC values of 60 mg/100 mL and is as much as 25-fold higher at 150 mg/100 mL compared with a non-intoxicated state.

Driving faults often depend on the following impairments:

– delayed reaction time
– excessive and inconsiderate speed caused by disinhibition and increased risk-taking
– inability of judgement of distance
– inability to perform more than one task at a time due to impaired distributive attention
– reduced vision field, visual acuity, and impaired light–dark adaptation
– hampered eye-hand co-ordination
– impaired vigilance
– alcohol-related drowsiness.

Although it is widely agreed that there is a direct correlation between BAC and biological effects, the interpretation of BAC may pose problems in specific conditions. If a significant proportion of the blood in the circulation is lost due to injury and replaced by transfusion, there will be a decrease in the blood alcohol level because of the dilution of the body water, as well as because of the metabolism which is proceeding concurrently. However, it is important to remember that the volume of water in the body in which ethanol is distributed is not only the 4 L or so of the blood volume but also the water in all other tissues. The vascularity of tissues, in fact, influences the distribution of alcohol, and their water content will determine the amount of alcohol present after equilibrium.

With regards to post-mortem samples, a few factors may alter the concentration of alcohol present in autopsy specimens. Post-mortem synthesis of alcohol may, indeed, occur due to ethanol production by microorganisms. This can be inhibited by adding a preservative to the samples and by storing them under refrigeration. In cases where putrefaction is present, it is recommended that, in addition to blood, other specimens are collected and analysed for the presence of alcohol (Winek and Esposito 1985). In this respect, the vitreous humour looks particularly suitable because of its seclusion from the sites where putrefaction starts.

23.6.3.1 Legislative measures Historically, the prevention of driving under the influence of alcohol was based on deterrence. Many European governments have established BAC limits when driving. Scientists have contributed to the establishment of BAC limits with data from experimental and epidemiological studies to identify the alcohol levels that produce driving skills impairment and increase road accidents rates. In Europe, after the introduction of the first legislation there was an immediate and substantial trend of reduction in traffic accidents following by stalling of this phenomenon. To hinder this, many countries have lowered their legally accepted blood alcohol limit from 80 to 50 mg/100 mL, and in some classes of drivers (e.g. professional drivers, drivers holding the driving licence for less than three years etc.), BAC should be 'not detectable'. Other countries have adopted a zero tolerance policy for all drivers. This trend reflects the international scientific consensus that there is no safe limit for alcohol consumption in relation to driving skills. Generally, the sanctions are withdrawal of a driving licence, mandatory alcoholism treatment, and licence plate or vehicle impoundment, but may also include gaol sentences.

23.6.4 Acute alcohol poisoning

Alcohol intoxication refers to a clinically harmful condition induced by ingestion of alcohol when alcohol and its metabolites accumulate in the blood faster than they can be metabolised by the liver (Jung and Namkoong 2014). When deaths are attributable to the acute excessive intake of alcohol, it is in general possible to distinguish between two main categories:

– acute alcoholic poisoning (uncomplicated)
– acute alcoholic poisoning associated with some form of obstructive asphyxia.

People dying from acute alcohol poisoning range from the very young to older age groups. They are predominantly male and may have a history of chronic alcohol abuse but, in some cases, it was their first episode of excessive consumption of alcohol.

As discussed in various sections of the present chapter, although alcohol has the potential to affect almost every organ, the major adverse effects of alcohol that gain clinical attention are the neurological, gastrointestinal, cardiovascular, and respiratory problems. Excessive alcohol ingestion not only causes medical complications, but has also been identified as a risk factor for suicide and injury. In acutely poisoned patients, there is a high prevalence of intentional suicide attempts (Woo et al. 2013).

23.6.4.1 Post-mortem findings in acute alcoholic poisoning Although the general appearance may prove non-specific after a death by acute alcohol poisoning, there are some findings that could appear explicit:

• asphyxial signs may be present, such as congestion and cyanosis, particularly in relation to the position of the body

- frequently the deceased is found in a prone position with the upper air passages blocked

- hypostasis is florid and dark, and contrasts markedly with the blanched areas which have been in contact with the underlying surface. These contact points on the face are commonly the tip of the nose, mouth, chin and parts of the side of the face, depending on how the head was inclined.
    Vomitus may be visible, but not infrequently regurgitated stomach contents are only found within the mouth with very little evidence that a significant amount has been deposited onto the face, clothing, and elsewhere. In such cases, it is important to assess:
    o whether the deceased had vomited and inhaled stomach contents, thus causing asphyxia and death
    o whether vomiting resulted as the terminal event in a person who was dying as a consequence of central respiratory depression per se
    o whether resuscitation, particularly positive pressure ventilation, propelled food particles to the smaller airways, thus leading the pathologist to erroneously attach significance to this finding.

Not infrequently, there is a distinct smell of 'alcohol'. However, it is surprising how often there is no such odour in cases where subsequent analysis reveals a high level of alcohol in the blood. In any case, detection and intensity of smell or its absence is of no guidance as to the degree of intoxication. Occasionally, the foetor of diabetic ketoacidosis may be confused with alcohol.

Alcoholics themselves, even after bingeing and no alcohol being found on analysis, may be ketotic.

Internal examination, on the other hand, will commonly reveal signs of central asphyxia, unless complicated by some form of airway obstruction, and cerebral oedema. In particular, the respiratory system may be involved in pulmonary oedema, congestion, and consequences of aspirated material in airways. Concerning gastrointestinal effects, reactive gastritis, sometimes with fresh or altered blood in the stomach or intestine, may be recorded. As previously mentioned, there may or may not be pathological changes to various organs (e.g. liver) if there is a history of chronic alcohol abuse.

23.6.4.2 The 'fatal level' in acute alcoholic poisoning
Fatal cases of acute alcohol intoxication may occur over a wide range of BAC. In particular, BAC in fatal cases of acute alcohol intoxication complicated by aspiration is often lower than in those cases where there is no evidence of aspiration at autopsy. Conversely, individuals with a history of alcohol abuse or evidence of alcoholic liver disease tend to have a higher BAC.

Fatal acute alcohol intoxication results when the alcohol concentration in the brain rises to a level paralysing the respiratory centre. According to a study conducted by Li et al. 149 deaths due to acute alcohol intoxication were recorded in the state of Maryland within eight years (2004–2012) (Li et al. 2017). Age distribution ranged from 16 to 65 years (mean 37 years) and 19.5% of the individuals were 16–25 years, three of them teenagers. A vast majority of the 149 cases (113) were found unresponsive in their residence. Alcohol analysis was carried out on different biological specimens collected at autopsy: in the heart, BAC ranged from 170 to 760 mg/100 mL (mean = 410 mg/100 mL), whereas the peripheral BAC ranged from 180 to 690 mg/100 mL (mean = 400 mg/100 mL) and in the vitreous humour alcohol concentration ranged from 250 to 700 mg/100 mL (mean = 480 mg/100 mL).

Cases of alcohol poisoning are occasionally seen in young children who may accidentally drink from a glass or bottle, particularly in households where alcohol is frequently abused and liquor may be left around. In these instances, the intoxication is particularly severe because:

- youngsters may rapidly drink large amounts of alcohol in relation to their body weight, causing high BAC

- the ability of under-fives to metabolise alcohol is limited as hepatic alcohol dehydrogenase activity is not mature.

Consequently, the potential for neurological depression is greater in this age group. Hypoglycaemia from alcohol ingestion is particularly common in young children because of inhibition of hepatic gluconeogenesis.

23.6.5 Alcoholic ketoacidosis

Alcoholic ketoacidosis (AKA) is an acute metabolic acidosis that typically occurs in people who chronically abuse alcohol and have a recent history of binge drinking, little or no food intake, and persistent vomiting. The suggestion by Dillon et al. (1940) that ketoacidosis might occur in non-diabetic, chronic alcohol abusers was not supported by further observations until 1970, when Jenkins et al. reported on three non-diabetic individuals with a history of chronic, heavy alcohol consumption and persistent ketoacidosis (Jenkins et al. 1971). Similar case studies were subsequently described with remarkably consistent features. all patients of these reports had a history of chronic alcohol abuse and recent particularly excessive intake, abruptly terminated some days prior due to abdominal pain and repeated vomiting (Palmiere and Augsburger 2014).

AKA is characterised by elevated serum ketone levels and a high anion gap. A concomitant metabolic alkalosis (secondary to vomiting and volume depletion) is common.

Although AKA most commonly occurs in adults with alcoholism, AKA has been reported in less-experienced drinkers of all ages. On physical examination, in addition to the typical signs of chronic alcohol abuse, these patients may present hyperventilation, tachycardia, hypotension, and signs of dehydration due to the decreased fluid intake and severe vomiting mentioned above. Though these subjects are in overall poor condition, the syndrome does not include any actual loss of consciousness and affected patients are usually alert and lucid despite the severity of the acidosis and marked ketonaemia (Rehman 2012).

AKA is a result of prolonged starvation with glycogen depletion, counter-regulatory hormone production, dehydration, and the metabolism of ethanol itself. When the dietary intake of carbohydrates is insufficient to supply glucose for the body's needs and hepatic glycogen stores are depleted by fasting, ketones are produced in the liver as an alternative source of energy. Moreover, decreased insulin activity, increased counter-regulatory hormone levels (primarily glucagon, but also cortisol, catecholamines, and growth hormone), and volume depletion all play a role in ketogenesis. Prolonged vomiting leads to dehydration, which decreases renal perfusion, thereby limiting urinary excretion of ketoacids. In addition, volume depletion increases the concentration of counter-regulatory hormones, further stimulating lipolysis and ketogenesis.

In the case of excessive consumption of alcohol, ethanol undergoes oxidisation to acetaldehyde, which is itself oxidised to acetate. A shift in the β-hydroxybutyrate (β-OH) to acetyl acetate (AcAc) equilibrium occurs towards β-OH. The latter is the predominate ketone in the AKA condition.

23.6.6 Causes of death directly related to chronic alcohol abuse

Alcohol affects many organ systems, most notably the central nervous system, the liver, and the cardiovascular system. From data obtained in autopsy studies, it appears that between 10 and 15% of alcoholics have cirrhosis at the time of death. Co-factors such as chronic infection with hepatitis C virus may increase the risk of the development of cirrhosis in an alcoholic. Amongst the typical organs affected by chronic alcohol abuse, the central and peripheral nervous system were identified by Carl Wernicke and Sergei Korsakoff at the end of the nineteenth century. Their observations were merged in the well-known Wernicke–Korsakoff syndrome, which, on the pathological side, is characterised by brain atrophy (in the mammillary bodies of the brain, thalamus, periaqueductal grey, third ventricle, cerebellum, and frontal lobe).

The cardiovascular system is also highly affected by sustained alcohol consumption, the alcoholic cardiomiopathy being its most typical pathological consequence, but other left ventricular dysfunctions, including hypertensive heart disease, ischemic cardiomyopathy, and heart valve disease, have been reported.

In general, women who drink an equal amount of alcohol to men are at higher risk than men for the development of alcohol-related diseases, possibly because of a decreased metabolism of alcohol.

Chronic alcohol abuse may cause death even without a concurrent acute ethanol intoxication. In fact, alcohol affects many organs, including the cardiovascular, endocrine, neurological, and metabolic systems, causing a variety of anatomic changes in the liver, heart, brain, and pancreas.

Accordingly, chronic alcoholics may be affected by a heterogeneous group of diseases associated with the effects of alcohol (e.g. acute and chronic pancreatitis, hepatic steatosis/cirrhosis with esophageal varices, alcoholic cardiomyopathy, gastritis, etc.), which can directly or indirectly cause death. Fatal bleeding from rupture of the oesophageal varices is a typical cause of death in alcoholics with severe hepatic cirrhosis with portal hypertension. In addition, prolonged alcohol abuse can provoke dilated cardiomyopathy, which may lead to sudden cardiac death. Sometimes, sudden death in chronic alcoholics may be due to sudden arrhythmic cardiac death (e.g. alcohol provokes prolongation of the QT interval) or alteration of the electrolytic/metabolic state (e.g. alcoholic ketoacidosis). In this case the only findings at post mortem are a fatty liver and a negative or low BAC. In fact, it is acknowledged that the presence of steatosis at post mortem is quite a sensitive indication of high alcohol consumption.

The diagnosis of associated metabolic derangements, including alcoholic ketoacidosis, may be aided with the analysis of vitreous electrolytes and hydroxybutyric acid. Alcohol can affect all body systems and a summary of such effects is given in Table 23.3.

23.6.7 Biomarkers of Chronic alcohol abuse

The need for objective methods allowing the diagnosis of alcohol abuse has always been of crucial importance in several contexts of forensic interest. The diagnosis of alcohol use disorders has long relied on the use of specific questionnaires (such as CAGE, AUDIT, or MAST) and clinical laboratory tests (including blood ethanol, serum γ-glutamyltransferase (GGT), carbohydrate-deficient

Table 23.3 Effects of alcohol on body systems.

Affected body system	Related effects
Blood	Thrombocytopenia
	Leucopenia
	Haemolytic anaemia
	Macrocytic sideroblastic anaemia
	Biochemical markers
Endocrine	Cushing's syndrome
	Thyroid
	Pituitary
	Hypoglycaemia
Vitamin deficiency	B1 (thiamine), B2, B6 eg beri beri (B1)
	Wernicke–Korsakoff (B complex, especially B1)
Respiratory	Lowered resistance to infection, e.g. tuberculosis
	Carcinoma of larynx (especially supraglottic)
Musculo-skeletal	Acute myopathy
	Chronic myopathy
	Dupuytren's contractures
	Neurogenic osteoarthropathy
Perinatal	Alcohol-foetal syndrome
	Spontaneous abortion
Skin	Hyperaemia
	Telangiectases
	Rhinophyma
	Erythema of palms and soles
	Spider naevi
	Porphyria cutanea tarda
Genital	Testicular atrophy
	Gynaecomastia
	Impotence

transferrin (CDT), and mean corpuscular volume of erythrocytes (MCV)). Since questionnaires depend on self-reports, they should be avoided in cases of forensic interest, when a diagnosis of alcohol abuse could lead to a limitation of the rights of the person. Laboratory tests based on biomarkers, on the other hand, are effective and objective in the determination of alcohol abuse (Niemelä 2007). The most common alcohol abuse biomarkers will briefly be described here.

23.6.8 Ethanol and its metabolites

Determining the presence of ethanol in biological fluids is the first approach when recent consumption of alcohol needs to be considered and as such requires the use of highly accurate, sensitive, and selective analytical methods. The gold standard for this determination is nowadays gas chromatography with flame ionisation detection subsequent to a headspace sample injection (HS-GC-FID). Ethanol determination can also be carried out on breath samples, providing a non-invasive, simple, and rapid approach, typically employed by police forces at roadside checkpoints, sometimes in conjunction with blood samples, to identify driving under the influence (DUI) drivers. In breath analysis, the corresponding BAC is indirectly estimated by applying a blood/breath conversion factor, which, in different studies, may vary between 2100:1 and 2300:1. This conversion factor was obtained from validation studies of breath analysers and is defined as the equilibrium that is created during the partitioning of ethanol in blood vessels to breath exhaled from the lungs. Variability in this ratio occurs not only between but within individuals, primarily due to arteriovenous differences in alcohol concentrations during the early stage of alcohol absorption in the body. During this stage, ethanol is found at higher concentrations in arterial blood transporting the newly absorbed alcohol to body tissues and in lower concentrations in venous blood carrying blood away from yet equilibrated tissues. Thus, the ratio of BAC to breath alcohol concentration (BrAC) will be lower in this early stage because BAC is drawn from venous blood and BrAC is measured using exhaled air from arterial blood in the lungs (Jaffe et al. 2013).

Qualitatively, ethanol may also be determined on an alternative biological matrix since a fraction of the ingested alcohol is excreted through sweat. Such an approach is more common when abstinence of the subject needs to be investigated. Sample collection occurs through water- and tamper-proof patches that are worn for days/weeks. Figure 23.1 shows the concentration/time ratio of ethanol determination in the most common biological matrices. One can appreciate how urine is the matrix in which ethanol may be determined for the longest time compared to other biological fluids.

In some cases, determining ethanol metabolites may also prove useful. Ethanol, similar to most xenobiotics, undergoes phase 1 and 2 metabolism reactions. In particular, the latter consists of the conjugation of the molecule with an endogenous substance, such as glucuronic acid and sulphate, with the final production of ethyl glucuronide (EtG) and ethyl sulphate (EtS), respectively. EtG and EtS require advanced analytical methods (GC–MS and LC–MS) for their determination in biological matrices where they are present at low concentrations. Such analysis is widely applied in forensic contexts where abstinence from alcohol needs to be proved, such as for the re-granting of a driving licence for DUI or for alcoholics undergoing programmed detoxification. Analogously to psychoactive drugs, when studying alcohol abuse histories the determination of EtG is widely applied in hair, where EtG can be determined at pg/mg concentrations (Kintz 2012).

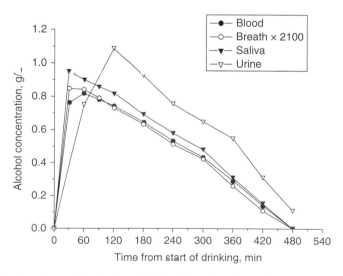

Figure 23.1   Mean concentration–time profiles of ethanol in blood, breath, saliva, and urine. Source: Adapted from Garriott, 2008.

Phosphatidylethanol (PEth) is a non-oxidative metabolite of ethanol that is employed as a valuable biomarker of alcohol abuse. Typically, the formation of PEth does not occur after consumption of a single dose of ethanol nor even after a weekend of heavy drinking. This characteristic makes PEth useful to investigate chronic abuse, independently from the alcohol concentration measured in blood or urine.

A different product of ethanol catabolism is represented by the fatty acid ethyl esters (FAEEs), derived by enzymatic reactions between the ingested ethanol and free fatty acids (both saturated and unsaturated). These can be detected in blood and other body organs after heavy consumption of alcohol. Interestingly enough, both FAEEs and the enzymes required for their synthesis are located in organs and tissues where hepatic damage tends to occur after a period of alcohol abuse (e.g. liver, brain, and pancreas). Alternative matrices for FAEE detection are hair and meconium; the latter, in particular, suggests that the foetus was exposed to alcohol during its development hence it becomes useful for postpartum health or for forensic parenting assessment.

23.6.9 Liver enzymes

Liver enzymes that are usually analysed in routine clinical tests in order to investigate a potential liver damage include GGT, aspartate aminotransferase (AST), and alanine aminotransferase (ALT). These parameters, although traditionally believed crucial for the diagnosis of alcohol abuse, are never determined alone because of a low diagnostic sensitivity. In fact, it is known that a heavy ingestion (>60 g/per day for a few weeks) of alcohol causes a leak of GGT from hepatocytes into the bloodstream. On the other hand, elevated values of GGT are also observed in cases of non-alcohol-related circumstances such as carcinoma, smoke, pregnancy, obesity, and diabetes. In a similar way, ALT and AST may or may not indicate alcohol-related liver pathologies. Additionally, the ALT/AST ratio is often employed as a screening approach in the general population or in follow-up investigations on alcoholics, being indicative of chronic alcohol abuse when it is higher than 2.0.

23.6.10 MCV

Liver enzymes results are often associated with another simple and cheap routine test that measures the mean corpuscular volume of erythrocytes. Red blood cells undergo enlargement (macrocytosis caused by folate deficiency) after a period of alcohol abuse (four to eight weeks). Although its diagnostic specificity is higher than the results of liver enzyme measurements, the MCV test is less sensitive as a biomarker of abuse of alcohol.

23.6.11 CDT

Transferrin (Tf), the main iron-transporting protein in plasma, has two glycosylation sites, composed of a bi- to tetra-antennary carbohydrate chain terminating with sialic acid residues. As a result of differences in glycosylation, normal human Tf occurs in a group of several glycoforms with zero to six (or more) sialic acid residues per molecule (Figure 23.2). The major human Tf glycoform in physiological conditions consists of four sialic acid residues (tetrasialo-Tf) and determines about 80% of total Tf. However, a regular consumption of 50–80 g of alcohol per day for at least one week is reflected in an increase of the less glycosylated forms of Tf known as CDT, such as asialo-Tf (no glycosylation) and disialo-Tf (Stibler 1991).

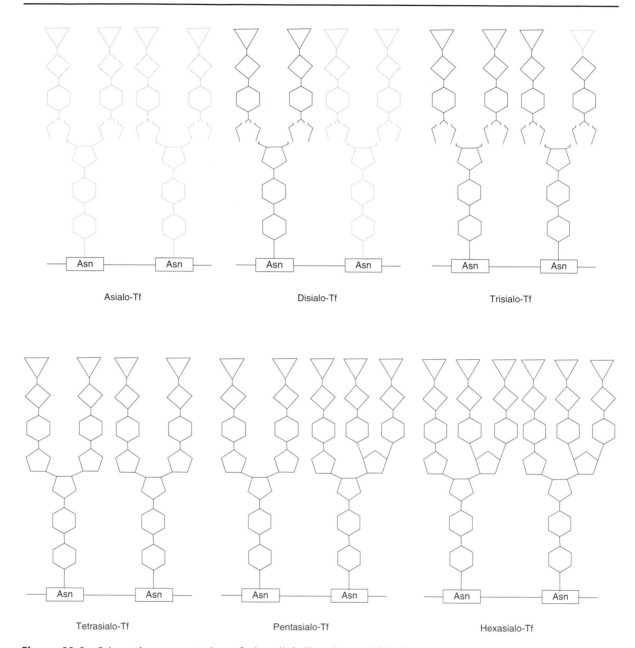

Figure 23.2 Schematic representation of the clinically relevant Tf isoforms. Asn, asparagine residue; hexagon, *N*-acetylglucosamine; pentagon, mannose; diamond, galactose; triangle, sialic acid. Source: de Jong (2016).

Unlike the traditional diagnostic approach to investigating alcohol abuse described above, CDT is not a marker of liver dysfunction or pathology and is therefore valuable to identify alcohol abusers in forensic contexts, where the aim is not clinical but focused on the risks for the public associated with alcohol abuse (e.g. traffic and workplace accidents). For this reason, CDT determination is now widely employed as the most specific biomarker of chronic alcohol abuse, particularly in traffic medicine, where it has proved to be an excellent marker of increased risk of alcohol-related road collisions (Bortolotti et al. 2015).

23.7   Alcohol withdrawal syndrome

When an individual reduces or stops alcohol consumption after a prolonged period of heavy drinking, it is likely that a specific set of symptoms will be reported. In fact, about 50% of alcoholics commonly develop clinically relevant symptoms of withdrawal, collectively known as alcohol withdrawal syndrome (AWS) (Brousse et al. 2012). On the other hand, alcohol-dependent patients often drink to relieve or avoid the unpleasant symptoms of withdrawal that are experienced after prolonged periods of excessive alcohol intake. In reality, drinking with the aim of achieving withdrawal relief is one of the diagnostic criteria for distinguishing between alcohol abuse and alcohol dependence (Cunningham et al. 2013). AWS typically occurs amongst alcoholics when they are hospitalised for other illnesses, since while in hospital they have no access to alcohol and consequently are forced into abstinence. On the other hand, severe AWS is less common amongst patients undergoing programmed detoxification because the application of these programmes includes measures to prevent AWS.

Three sets of symptoms describe the chronological and clinical stages of AWS:

- autonomic hyperactivity, with symptoms such as nausea, vomiting, anxiety, trembling, sweating, and agitation, occurs within hours of the last drink and has its peak within 24 hours

- within 24–48 hours of abstinence neuronal excitation with seizures and global confusion occurs

- finally, *delirium tremens* and alcohol withdrawal delirium (AWD), which consist of auditory and visual hallucinations, disorientation, pronounced autonomic hyperactivity, confusion, and impaired attention, occur and can be more protracted.

AWD may culminate, if untreated, in death subsequent to respiratory and/or cardiovascular failure.

Table 23.4   Summary of interactions of alcohol with other drugs.

Drugs	Effect of combination with alcohol
Amphetamines	Complex interaction between a stimulant and a depressant drug
	Net effect depends on the dose of each drug and the activity involved
Antidepressants	Possibility of hypertension due to tyramine content of some beverages
	Mono-amine oxidase inhibitors may inhibit the metabolism of alcohol
	Increased impairment of psychomotor skills
Antihistamines	Enhancement of drowsiness caused by some antihistamines
Cannabis	Additive deleterious effects on psychomotor performance
Cocaine	Both ethanol and cocaine increase the amount of dopamine in the brain
	The concurrent use of cocaine and alcohol produces another psychoactive substance, cocaethylene, showing biological activity similar to that of cocaine, but with a plasma half-life three to five times higher
	Cocaethylene has been associated with seizures, liver damage, and an 18- to 25-fold increase over cocaine alone in risk for immediate death
Paracetamol	Danger of severe liver damage
	Lowering of lethal dose of paracetamol

23.8 Alcohol interaction with other drugs

Alcohol can have different effects with both legal and illegal drugs, for example it may enhance the sedating effect of sleeping tablets and opiate-based pain relief or increase the possibility of paracetamol causing liver damage. A summary of the interaction of alcohol with other drugs is shown in Table 23.4

References

Baselt, R.C. and Cravey, R.H. (1995). *Disposition of Toxic Drugs and Chmicals in Man*, 4e. Foster City, CA: Chemical Toxicology Institute.

Bortolotti, F., Micciolo, R., Canal, L., and Tagliaro, F. (2015). First objective association between elevated carbohydrate-deficient transferrin concentrations and alcohol-related traffic accidents. *Alcoholism: Clin. Exper. Res.* 39 (11): 2108–2114. https://doi.org/10.1111/acer.12879.

Brousse, G., Arnaud, B., Vorspan, F. et al. (2012). Alteration of glutamate/GABA balance during acute alcohol withdrawal in emergency department: a prospective analysis. *Alcohol Alcohol* 47: 501–508.

Canfield, D.V., Dubowski, K.M., Cowan, M., and Harding, P.M. (2014). Alcohol limits and public safety. *Foren. Sci. Rev.* 26: 10–19.

Cunningham, C.L., Fidler, T.L., Murphy, K.V. et al. (2013). Time-dependent negative reinforcement of ethanol intake by alleviation of acute withdrawal. *Alcohol and Alcoholism* 73: 249–255.

Dillon, E.S., Dyer, W.W., and Smelo, L.S. (1940). Ketone acidosis in nondiabetic adults. *Med. Clin. North Am.* 24: 1813–1822.

Ferner, R.E. (2008). Post-mortem clinical pharmacology. *Br. J. Clin. Pharmacol.* 66 (4): 430–443.

Garriott, J.C. (2008). *Garriot's Medicolegal Aspects of Alcohol*, 5e. Lawyers & Judges Publishing Company.

Hickley, M. (2007) 'Binge-drinking epidemic increases as alcohol related A&E admissions soar', Daily Mail Online.

Hingson, R. and Howland, J. (1987). Alcohol as a risk factor for injury or death resulting from accidental falls: a review of the literature. *J. Stud. Alcohol.* 48 (3): 212–219. doi:10.15288/jsa.1987.48.212.

Jaffe, D.H., Siman-Tov, M., Gopher, A., and Peleg, K. (2013). Variability in the blood/breath alcohol ratio and implications for evidentiary purposes. *J. Forensic Sci.* 58 (5): 1233–1237. https://doi.org/10.1111/1556-4029.12157.

Jenkins, D.W., Eckel, R.E., and Craig, J.W. (1971). Alcoholic Ketoacidosis. *JAMA* 217 (2): 177–183.

de Jong, G. (2016). *Capillary Electrophoresis–Mass Spectrometry (CE-MS): Principles and Applications*. Wiley-VCH.

Jung, Y. and Namkoong, K. (2014). Alcohol: intoxication and poisoning – diagnosis and treatment. In: *Handbook of Clinical Neurology*, 115–121. Elsevier.

Kintz, P. (2012). Consensus of the society of hair testing on hair testing for chronic excessive alcohol consumption 2011. *Forensic Sci. Int.* 218 (1–3): 2.

Klaassen, C.D. and Watkins, J.B. III (2010). *Casarett & Doull's Essentials of Toxicology*. McGraw Hill Lange.

Launiainen, T. and Ojanperä, I. (2014). Drug concentrations in post-mortem femoral blood compared with therapeutic concentrations in plasma. *Drug Test. Anal.* 6: 308–316.

Li, R., Hu, L., Hu, L. et al. (2017). Evaluation of acute alcohol intoxication as the primary cause of death: a diagnostic challenge for forensic pathologists. *J. Forensic Sci.* 62 (5): 1213–1219. https://doi.org/10.1111/1556-4029.13412.

Niemelä, O. (2007). Biomarkers in alcoholism. *Clin. Chim. Acta* 377: 39–49.

Palmiere, C. and Augsburger, M. (2014). The postmortem diagnosis of alcoholic ketoacidosis. *Alcohol Alcohol.* 49 (3): 271–281.

Rehman, H.U. (2012). A woman with ketoacidosis but not diabetes. *BMJl* 344: 1535–1536.

Saukko, P. and Knight, B. (2004). *Knight's Forensic Pathology*, 3e. London: CRC Press.

Sjögren, H., Eriksson, A., and Ahlm, K. (2000). Alcohol and unnatural deaths in Sweden: a medico-legal autopsy study. *J. Stud. Alcohol.* 61 (4): 507–514. doi:10.15288/jsa.2000.61.507.

Smith, G., Branas, C., and Miller, T. (1999). Fatal nontraffic injuries involving alcohol: a metaanalysis. *Ann. Emerg. Med.* 33 (6): 659–668.

Stibler, H. (1991). Carbohydrate-deficient transferrin in serum: a new marker of potentially harmful alcohol consumption reviewed. *Clin. Chem.* 37 (12): 2029–2037.

Turk, E.E. (2010). Hypothermia. *Forensic Sci. Med. Pathol.* 6 (2): 106–115. https://doi.org/10.1007/s12024-010-9142-4.

Winek, C.L. and Esposito, F.M. (1985). Blood alcohol concentrations: factors affecting predictions. *Legal Med.* 1985: 34–61.

Woo, S.H., Woon J.L., Won J.J., Yeon Y.K. and Se M.C. (2013). Blood alcohol concentration and self-reported alcohol ingestion in acute poisoned patients who visited an emergency department. *Scand. J. Trauma. Resus. Emerg. Med.* 21: 24. https://doi.org/10.1186/1757-7241-21-24.

24
Illicit Drug Use

Giovanni Serpelloni[1] and Claudia Rimondo[2]

[1] UOC Addiction Department, Verona, Italy

[2] Department of Diagnostic and Public Health, University of Verona, Verona, Italy

In this chapter the main substances of abuse which may have effects on the human being and are responsible for clinical intoxications are discussed, including related legislation to control them.

24.1 Definitions

Some pertinent definitions in relation to drug abuse are set out below.

24.1.1 Illicit drug use

Illicit drug use includes the non-medical use of several drugs that are prohibited by international law, that is, substances listed in the schedules for the 1961 and 1971 Conventions and tables for the 1988 Convention. These drugs include cannabis, heroin and other opioids, cocaine, amphetamine-type stimulants, and MDMA (ecstasy) (Degenhardt et al. 2004).

24.1.2 Substance abuse

According to the World Health Organization, substance abuse relates to harmful or hazardous use of psychoactive substances, alcohol, and illicit drugs (WHO 2018). In this respect, harmful use is a pattern of psychoactive substance use that is causing damage to health, physical (e.g. hepatitis following injection of drugs) or mental (e.g. depressive episodes secondary to heavy alcohol intake). Harmful

Essential Forensic Medicine, First Edition. Edited by Peter Vanezis.
© 2020 John Wiley & Sons Ltd. Published 2020 by John Wiley & Sons Ltd.

use commonly has adverse social consequences. In the context of international drug control, drug abuse constitutes the use of any substance under international control other than for therapeutic indications, in excessive dose levels, or over an unjustified period of time (UNODC 2003a,b).

24.1.3   Drug misuse

Drug misuse refers to the use of a substance with an aim not consistent with legal or medical rules (WHO 2018). It has a negative impact on health or functioning and may take the form of drug dependence or be part of a wider spectrum of problematic or harmful behaviour (National Collaborating Centre for Mental Health 2008). In the UK, the Advisory Council on the Misuse of Drugs (ACMD) defines problem drug use as a condition that may lead an individual to experience social, psychological, physical or legal problems related to intoxication and/or regular consumption, and/or dependence (National Collaborating Centre for Mental Health 2008).

24.1.4   Recreational drug use

Recreational drug use is the use of psychoactive substances to 'have fun' in nightlife settings (EMCDDA 2002). The main reasons people take drugs occasionally is to enjoy dancing and have fun, to boost confidence and energy or offer new experiences (Calafat et al. 2001). Alcohol remains the psychoactive substance most frequently and widely used for recreational purposes, and t is often associated with drug use in recreational circumstances.

24.1.5   Problem drug use

Problem drug use is defined by the European Monitoring Centre for Drugs and Drug Addition (EMCDDA) as 'injecting drug use or long duration or regular use of opioids, cocaine and/or amphetamines'. This definition specifically includes regular or long-term use of prescribed opioids but it does not include their rare or irregular use nor the use of ecstasy or cannabis (EMCDDA 2018). Godfrey et al. (2004) stated that problem drug users are generally those whose drug use is no longer controlled or undertaken for recreational purposes and where drugs have become a more essential element of an individual's life. The United Nations Drug Control Programme (UNDCP) identifies 'problem drugs' based on 'the extent to which the use of a certain drug leads to treatment demand, emergency room visits (due to overdose), drug-related morbidity (including HIV/AIDS, hepatitis etc.), mortality and other drug-related social ills' (UNDCP 2000).

24.1.6   Tolerance

According to the United Nations Office on Drugs and Crime (UNODC), tolerance is a decrease in response to a drug dose that occurs with continued use. In other words, increased drug doses are required to achieve the effects originally produced by lower doses (UNODC 2016). Similarly, according to the National Institute on Drug Abuse, tolerance occurs when a person no longer responds to the drug in the way s/he initially responded. That is, it is necessary to assume a higher dose of the drug to reach the same level of response achieved initially (NIDA 2007). The development of tolerance is not the same as addiction, although many drugs producing tolerance may have addictive potential. Tolerance to drugs can be produced by several different neurobiological mechanisms (NIDA 2007). Tolerance and dependence may only be incidentally associated with addiction as a result of a non-specific adaptation by the body to the presence of a drug (Miller et al. 1987).

24.1.7 Chronic drug use

Chronic drug use is the prolonged, continuous, frequent, long-term or heavy use of a substance over a certain period of time, leading to severe adverse health effects (UNODC 2003a,b).

24.1.8 Addiction

Addiction is defined as a chronic, relapsing brain disease that is characterised by compulsive drug seeking and use, despite harmful consequences. It is considered a brain disease because drugs change the brain; they change its structure and how it works. These brain changes can be long lasting and can lead to many harmful, often self-destructive, behaviours (NIDA 2016). According to the American Psychiatric Association 1994 and the World Health Organization 1992, drug addiction is a chronically relapsing disorder that is defined by both a compulsion to take the drug with a narrowing of the behavioural repertoire towards excessive drug intake, and a loss of control in limiting intake (Koob and Le Moal 2001). The UNODC refers to addiction as the repeated use of a psychoactive substance or substances to the extent that the user is periodically or chronically intoxicated, shows a compulsion to take the preferred substance (substances), has great difficulty in voluntarily ceasing or modifying substance use, and exhibits determination to obtain psychoactive substances by almost any means (UNODC 2003a,b).

24.1.9 Craving

Over the past 40 years, drug craving has been a controversial topic. In the current version of the International Classification of Diseases (ICD-10-2016), craving is listed as one of the six features of psychoactive substance dependence. Most researchers assume that craving is a subjective experience of wanting to use a drug. This definition has three distinct elements: craving is conscious, craving is best captured by an expression of desire, and that desire is directed towards the use of a specific drug (Drummond 2001; Tiffany et al. 2008).

24.2 Type of substances

The main substances of abuse that may have effects on the human body and which are responsible for clinical intoxications are described in the following sections.

24.2.1 Cannabis

The cannabis plant and its products are made of many chemical components with more or less known biological activity, including over 60 phyto-cannabinoids (cannabinoids of vegetal origin). The main phyto-cannabinoids are tetrahydrocannabinol (THC), cannabidiol (CBD), cannabinol (CBN), cannabigerol (CBG), and cannabichromene (CBC) (ElSohly and Slade 2005; Brenneisen 2007). THC is the main psychoactive constituent. The concentration (%) of THC contained in the plant is generally the measure of the power of cannabis and, consequently, of its effects (Murray et al. 2008). Cannabis is usually smoked but can also be taken orally, sometimes mixed with tea or food. Cannabis (especially marijuana) can be mixed and smoked with opiates and phencyclidine (PCP) to get more intense effects (Ellenhorn et al. 1997). It is often also taken with other substances like nicotine, alcohol, and cocaine.

Cannabis products fall into three main categories: marijuana, hashish, and liquid cannabis (cannabis oil). They may have different percentages of Δ9-THC. Marijuana is the term used to describe the substance obtained from the dried female inflorescence of cannabis plants. The percentage of Δ9-THC varies between 2 and 12% (UNODC 2009). Hashish is the name attributed to the products obtained by processing cannabis resin. It contains a percentage of Δ9-THC oscillating between 4 and 21% (UNODC 2009). Liquid cannabis, also known as hash oil, and shatter (Bell et al. 2015; Romanowski et al. 2017), is a concentrated liquid extract of both cannabis and cannabis resin material reaching a concentration of THC greater than 60% (UNODC 2009). THC extraction from cannabis can also be achieved by means of butane gas, which gives a product called butan hash oil (BHO, dabbing) (Chan et al. 2017).

24.2.2   Cocaine

Cocaine is an addictive stimulant drug made from the leaves of the coca plant native to South America. For thousands of years people in South America have chewed and ingested coca leaves (*Erythroxylon coca*), the source of cocaine, for their stimulant effects (Calatayud and González 2003; Goldstein et al. 2009). Cocaine hydrochloride, the purified chemical, was isolated from the plant more than 100 years ago. Before the development of synthetic local anaesthetic, surgeons used cocaine to relieve pain (Calatayud and González 2003). However, research has since shown that cocaine is a powerfully addictive substance that can alter brain structure and function when used repetitively (NIDA 2016a). As a street drug, cocaine looks like a fine, white, crystalline powder. It has several names: Coke, C, Snow, Powder, or Blow. Street dealers often dilute it with non-psychoactive substances such as corn-starch, talcum powder, flour, or baking soda to increase their profits. They may also adulterate cocaine with other drugs like procaine (a chemically related local anaesthetic) or amphetamine (another psychoactive stimulant) (Goldstein et al. 2009; Drent et al. 2012). Some users combine cocaine with heroin, a mixture called Speedball (Goldstein et al. 2009).

People usually use two chemical forms of cocaine: the water-soluble hydrochloride salt and the water-insoluble cocaine base (or freebase, processed to make a rock crystal). Users usually inject or snort the hydrochloride salt, which is a powder. The base form of cocaine is created by processing the drug with ammonia or sodium bicarbonate (baking soda) and water, then heating it to remove the hydrochloride to produce a smokable substance. The term *crack*, which is the street name given to freebase cocaine, refers to the crackling sound heard when the mixture is smoked (CESAR 2018; Goldstein et al. 2009).

Cocaine users often take it in binges, that is they take the drug repeatedly within a short time, at increasingly higher doses, to maintain their 'high' (John and Wu 2017).

24.2.3   Heroin

Heroin is a synthetic substance with a strong anti-pain effect. It is an opioid drug made from morphine, a natural substance coming from the seed pod of opium poppy plants grown in Southeast and Southwest Asia, Mexico, and Colombia (LeVert 2006). The heroin appears as a fine or granular powder of white, brown or reddish colour, water-soluble. Heroin can be inhaled, smoked or injected into the vein or muscle. Usually sold on the street, heroin is known by the names stuff, rubber, black tar, big H, horse, hell dust, and smack (Dipartimento Politiche Antidroga 2009b). Some people mix heroin with crack cocaine, a practice called speedballing (Platt 2000).

24.2.4 Amphetamine/Methamphetamine

Amphetamine is a stimulant, mostly available in the form of tablets that are ingested. It is generally used for medical purposes to treat pathologies such as attention deficit syndrome (ADHD) or narcolepsy. However, it can be used improperly or with no prescription (Heal et al. 2013). Methamphetamine is also a potent stimulant with a chemical structure similar to that of amphetamine. Methamphetamine is usually a white, bitter-tasting powder or pill. Crystal methamphetamine looks like glass fragments or shiny, bluish-white rocks. Methamphetamine can be easily dissolved in water or in alcohol. It may be ingested, smoked, sniffed or injected. Its most common names are chalk, crank, crystal, ice, meth, and speed (Dipartimento Politiche Antidroga 2009a). Both amphetamine and methamphetamine can be produced in illegal laboratories with toxic compounds under very poor hygienic conditions (EMCDDA–Europol 2009). As the 'high' produced by the drug starts and fades quickly, people often take repeated doses of methamphetamine. In some cases, people take the substance in binges known as a 'run', giving up food and sleep while continuing to take the drug every few hours for up to several days (NIDA 2016b; NIDA 2018c). Amongst methamphetamines, is ecstasy, a common term for MDMA or 3,4-methyldioxymethanphetamine. A substance of synthetic origin, ecstasy produces effects similar to those of other stimulants. It is usually taken in the form of tablets or capsules of various colours that portray images of various types. Some swallow it in liquid form or snort the powder. Tablets generally do not contain only MDMA but also combinations of MDMA with other substances such as caffeine, dextromethorphan, amphetamine, PCP or cocaine. Purity is therefore always doubtful (NIDA 2016d).

24.2.5 Hallucinogens

Hallucinogens are a wide group of substances able to alter perception, thoughts, and feelings. People have used hallucinogens for centuries, mostly for religious rituals (Cunningham 2008). They can be found in plants and mushrooms (or their extracts) or can be human-made. Common hallucinogens include the following (Laing 2003):

- Ayahuasca (Hoasca, Aya, Yagé), a tea made from Amazonian plants containing dimethyltryptamine (DMT), the primary mind-altering ingredient. DMT (or Dimitri) is a chemical found in nature or produced in the laboratory, usually available in the form of a white crystalline powder.

- Salvia divinorum (Diviner's Sage, Maria Pastora, Sally-D, Magic Mint) is a plant common to southern Mexico and Central and South America whose active ingredient, salvinorina A, is mainly responsible for the plant's psychoactive effects.

- Peyote (Buttons, Cactus, Mesc) is a small, spineless cactus with mescaline as its main ingredient. Peyote can also be synthetic.

- 4-phosphoryloxy-*N*,*N*-dimethyltryptamine (Psilocybin or Little Smoke, Magic Mushrooms, Purple Passion, Shrooms) comes from some mushrooms living in tropical regions of South America, Mexico, and the United States.

- D-lysergic acid diethylamide (LSD, Acid, Blotter, Dots, Yellow Sunshine) is a clear or white odourless material made from lysergic acid, which is found in a fungus growing on rye and other grains. Available in liquid form, LSD is absorbed onto small pieces of paper (stamps, blotters) or on tablets.

- Ketamine (K, Special K, Cat Valium) is used as a surgery anaesthetic for humans and animals. While available as an injectable liquid, manufacturers mostly sell it as a powder or pills.

- Phencyclidine (PCP, Angel Dust, Hog, Love Boat, Peace Pill) was a general anaesthetic for surgery in the past, but is no longer used for this purpose due to serious side effects. PCP can be found in tablets or capsules, as a liquid or as a white crystal powder.

Hallucinogens may be used in several ways, according to the type of substance, with the best known being swallowing as tablets, pills or liquid, consuming moist or dried, brewing into tea, snorting, injecting, inhaling, vaporising or smoking, and absorbing through the lining in the mouth using drug-soaked paper pieces (NIDA 2016c).

24.2.6 Inhalants

The term 'inhalants' refers to several substances typically taken by inhalation showing psychoactive properties when administered, giving a sensation of 'high'. These substances include solvents, aerosol sprays, gases, and nitrites (Sherry 2001). People usually breathe them in through the mouth (huffing) or nose (NIDA 2017b) as follows:

- sniffing or snorting fumes from a dispenser (i.e. glue bottle or marking pen)

- spraying aerosols (i.e. computer cleaning dusters) directly into the nose or mouth

- 'huffing' from a chemical-soaked rag in the mouth

- sniffing or inhaling fumes from chemicals sprayed or put inside a plastic or paper bag (bagging)

- inhaling from balloons filled with nitrous oxide.

Although the high that inhalants produce usually lasts just a few minutes, people often try to make it last by continuing to inhale again and again (NIDA 2017b).

24.2.7 New psychoactive substances

Over the past 10 years there has been an unprecedented increase in the number, type, and availability of new psychoactive substances (NPS) in Europe. NPSs represent a very large group of molecules, mainly synthetic, characterised by pharmacological and toxicological properties that are particularly dangerous to consumer health (Serpelloni 2013; UNODC 2013a,b; EMCDDA 2015a). The main structural groups of NPS reported are the following (Serpelloni 2013; EMCDDA 2015a):

- *Synthetic cannabinoids*: synthetic chemicals that are either sprayed on dried, shredded plant material so they can be smoked (herbal incense) or sold as liquids to be vaporised and inhaled in e-cigarettes and other devices (liquid incense). They are related to chemicals found in the marijuana plant. Because of this similarity, synthetic cannabinoids are sometimes misleadingly called 'synthetic marijuana'.

- *Synthetic cathinones*: related to the parent compound cathinone, one of the psychoactive principals in khat (Catha edulis Forsk). Since the mid-2000s, unregulated ring-substituted cathinone derivatives have appeared in Europe, the most commonly known being mephedrone and methylone. These products are usually available as highly pure white or brown powders.

- *Phenethylamines*: a wide class of molecules with psychoactive stimulant activity which includes amphetamine, methamphetamine, and 3,4-methylenedioxymethamphetamine. They are divided into different sub-groups according to the different substitution on the aromatic ring, the alkyl chain, and the nitrogen.

- *Piperazines*: a large class of chemical compounds in which different chemical portions are linked to the main piperazine molecule. Known as stimulants, piperazine derivatives are synthesised in laboratories and are available in the form of capsules or tablets with various shapes and logos, and more rarely in the form of powder. They are often sold in place of MDMA.

- *Tryptamines*: molecules in which the main skeleton is constituted by a tryptamine, a natural alkaloid. Some are natural neurotransmitters (e.g. serotonin) and others are present in plants and have hallucinogenic activity (i.e. DMT and psilocybin). Natural tryptamines circulate as dried vegetable preparations (i.e. dried mushrooms), while synthetic tryptamines may be in the form of capsules, tablets, powders, or liquid. Generally, they are ingested, snorted, smoked or injected.

- *Azepanic analogues*: a group of molecules in which the main skeleton is an azepan structure. Examples are the benzothiazepines diltiazem and quetiapine, and the benzodiazepine etizolam, which are active ingredients of pharmaceutical drugs circulating on the illicit drug market for non-medical purpose.

- *Fentanyl and analogues*: a potent narcotic analgesic, fentanyl and its derivatives (alfentanyl, sufentanyl, remifentanil, and carfentanyl) are used as anaesthetics and analgesics in humans and in veterinary medicine. The structural analogue 3-methylfentanyl is illegally synthesised and sold as 'synthetic heroin' or mixed with heroin itself. The non-medical use of fentanyl is reported through routes unrelated to the pharmaceutical formulation: by injection, ingestion of tablets (trans-mucosal assumption), and the use of patches. Fentanyl powder or from patches is also smoked or assumed intranasally (sniffing).

- *Synthetic opioids*: substances binding to the same receptors in the brain as morphine, stimulating the activity of dopamine in the limbic system. Heroin and morphine are the best-known opioids.

In recent years, several new synthetic opioids have appeared on the illicit drug market. Amongst these are methorphan, demerol (pethidine), propoxyphene, AH-7921, and dipipanone.

- *Phencyclidine analogues*: molecules with the basic skeleton of phencyclidine (PCP), which was used as anaesthetic drug in the past but withdrawn from the market for its side effects. PCP analogues are the eticyclidine (PCE), the rolicyclidine (PHP, PCPY), the 3-methoxyeticyclidine (3 MeO-PCE), and the 4-methoxyphencyclidine (4-MeO-PCP). 3-MeO-PCE and 4-MeO-PCP are often sold as 'reagents for research', in the form of powder.

24.3   The legal scenario of drug use

24.3.1   International law

Narcotic drugs are classified and placed under international control by the United Nations Single Convention on Narcotic Drugs, as amended in 1972. This convention aims to combat drug abuse through co-ordinated international action. In fact, there are two forms of intervention and control that must work together. First, the Convention aims to restrict the possession, use, trade, distribution, importation, exportation, manufacture, and production of drugs exclusively for medical and scientific purposes (Article 4c). Second, the Convention wants to combat drug trafficking through international cooperation to deter traffickers. The annex to the 1961 Convention classifies the narcotics in four tables, as shown in Table 24.1.

Psychotropic substances were placed under international control by the 1971 United Nations Convention. The objectives of this Convention are to limit the use of these substances for medical and scientific purposes (Articles 5 and 7). In fact, while some psychotropic substances may have therapeutic value, they may also present a dangerous risk of abuse (EMCDDA 2016).

Table 24.1 Classification of drugs according to the 1961 UN Convention, amended in 1972.

Table	Harmfulness	Degree of control	Examples
I	Substances capable of producing addiction, which present a serious risk of abuse	Very severe; the substances included in Table I are subject to all control measures applicable to drugs pursuant to this Convention (Article 2.1)	Cannabis and its derivatives, cocaine, heroin, methadone, morphine, opium
II	Substances normally used for medical purposes and with lower risk of abuse	Less severe	Codeine, dihydrocodeine, propiram
III	Preparations based on substances listed in Table II, as well as cocaine preparations	Mild; according to the WHO, these preparations do not present any risk of abuse	Preparations based on codeine, dihydrocodeine, propiram
IV	The most dangerous substances, already listed in Table I, which are particularly harmful and of extremely limited medical or therapeutic value	Very severe, leading to a total ban on the production, manufacture, export and import, trade, possession or use of such substances except for quantities that may be necessary for medical and scientific research (Article 2.5.b)	Cannabis and cannabis resin, heroin

Table 24.2 Classification of drugs according to the 1971 UN Convention.

Table	Harmfulness	Degree of control	Examples
I	Substances with a high risk of abuse, which present a particular, serious threat to public health and which are of little or no therapeutic value	Very severe; use is prohibited except for scientific or limited medical purposes	LSD, MDMA (ecstasy), mescaline, psilocybin, tetrahydrocannabinol (including isomers and stereochemical variants)
II	Substances presenting a risk of abuse, posing a serious threat to public health and having a low or moderate therapeutic value	Less severe	Stimulants and stimulants of the amphetamine type, including Dronabinol Δ9-tetrahydrocannabinol, and its stereochemical variants
III	Substances presenting a risk of abuse which pose a serious threat to public health and which are of moderate or high therapeutic value	These substances are available for medical purposes	Barbiturates, including amobarbital, buprenorphine
IV	Substances presenting a risk of abuse which represent a minor threat to public health, with a high therapeutic value	These substances are available for medical purposes	Tranquillisers, analgesics, narcotics, including allobarbital, diazepam, lorazepam, phenobarbital, temazepam

More specifically, the Convention establishes an international control system for psychotropic substances. It responds to the diversification and expansion of the spectrum of substances of abuse and introduces controls on numerous synthetic substances according to their potential abuse, on the one hand, and their therapeutic value, on the other. The 1971 United Nations Convention on Psychotropic Substances classifies substances in four sections, as shown in Table 24.2.

Finally, the 1988 UN Convention against Illicit and Psychotropic Drugs Traffic aims to promote cooperation between states so that they can deal more effectively with the various aspects of illicit drug and psychotropic substances trafficking having an international dimension. In carrying out their obligations under the Convention, states should take the necessary measures, including legislative and administrative measures, in accordance with the fundamental provisions of their respective national legislative systems.

The three main international drug control treaties are mutually supportive and should be considered complementary to each other. An important objective of the first two treaties is to codify the control measures applicable at international level to ensure the availability of drugs and psychotropic substances for medical and scientific purposes, and to prevent them being diverted to illicit channels. With the third Convention, on the other hand, aspects of co-operation for the fight against trafficking and dealing are strengthened.

It is important to note that the Conventions do not specify that the use of drugs per se should be a punishable crime, even if each country can independently establish that the use of drugs is a real crime within its own borders. Furthermore, it is important to highlight that the Conventions do not indicate any link between the type of drugs and the penalties established by national law. While the tables influence the different regulatory mechanisms that countries are required to apply to the distribution of drugs, the same countries are not obliged to use these mechanisms for the definition of national criminal sanctions.

24.3.2   EU drug policy

To complete the legal framework that regulates drugs in Europe, it is necessary to mention the European Drugs Strategy 2013–2020 and the related 2017–2020 Action Plan. In fact, the two European documents confirm the adherence to the UN Conventions described above, without proposing any changes to the international approach currently in force.

The European Drug Strategy and the related Action Plan do not impose legal obligations on Member States but promote a strategic model with priorities, objectives, actions, and indicators to measure performance. They represent the context within which each Member State can define its own drug strategy, respecting the priorities identified at national level (EMCDDA 2015b).

In general, the EU drug strategy is aimed at coordinating European policies amongst Member States and promoting a shared European approach. The existing strategy (2013–2020) presents the current drug policy position of the Member States, the common objectives to reduce drug demand, addiction, drug-related health, and social risks and to reduce drug supply.

The Action Plan serves to translate the priorities indicated in the strategy into actions, with defined timing, implementing actors, and evaluation indicators. The current plan (2017–2020) is aimed at strengthening the co-ordination and co-operation of law enforcement agencies and fortifying judicial co-operation and legislation in Europe to respond to emerging issues, such as the appearance of NPS or the increasing use of the Internet for drug trafficking. In this regard, the European strategy, and the related Action Plan, promote the adoption of new forms of contrast to trafficking and dealing alternative to traditional ones, to better address the emerging phenomena currently characterising the drug scene in Europe and around the world.

The strategy, in addition to reducing the demand and supply of drugs, also aims to reduce health and social risks and harms caused by drugs. Furthermore, for the first time, the need to guarantee the quality of intervention policies has been included in the European documents, adopting minimum quality standards and evaluation indicators. Civil society is gaining more and more importance in the policy-making process at European level, participating at international tables and giving voice to the positions of drug users, community leaders, operators, etc. The new strategy aims at social reintegration and recovery of drug users, through more effective and efficient drug treatment services, and the guarantee of adequate treatment for drug users in prisons.

For the first time, the new EU strategy emphasises the need to adopt an empirical and evidence-based approach in the definition of decision-making and maintains the indication, contained in the 2009 UN political declaration on drugs, about the definition of an integrated (combining all aspects of drug activities) and balanced (concentrated on both demand reduction and supply reduction measures) approach (EU Council Recommendations 402/01 2012).

According to the laws of the EU, the criminal or administrative response to crimes related to drug use are the responsibility of Member States and not of the EU. Regarding drug trafficking, the 2004 EU Council Framework Decision (2004/757/JHA) established minimum rules on the constituent elements of illicit drug trafficking and precursor crimes to allow a common approach at European level to combat drug trafficking. Possession for personal consumption of substances is specifically excluded from this framework decision. Member States are required to take the necessary measures to ensure that crimes are punishable by 'effective, proportionate and dissuasive criminal penalties'. In addition to this general obligation, the minimum and maximum levels of sanction are indicated (Article 4). Aggravating circumstances include crimes involving 'drugs that cause harm to health' (Article 4 (2) (b)), but the specific definition of such drugs has been left to the Member States (EU Council Framework Decision 2004).

Clearly, outside Europe, other international organisations have their own drug strategies and action plans. For example, the Organization of American States (OAS) defined the Hemispheric Drug Strategy in 2010, the Andean Community adopted a 2012–2019 drug strategy, the African Union (AU) promoted the Action Plan on Drug Control 2013–2017, the Association of Southeast Asian Nations (ASEAN) promotes the Work Plan on Combating Illicit Drug Production, Trafficking, and Use 2009–2015, etc. (EMCDDA 2015b). All these strategies differ from one another based on different drug situations and available resources. However, similarities can be identified in some areas, such as a comprehensive approach to reducing drug demand and supply. However, it has been internationally understood that the drug problem cannot be tackled at the individual country level but that a broader and more coordinated approach is needed to develop more effective common strategies and actions, and to protect public health and safety.

24.3.3 UK level

The Misuse of Drugs Act 1971 is the main law regulating drug control in the UK. It subdivides substances into three classes (A, B and C) to which it attributes different levels of penalties for the crimes committed.

Maximum penalties vary according to the class of substance and according to whether the conviction is made at a magistrates' court for a summary offence or on indictment, after a trial at a Crown Court. Table 24.3 summarises the penalties provided for possession, supply, and production of drugs, depending on the class to which the substance belongs (GOV.UK 2018).

Table 24.3 Penalties provided for possession, supply, and production of drugs in the UK.

Class	Drug	Possession	Supply and production
A	Crack cocaine, cocaine, ecstasy (MDMA), heroin, LSD, magic mushrooms, methadone, methamphetamine (crystal meth)	Up to 7 years in prison, an unlimited fine or both	Up to life in prison, an unlimited fine or both
B	Amphetamines, barbiturates, cannabis, codeine, ketamine, methylphenidate (Ritalin), synthetic cannabinoids, synthetic cathinones (e.g. mephedrone, methoxetamine)	Up to 5 years in prison, an unlimited fine or both	Up to 14 years in prison, an unlimited fine or both
C	Anabolic steroids, benzodiazepines (diazepam), γ-hydroxybutyrate (GHB), γ-butyrolactone (GBL), piperazines (BZP), khat	Up to 2 years in prison, an unlimited fine or both (except anabolic steroids – it is not an offence to possess them for personal use)	Up to 14 years in prison, an unlimited fine or both
Temporary class drugs[a]	Some methylphenidate substances (ethylphenidate, 3,4-dichloromethylphenidate (3,4-DCMP), methylnaphthidate (HDMP-28), isopropylphenidate (IPP or IPPD), 4-methylmethylphenidate, ethylnaphthidate, propylphenidate) and their simple derivatives	None, but police can take away a suspected temporary class drug	Up to 14 years in prison, an unlimited fine or both

[a] The government can ban new drugs for one year under a temporary banning order while they decide how to classify them.

The Misuse of Drugs Act 1971 does not consider drug use per se an offence. Rather, it is the possession of the drug that represents an offence. Under this law, a distinction is made between the possession of controlled drugs and the possession with intent to supply them to someone else. The latter case precisely refers to drug-trafficking offences.

Another important law to consider when dealing with drugs in UK is the Drug Trafficking Act 1994, which defines drug trafficking as transporting or storing, importing or exporting, manufacturing or supplying drugs included in the Misuse of Drugs Act 1971. The penalties applied depend on the classification of the drug and the penal procedure adopted (magistrate level or Crown Court level). For Class A drugs, the maximum penalty for trafficking is life imprisonment; for Class B and Class C drugs, that penalty can reach up to 14 years in prison. Moreover, temporary class drug orders were introduced through the Police Reform and Social Responsibility Act 2011 to speed legislative response to NPS supply offences.

In 2016, the Psychoactive Substances Act criminalised the production, supply or possession of substances when those same substances were meant to be used for their psychoactive effects.

Finally, it is also important to consider the Medicine Act 1968, which governs the manufacture and supply of medicine. The Medicine Act 1968 organises medical drugs into three categories:

- prescription-only medicines: these can be sold or supplied only by a pharmacist and only if prescribed by a doctor

- pharmacy medicines: these can be sold without a prescription but only supplied by a pharmacist

- general sales list medicines: these can be sold by any shop, but advertising, labelling, and production restrictions remain.

In order to comply with EU legislation, in 2012 Section 10(7) of the Medicines Act 1968 was repealed. It provided an exemption from the obligation for a pharmacist to hold a wholesale dealer's licence if he/she trades in medicines under certain circumstances.

24.4   The drug scene today

24.4.1   Drug demand

According to the UNODC World Drug Report 2017, around 5% of the global adult population 15–64 years old (about 250 million) used drugs at least once in 2015 (UNODC 2017). Cannabis represents the most widely used drug: 183 million adult people consumed it in the past 12 months. Amphetamine is the second most consumed drug (35 million past-year users). In 2015, opiates and misuse prescription opioids have been used by 35.1 million people, of whom 17.7 million used heroin and opium. The misuse of pharmaceutical opioids is a key issue in several countries, where it has been associated with an increase in morbidity and mortality related to opioids. Cocaine is consumed by nearly 17 million people all over the world and the trend seems to be increasing (UNODC 2017).

Nearly 30 million (0.6%) of the global adult population suffer from drug use disorders requiring treatment or resulting in premature death. This number has been increasing in the last 10 years while access to services for the treatment of drug use disorders is provided to only 17% of drug users. In 2015, 70% of global drug-related diseases was attributable to opioids, with just under 40 million deaths per million in people aged 15–64 years. Most deaths are concentrated in North America (UNODC 2017).

In the last 10 years, women have been the most affected by the negative health consequences of drug use. At the global level, men are three times more likely than women to use drugs (especially cannabis, cocaine or amphetamines). By contrast, women are more likely than men to misuse prescription drugs (prescription opioids and tranquillizers) (Grella 2008). Moreover, women usually begin to use drugs later in life than men, but once they have begun they tend to increase their rate of consumption more rapidly than men and may progress faster to the development of drug use disorders (Van Etten and Anthony 2001).

The number of people worldwide who injected drugs in 2015 was 11.8 million (0.25% of the total from 15 to 64 age group population) (UNODC 2017). HIV infections amongst injecting drug users increased from 114.000 in 2011 to 152.000 in 2015. In 2015, hepatitis C infections were found in 6.1 million injecting drug users, leading to co-infection of HIV-hepatitis C of 82.4% (Platt et al. 2016).

24.4.2 Drug supply

Recently, the number and type of substances available on the drug market have been significantly increasing. The use of multiple drugs (polydrug use) has become a common use pattern, becoming more and more dangerous due to the high number of substances available and their many combinations, resulting in unknown and often unexpected health consequences. For instance, a combination of heroin and synthetic opioids and many analogues of fentanyl has been observed (UNODC 2017).

Illicitly manufactured synthetic opioids are becoming widely available, posing serious public health concerns, including opioid related deaths (UNODC 2017).

Data show that drug trafficking has increased in the last five years, especially with reference to synthetic drugs markets and cocaine. Opium production has increased as well: by 33% over 2015. This may be related to the improvement in opium poppy yields in Afghanistan compared with the previous year. However, global opium production is still lower than it was in 2014. Seizures of both opium and heroin have remained quite stable, suggesting a regular supply of heroin despite changes in opium production.

24.4.3 New psychoactive substances

Since 2005, several NPS, belonging to different chemical groups, have been registered worldwide on the drug market. These substances are not covered by international drug controls and represent a broad range of drugs such as synthetic cannabinoids, stimulants, opioids, and benzodiazepines. In most cases they are marketed as 'legal' replacements for illicit drugs, while others are aimed at consumers who wish to explore novel effects (Serpelloni et al. 2013).

Steps have been taken by the international community to schedule NPSs under international control but the speed with which they appear on the drug market makes it difficult to control them (UNODC 2017). In many cases, new substances are produced in bulk quantities by chemical and pharmaceutical companies in China. From there, they are shipped to Europe, where they are processed into products, packaged, and sold. In addition, some new substances may be sourced as medicines, either diverted from the legitimate supply chain or sourced illegally. These substances may be produced in clandestine laboratories (EMCDDA 2015b).

In the last couple of years, synthetic cannabinoids have increasingly appeared amongst NPSs. They represent a diverse group of psychoactive substances, usually used as substitutes for natural cannabis, although cannabis consumers seem to continue to prefer natural cannabis, perceived as less harmful. Noteworthy is that synthetic cannabinoid-related intoxications have been associated with the same severe adverse health events as those associated with natural cannabis use, including hospitalisations and fatalities (Serpelloni et al. 2013).

Unlike heroin and cocaine markets, the production of synthetic drugs is not bound to a geographic region because the molecules responsible for the psychoactive effect are not found in plants that need to be cultivated in specific areas and under certain conditions. As information on the extension of the synthetic drug market remains limited, it is difficult to estimate the actual production of this kind of drug worldwide. However, data on seizures and use suggest a growing supply. More and more countries are reporting NPS seizures (over 20 tons seized globally in 2015 alone) as well.

24.4.4 Internet and cybercrime

The increasing availability of digital technologies and Internet connectivity has allowed the development of online drug trafficking. Within the 'deep web' it is not possible to trace any user or movement, therefore this form of anonymity has allowed the development of illicit online activities that are difficult to detect (EMCDDA 2016, 2017b). According to the Global Drug Survey, the proportion of drug users who obtained drugs over the 'dark net' in the previous 12 months (mainly ecstasy, cannabis, LSD, and NPSs) increased by 70% from 2014 to 2017 (Winstock et al. 2017).

The dark net is a new drug traffic route that, although not yet completely replacing traditional traffic routes, is an extremely profitable and relatively secure sale form, given the difficulty of tracking and tracing transactions, and it is likely to become more important in the drug market in the future.

24.4.5 Fentanyl-related intoxications and deaths

Fentanyl, one of the most potent opioids, has been increasingly reported amongst drugs, especially in the United States. Mixed with other opioids or with heroin, it has been recently associated with an increase in mortality. Fentanyl has been controlled under Schedule I of the 1961 UN Single Convention on Narcotic Drugs since 1964. The lethal dose for humans is approximately 2 mg. It is contained in several pharmaceutical products and may cause severe harm if users increase the dose or modify the route of administration. Since 2013, the number of substances containing fentanyl reported to UN has been increasing, and it became dramatically high over the period 2014–2015 (US DEA 2016).

In addition, the number of reports regarding fentanyl found in combination with other drugs, within the same compound, has increased: in 93% of cases, fentanyl was found in combination with heroin. However, while in the United States the use of fentanyl is diverted by the pharmaceutical one, in most other countries the substance is clandestinely produced and trafficked. In Canada, the United States, and Europe, several cases of intoxication have been reported in association with the use of fentanyl or other synthetic opioids (US DEA 2015).

24.4.6 Debate on cannabis legalisation

Most jurisdictions in the United States now permit access to medical cannabis while nine allow the cultivation of cannabis for recreational use. In 2016, the legalisation of cannabis for recreational use was voted for in four more states.

According to the Monitoring the Future Survey promoted by the National Institute on Drug Abuse since 1975, in the United States at federal level, consumption of all substances except marijuana is declining amongst the juvenile population. The consumption of marijuana, on the other hand, is stable, focusing mainly on young people resident in states where marijuana has been legalised for medical purposes. In states that have legalised marijuana for recreational purposes, there has been a general increase in marijuana consumption in all age groups considered (12–17 years, 18–26 years, >26 years) and in particular in the 18–26 population (Johnston et al. 2016). The perception of the risk arising from the use of marijuana in all age groups considered (12–17, 18 26, >26) has decreased, especially in the range 18–26 years (CDC 2014; Center for the Study of Health and Risk Behaviors 2015).

There has been an increase in cases of acute intoxication registered at emergency departments and an increase in hospitalisation in relation to marijuana intake. Likewise, the number of calls to poison control centres has significantly increased for cannabis-related acute poisoning. It is worth noting the high level of intoxication that occurred in the age range of 0–10 years, probably due to accidental intake of cannabis but also because of the ever-growing availability of edible products containing THC within the reach of children (CHA 2016). There has also been an increase in the prevalence of suicide victims found positive for THC (Colorado), with positive percentages (16%) higher than those of alcohol (77%) and cocaine (1.9%) (Colorado Department of Public Health and Environment 2016).

After legalisation, there was a very strong increase in THC positivity in traffic road accidents, ranging from 14.1% in 2011 to 21% in 2015 in Colorado (Colorado Department of Transportation 2015). This figure is also confirmed by the simultaneous increase in the number of marijuana-related deaths, especially in the state of Washington. Additionally, there has been a marked increase in THC prevalence amongst workplace drug testing (Quest Diagnostics 2018)

Another aspect to consider when dealing with the legalisation of cannabis is the increase in the percentage of potency (THC) in the plant and its consequences on health and patterns of consumption. Analysis of trends in the EU consistently shows a large increase in THC of both herbal cannabis and cannabis resin between 2006 and 2014, stabilising in 2015. Reasons for this phenomenon may include the introduction of intensive production techniques and the introduction of high-potency plants and new techniques in Morocco (UNODC 2017).

Although still controversial, the question of cannabis legalisation is also generating wide interest in Europe, where considerable diversity in attitudes exists, with approaches ranging from restrictive models to the tolerance of some forms of personal use. The main issues on which the European debate is focusing concern permitting the production of cannabis for personal use and making cannabis available for treating medical conditions. From a commercial point of view, the cannabis market is seeing new impulses through sales of vaporisers, E-liquids, and edible products, making the substance more and more available to everyone (SAM 2016). Therefore, beyond the political aspects, it will be important to assess how legalisation will affect consumers (and non-consumers), especially from a health point of view.

24.5 Consequences of drug use

24.5.1 Effects on mental health

Long-term use of drugs may cause short- and/or long-term changes in the brain. These changes may lead to mental health issues like depression, anxiety, aggression, hallucinations, etc. People with drug addiction are often diagnosed with mental disorders: they have twice the probability of developing mood and anxiety disorders, and vice versa. While substance use disorders usually arise together with other mental illnesses (comorbidity), it is not clear yet whether one caused the other or if common risk factors contribute to both disorders. The type of mental disorder associated with the use of drugs may change depending on the substance being consumed. The main mental health effects for each of the substances described in the previous paragraphs are described below.

24.5.1.1 Cannabis Over the last decade, several studies have reported data on the alteration of cognitive function resulting from the use of cannabis, even after a period of abstinence. In general, compared to non-consumers, cannabis consumers show worse performance in neuropsychological functions, particularly in executive functions, attention, learning and long-term memory, motor skills, and verbal abilities (Grant et al. 2003; Ranganathan and D'Souza 2006; Puighermanal et al. 2009). A review of the chronic effects of cannabis consumption on memory has reported that chronic consumers, in a state of detoxification, show an immediate effect on working memory and verbal episodic memory (conscious recall of facts) (Solowij and Pesa 2012). In particular, a delay in the call for verbal information, a recurrence of memory problems, a difficulty in processing the contents of work memory, and difficulties in problem solving and decision-making have been highlighted. The deterioration of the brain functions persists even after the acute phase of intoxication. This is also confirmed for teenage consumers who have used cannabis frequently (Schweinsburg et al. 2008), for which there has also been a reduced psychomotor speed, poorer performance of episodic memory, planning and sequencing of activities, non-verbal memory and learning, even after a month of abstinence (Tapert et al. 2002; Harvey et al. 2007; Medina et al. 2007). Evidence also suggests that the magnitude of neuropsychological impairment and the extent to which it persists after abstinence may depend on the frequency and duration of the use of cannabis, the length of the withdrawal period, and the age of onset (Solowij and Pesa 2012).

People who regularly use cannabis often report lethargy, both physical and mental. Long-lasting consumption of cannabis causes the appearance of indolence, unproductiveness, and neglect in hygiene, becoming increasingly noticeable until social relations are unacceptable. There is a kind of apathy and anhedonia, that is, inability to feel pleasure, even in circumstances and activities that are normally rewarding such as eating, sleep, having social contacts, and sexual intercourse. These symptoms characterise what is defined as cannabis-related amotivational syndrome (McGlothlin and West 1968; Johns 2001), which manifests itself with apathy and reduced ability to concentrate, follow up routine activities, and manage new stimulation with success (Volkow et al. 2016). In young people, these symptoms may appear even after a short time (Lynskey and Hall 2000).

Reliable population studies have concurrently found an increased risk of depression in heavy cannabis users or in those who are dependent on it (Chen et al. 2002; Degenhardt et al. 2003), also highlighting a risk of having a depressive episode six times higher than healthy subjects and bipolar disorders (Henquet et al. 2006; Hayatbakhsh et al. 2007; van Laar et al. 2007). When taken at high doses, cannabinoids have psychoactive effects similar to those of hallucinogens, such as LSD, and cannabinoid users may experience adverse mental effects that look like 'bad trips', a slang expression that refers to the unpleasant and negative effects resulting after the consumption of hallucinogens. These effects range from moderate levels of anxiety to severe anxiety reactions with panic attacks, suspicion, and delusions with hallucinations. Depression has also been reported (sensation of detachment or self-extraneousness) and derealization (a feeling of perceiving the outside world in a distorted way and sometimes perceiving known individuals as strangers). Longitudinal studies have shown strong association between the use of cannabis amongst adolescents and the onset of psychosis and schizophrenia (Arsenault et al. 2002; Volkow et al. 2016).

The use of cannabis also appears to influence the intellectual quotient (QI). Indeed, a study by Meier et al. (2012) investigated the association between cannabis use and neuropsychological decline in over 1000 individuals, followed for 38 years. The results of the study showed that IQ declined from adolescence to adulthood as a function of cannabis use by up to –8 points. In particular, the longer and heavier the use of the substance, the greater the reduction in IQ as age increased. Conversely, those who had never used cannabis showed higher QI values over time (Meier et al. 2012). Subsequent studies seem to confirm these results (Moffitt et al. 2013).

The use of cannabis can lead to addiction (Gessa et al. 1998; Bossong et al. 2008) and abstinence (Diana et al. 1998). Abuse and addiction to cannabis generally develop over an extended period, though progression may be more rapid in young people with behaviour disorders. Most of those who become addicted typically set up a chronic use mode that gradually increases in both frequency and quantity. Symptoms of a possible irritability or anxious mood, accompanied by physical modifications such as tremor, sweating, nausea, appetite modification, and sleep disturbances, have been described in association with the use of very high doses of substance (Budney and Hughes 2006; Quickfall and Crockford 2006).

24.5.1.2 Cocaine

When exposure to cocaine is repeated, the brain begins to adapt to this kind of stimulus so that the reward pathway becomes used to it and loses sensitivity to natural reinforcers (Wolf 2010; Büttner 2012). Simultaneously, circuits involved in stress become more and more sensitive. That leads to increased irritation and negative moods when the drug is not taken, which are typical signs of withdrawal. These combined effects make the user more likely to concentrate on seeking and taking the drug rather than seeking relationships, food, or other natural rewards.

With regular use of cocaine, tolerance may develop. In this case, higher doses, more frequent use of the substance or both are needed to obtain the same level of reward and relief. At the same time, cocaine users may also develop sensitization in which less cocaine is needed to produce anxiety, convulsions, or other toxic effects. In a regular user, risk of overdose can be increased by tolerance to cocaine reward and by sensitization to cocaine toxicity (Riezzo et al. 2012).

Cocaine users usually take cocaine in binges. Such behaviour is associated with restlessness, irritability, panic attacks, paranoia, and psychosis. The person loses their perception of reality and experiences auditory hallucinations (Goldstein et al. 2009).

The higher the doses or the higher the frequency of use, the higher the risk of adverse psychological or physiological effects (Goldstein et al. 2009; Riezzo et al. 2012).

Due to brain impairment associated with cocaine use and to brain sensitization matured with a prolonged use of the substance, people who used cocaine in the past show a high risk for relapse, even after long periods of abstinence (Sinha 2013).

Finally, studies have reported that long-term cocaine use can lead to the impairment of several cognitive functions, like sustaining attention, memory, impulse inhibition, taking decisions about punishments or rewards, and accomplishing motor tasks (Spronk et al. 2013).

24.5.1.3 Heroin

Like other drugs, repeated use of heroin changes brain physical structure and physiology. These modifications can create long-term impairment in neuronal and hormonal systems (Wang et al. 2012), which can rarely be restored (Krook et al. 1984). Scientific studies have shown a decrease in brain's white matter related to heroin use. This has been associated with impairment of decision-making and the ability to control behaviour and to respond positively to stressful situations (Qiu et al. 2013; Li et al. 2013).

Heroin, which is an extremely addictive substance, can cause deep tolerance and physical dependence. Withdrawal can occur rapidly after last drug intake. Its main symptoms are restlessness, insomnia, muscle and bone pain, vomiting, diarrhoea, cold feeling, and goose skin. Symptoms reach their peak 24–48 hours after the last consumption of heroin and can last up to one week (although there are cases of withdrawal lasting for months) (Kreek et al. 2012). Heroin addiction is a chronic disorder with frequent relapses.

A strong association between mental illness and prescription opiate abuse has been reported and neurobiological processes involved in psychosis and opiate abuse may partially explain this association. Prescription opiate abuse often leads to daily heroin use (Kern et al. 2014).

24.5.1.4 Methamphetamine

Dopamine plays an important role in regulating body movement, pleasure, motivation, and reward. When consumed, methamphetamine increases the amount of natural dopamine in the brain, causing the release of large amounts of dopamine in brain reward areas. That produces a feeling of euphoria ('rush', 'flash'), which is associated with an alteration of judgement and decision-making leading to risky behaviours, dangerous for the well-being of the consumers and those close to him/her. For instance, behaviours like unprotected sex may worsen the evolution of HIV/AIDS and its consequences. In this regard, studies have shown that injury to nerve cells and cognitive problems are more frequently registered amongst HIV-infected people who use methamphetamine rather than amongst HIV-infected people not using the substance (Skowronska et al. 2018). Cognitive problems include the ability to think, understand, learn, and remember (Chang et al. 2005).

Changes in the brain dopamine's system are associated with reduced co-ordination and verbal learning. Changes may also occur in those brain areas involved in emotion and memory (Volkow et al. 2001). Although some of these brain changes can be reversible with abstinence, others cannot. Indeed, it has been shown that people who made use of methamphetamine have a greater chance of developing diseases such as Parkinson's than non-consumers (Wang et al. 2004; Curtin et al. 2015). In the long term, methamphetamine consumption can also cause sleeping problems, anxiety, confusion, violent behaviour, hallucinations, and paranoia.

24.5.1.5 Hallucinogens

Several drugs belong to the group of hallucinogens. One of their common properties is to alter the perception of reality, thoughts, and feelings. They can cause hallucinations or feelings and images that are apparently real. Studies suggest that these substances can temporarily disrupt the communication amongst cerebral chemical systems, through the brain and the spinal cord, and that is the basis of hallucinations and mental problems associated with the use of hallucinogens (De Gregorio et al. 2016). Some hallucinogens impair the action of serotonin, altering mood, sleep, sensory perception, body temperature, hunger, muscle control, and sexual behaviour. Other hallucinogens alter the action of glutamate, which regulates response to the environment, pain perception, emotion, learning, and memory (Kyzar et al. 2017).

Although more research is necessary to define the long-term effects of hallucinogens, scientists know that repeated use of PCP can lead to memory loss, speech problems, anxiety, and depression and that these effects may last over one year after abstinence (Morris et al. 2005). Other long-term effects associated with the use of hallucinogens are (NIDA 2016c):

- persistent psychosis, with disorganised thinking, paranoia, and mood changes

- flashbacks, that is, recurrence of experiences associated with drug consumption, which may occur suddenly, even after one year of abstinence; in the worst cases, hallucinations occur daily, preventing the subject from living normally

- tolerance and addiction, for instance LSD can produce tolerance and push the drug user to take more and more drug at higher doses to reach the same effect. Although LSD is not considered addictive itself, it can produce tolerance to other hallucinogens. Instead, PCP can be addictive and people who stop its use can experiment cravings, headaches, sweating, and other symptoms common to withdrawal.

24.5.1.6 Inhalants

Most inhalants disturb the central nervous system and reduce brain activity speed. Short-term effects include altered speech, lack of coordination, dizziness, and euphoria. Some people may experiment hallucinations or delusions. Repeated inhalations can lead people to feel less self-conscious and less control, with episodes of vomiting, drowsiness, and headache (Balster 1998; Larrimore and Powell 2015).

Long-term effects on mental health can include loss of co-ordination and limb spasms due to nerve damage, delayed behavioural development due to brain problems, and direct brain damage due to cut-off oxygen flow to brain areas (Balster 1998; Larrimore and Powell 2015; Wayman and Woodward 2017).

24.5.1.7 New psychoactive substances

As described in the previous paragraphs, the NPSs available on the drug market are very different. Their number and diversity make it difficult to establish a single category of effects. The difficulty in predicting the effects of NPS on humans is especially due to the fact that the very composition of these substances varies, therefore their components may be able to cause effects that are not expected by the consumer.

What it is known is that synthetic cannabinoids act on the same brain cell receptors as THC, the active ingredient of cannabis. There are a few scientific studies on the mental effects caused by synthetic cannabinoids and on their effects on human brain. However, it is known that their capacity to bind to cannabis receptor is higher than THC and therefore they can produce stronger effects. To date, the mental effects recorded after the consumption of synthetic cannabinoids have been feelings of relaxation, elevated mood, altered perception, delusional or disordered thinking detached from reality, anxiety, confusion, hallucinations, and suicidal thoughts (Davidson et al. 2017).

Several deaths related to synthetic cannabinoids use have been registered across the world (UNODC 2017).

Synthetic cannabinoids can be addictive and when users quit their use they can experience withdrawal symptoms such as anxiety, irritability, and depression (NIDA 2018a).

Further studies are needed to understand the effects of synthetic cathinones on the brain. To date, scientific literature shows that synthetic cathinones are chemically similar to amphetamine, methamphetamine, and cocaine (Baumann et al. 2013), therefore it is expected that synthetic cathinones will be able to cause similar effects, such as anxiety, depression, and loss of control (NIDA 2018b).

24.5.2 Effects on the organism

24.5.2.1 Cannabis

The systems most affected by cannabis use are the cardiovascular system, the respiratory system, the reproductive system, and the immune system.

In some studies, the high carcinogenic and mutagenic risk of cannabis has been highlighted (Sidney et al. 1997), as well as the formation of pulmonary cells equal to those that precede tumour development in tobacco smokers (Zhang et al. 1999). Tumours occur especially in the lungs and in the respiratory tract (Zhang et al. 1999). The oncogenic, teratogenic, and mutagenic effects of cannabis depend on the amount of substance smoked and the duration of intake (Reece 2009). There have been rare cases of cancer of oropharynx in young people smoking cannabis chronically. In addition, chronic cannabis smoking is often associated with inflammation of bronchial mucosa, acute bronchitis, pulmonary density reduction, and pulmonary cysts (Reece 2009; Lutchmansingh et al. 2014).

The physiological effects of cannabis smoke on the cardiovascular system mainly include tachycardia and increased blood pressure, thus reducing the ability to transport oxygen to the blood (Sidney et al. 1997; Franz and Frishman 2016). In addition, the use of cannabis has been associated with myocardial infarction in young male patients (Mittleman et al. 2001) and angina in patients with pre-existing cardiac disorders (Gottschalk et al. 1997). An increasing number of case reports link cannabis consumption to cerebrovascular events (Hackam 2015).

Regarding the reproductive system, the effects of cannabis use on male fertility include reduction of serum levels of luteinising hormone (LH) and testosterone, induction of gynecomastia, decreased spermatogenesis and mobility (oligospermia), induction of sperm abnormalities, and blockade of acrosomal reaction. Concerning the effects on female fertility, studies report impairment of LH levels, inhibition of prolactin secretion, increased levels of testosterone, menstrual cycle changes, premature birth, and low birth weight of foetus (Murpy 2001).

THC damages the ability of the immune system to combat infectious diseases and cancer (Hollister 1992; Hall and Degenhardt 2009). In addition, it has immunomodulatory effects that can alter the normal functions of B and T lymphocytes, natural killer cells (NK), and macrophages (Friedman et al. 2003). An important risk associated with the use of cannabis concerns the suppression of infection resistance in the host (McGuinness 2009).

Finally, cannabis is known for its influence on bone metabolism: cannabis use has been associated with reduced bone formation and bone resorption (Reece 2009).

24.5.2.2 Cocaine

Immediately after intake, cocaine can generate a strong sense of pleasure, increased vigilance, increased loquacity, and energy. Other short-term effects include increased body temperature, heart rate, and blood pressure, pupil dilation, nausea, blurred vision, muscle spasms and confusion, but also anxiety and irritability.

Adverse effects related to cocaine consumption vary according to the route of administration. When snorted regularly, cocaine can cause loss of sense of smell, problems with swallowing, nosebleeds, hoarseness, and a general irritation of the nasal septum with a frequently inflamcd nose

(Bussi et al. 2011; Advokat et al. 2014). When smoked (crack), cocaine can provoke damage to the lungs and make asthma worse (Drent et al. 2012). When injected, cocaine users show puncture marks, usually in their forearms, and run the risk of contracting infectious diseases such as HIV and hepatitis (Riezzo et al. 2012). Allergic reactions to the substance itself or to additives may occur as well, leading to death in severe cases (NIDA 2016d).

In humans, cocaine reduces blood flow in the gastrointestinal tract, leading to possible ulcerations (Riezzo et al. 2012). Because of the loss of appetite, cocaine users can show loss of weight and malnourishment. Moreover, cocaine use can produce important toxic effects on the cardiovascular system: chest pain, stroke, inflammation of the heart muscle, reduction of heart contract ability, rupture of aortic (Fonseca and Ferro 2013; Maraj et al. 2010).

Amongst neurological problems, studies show that cocaine use is associated with seizures, intracerebral haemorrhage, intracranial bleeding, and swellings in the walls of cerebral blood vessels (Büttner 2012). Prolonged cocaine use may lead to impaired movement and Parkinson's diseases (Riezzo et al. 2012).

24.5.2.3 Heroin Heroine, like other opiates, acts on the following brain and nervous areas:

- the limbic system (responsible for controlling emotions and feelings): heroin leads to an increase in feelings of pleasure, relaxation, and fulfilment

- the trunk of the brain (controlling the automatic actions of the body): heroin causes a slowing of breathing

- the spinal cord (transmitting pain signals to the body): heroin blocks painful sensations.

Heroin intake has a sedative effect on the nervous system, giving an immediate feeling of well-being and a reduction in anxiety and pain. This follows a blur of mental functions with lowering heart and respiratory rates (Dipartimento Politiche Antidroga 2009b).

When people take heroin, they feel a so-called 'rush' (a pleasure or euphoria flow). Other short-term effects are warm flushing, feeling of heavy limbs, dry mouth, itching, nausea, sensation of mental blurring, and state of semi-consciousness (NIDA 2017a).

In the long term, heroin users can experience collapsed veins (from injection), damaged tissue in the nose (from sniffing), insomnia, heart infection, liver and kidney disease, lung infection, abscesses, constipation, mental disorders, sexual dysfunction, and irregular menstrual cycle (NIDA 2017a).

Heroine is often enriched with additives like sugar, starch, powder milk, etc. Those additives can obstruct blood vessels, reducing blood circulation capacity towards brain, lungs, liver, kidneys. The exchange of syringes while having impaired judgement also can be a vehicle for hepatitis and HIV.

The use of heroin poses serious health hazards, especially if the intake is injected. The substance is absorbed immediately and can block the respiratory centres, causing death. In such cases, the respiratory rate will either be very slow or breathing will be undetectable. The amount of oxygen reaching the brain is reduced (hypoxia) and in survivors this condition can lead to several health consequences (short- and long-term), including permanent brain damage.

24.5.2.4 Amphetamine/Methamphetamine In the short term, amphetamine/methamphetamine cause an intense sensation of cheerfulness and vigilance. Those who consume these substances become very quirky, energetic, active, curious or even irritable. Other short-term effects include increased body temperature, heart rate, blood pressure, and respiratory rate, pupil dilation, nausea, muscle spasms, mental confusion, blurred vision, and decreased appetite.

Continued use of amphetamine/methamphetamine causes many harmful effects, including dependence (Dipartimento Politiche Antidroga 2009a; NIDA 2018c). Other long-term effects include paranoia, aggression, strong anorexia, difficult thinking, visual and auditory hallucinations, severe teeth problems, weight of loss, itching, and mental disorders. These substances can cause several cardiovascular problems, including accelerated heart rate, increased blood pressure, and irreversible damage to the small blood vessels of the brain with the risk of apoplectic stroke. In case of overdose, hyperthermia and seizures may occur, which, if not treated immediately, can lead to death (Dipartimento Politiche Antidroga 2009a; NIDA 2018c).

Amphetamine/methamphetamine can lead to dependence, with the manifestation of the usual withdrawal symptoms when the substance is not taken. Overdose may occur when a person takes too much drug and show a toxic reaction, possibly leading to stroke, heart attack, and organ problems caused by high temperature. Such a reaction can lead to death.

24.5.2.5 Hallucinogens Due to the sharp change in sensory perceptions and the deep distortion of reality that the consumption of hallucinogens causes, consumers experience a serious state of loss of contact with reality and judgement, which leads to underestimating dangerous situations. It has happened that some people under the influence of hallucinogens, thinking they can fly, have thrown themselves from high places resulting in injuries causing death or serious disability. Hallucinogens can also cause death directly due to acute intoxication, kidney or cardiovascular failure, and more often indirectly, due to accidents.

The effects of hallucinogens occur after about half an hour from intake and can last up to 12 hours, depending on the substance and the amount taken. Consumers define sensory experiences caused by the assumption of hallucinogens as 'trips' ('bad trips' in case of unpleasant experience). In addition to the actual hallucinations, short-term effects include increased heart rate, increased blood pressure, increased temperature, altered time perception, nausea, dry mouth, and excessive sweating (Dipartimento Politiche Antidroga 2009c; NIDA 2016c).

Knowledge about long-term effects is still limited. However, it is well known that ketamine can cause bladder ulcers, kidney problems and reduced mnemonic capacity, and that PCP can lead to memory loss, weight loss, speaking problems, and mental disorders (Dipartimento Politiche Antidroga 2009c; NIDA 2016c).

24.5.2.6 Inhalants Inhalants have psychoactive effects similar to those caused by alcohol: difficulty in speaking, lack of coordination, euphoria, and dizziness. Repeated inhalations cause disinhibition, loss of control, drowsiness, and prolonged headaches.

Some chemical components of the inhalants are quickly discharged from the body, others may be absorbed by the fatty tissues of the brain and the nervous system (myelin sheath). Prolonged use of these substances can therefore damage the neuronal myelin sheath, responsible for the transmission of pulses from/to the brain, with effects similar to multiple sclerosis: motor disturbances, tremors, and muscle spasms. Long-term effects also cause liver failure, cardiac infarction, permanent brain and spinal cord damage, and permanent nerve dysfunction (polyneuropathy) (NIDA 2017b).

24.5.2.7 New psychoactive substances The effects of NPSs vary significantly depending on the type of substance, the amount taken, and the mixture of components that is being consumed. Therefore, given the wide range of substances available, it is difficult to draw up a precise list of the effects on the organism for each substance. However, cases of poisoning registered in Europe and across the Atlantic have allowed some common and other specific effects per substance group to be identified (Serpelloni et al. 2013).

The most common adverse effects are nausea, vomiting, anxiety, and palpitations. NPSs may also cause epileptic seizures, psychotic episodes, addiction, and withdrawal symptoms.

For synthetic cannabinoids, the effects are similar, if not greater, than those caused by cannabis consumption. Their intake generates short-term conjunctivitis, tachycardia, xerostomia, and an alteration in perception and mood. These effects can last up to six hours. In addition, the literature reports cardiovascular system disorders (i.e. acute coronary syndrome, severe and prolonged bradycardia or tachycardia) and disorders of the nervous system such as temporary loss of knowledge, psychomotor agitation, panic attacks and confusional states, seizures.

For synthetic cathinones, the most commonly reported clinical effects are anxiety, decreased concentration and short-term memory, nasal membrane irritation, headache, tachycardia, hypertension, hyperhidrosis, midriasis, trisma, bruxism, hallucinations, severe psychomotor agitation and aggression, and seizures.

Phenethylamines cause an increase in heart rate, respiration, blood pressure, and body temperature. This last effect can cause seizures and coma. However, the effects vary from substance to substance and include high blood pressure associated with seizures, confusion, cardiovascular disorders, dehydration, confusion, central nervous system depression, panic attacks, vomiting, delirium, memory loss, and muscle stiffness.

In addition to the analgesic effect, fentanyl is able to produce drowsiness and euphoria, although the euphoric effect is less pronounced than that produced by heroin and morphine. The main side effects include nausea, dizziness, emesis, fatigue, headache, constipation, anaemia, and peripheral oedema.

Synthetic opioids may have stimulant effects mediated by the inhibition of dopamine or norepinephrine transporter. In addition to the side effects common to all opiates (constipation, dry mouth, dizziness, muscle contractions, and nausea), repeated administration of synthetic opioids can lead to neurotoxic effects.

24.5.3 Drug use and related infectious pathologies

Drug use increases viral infection risk because some viruses can spread widely through blood or body fluids. This happens when drug users inject the substance and then share needles (or other drug equipment that has been in contact with their blood) or when, under the effect of drugs, people take risky behaviours like unprotected sex with infected partners. Moreover, infected women can pass the virus to their baby during pregnancy or during breastfeeding, even if they do not take drugs.

The viral infections of most concern are HIV and hepatitis B and C. It is important to notice that drug use can worsen the symptoms rising from a viral infection. In case of HIV symptoms, drug use can cause greater nerve cell injury and impairment of functions like thinking, learning, and memory. Amongst people infected with hepatitis B or hepatitis C virus, drug use can also directly damage the liver, increasing the risk for chronic liver disease and cancer (NIDA 2018d).

Drug users who inject drugs are exposed to frequent transient bacterium episodes, which may become sepsis when they generate infectious outbreaks that are able to infuse microbes in circulation, in a continuous or intermittent way, causing the onset of septicaemia. Endocarditis is one of the most frequent and serious infectious diseases in the drug user and, together with sepsis, is often linked to an infection of the skin and soft tissues or thrombophlebitis at the injection sites (Russo and Rezza 2012).

Injecting cocaine, usually mixed with heroin (speedball), is often complicated by skin necrosis due to the powerful vasoconstrictive effect. Booting consists of repeatedly aspirating blood into the syringe before downloading the entire content into the vein. Drug users sometimes fragment capsules or tablets with the teeth before injecting the material, exposing themselves to bacterial infections of the oral cavity (streptococci, Gram-negatives, anaerobes). Needle licking is not uncommon. Direct injection into the intramuscular or subcutaneous site may be affected by the lack of peripheral vascular veins or poor injecting technique. This facilitates the onset of infections of the skin and soft tissues as well (Mengoli 2012).

Injecting drug use is also related to osteoarticular infections. These include acute bacterial arthritis, chronic arthritis, tuberculous arthritis, and osteomyelitis. Acute bacterial arthritis is the most common form amongst drug users. Microorganisms reach the articulation predominantly by the hematogenic route, or by spreading from contiguous infectious processes or direct joint injury. Chronic arthritis in drug users is supported by michets and in particular by *Candida* spp., which cause fungal infection. In immunocompromised patients with acquired immune deficiency syndrome, Cryptococcus and Micobacteria are also recognised. These are typically conditions which present few symptoms and evolve slowly, but if untreated inevitably lead to the destruction of the joint, with loss of function and mobility. Tuberculous arthritis can be found in about 10% of all extrapulmonary tuberculosis forms. The major risk factors are the abuse of alcohol and injecting drugs, malnutrition, and acquired immunodeficiency syndrome. Osteomyelitis is the inflammation of bone tissue caused by an infection sustained by multiple microorganisms (Wilson and Winn 2008).

In patients who use intravenous or inhaled drugs, insults on the lung tissue may be of two types, infectious or inflammatory, often co-existent in their clinical presentation. Double-pathogenesis has a 10-fold greater risk of lung infection than in other patients (Hind 1990) and, in coinfection with the HIV virus, an increased incidence of infection, despite the effectiveness of antiretroviral treatment (Le Moing et al. 2006). Amongst the causes of increased risk are altered clearance of secretions, reduced systemic and local immune function, frequent coinfection with other parenteral pathologies (HCV and HIV), and poor living conditions.

Endogenous endophthalmites account for 5–7% of all endophthalmitis and in most cases they are associated with one or more risk factors, including intravenous drug use and immunosuppressive diseases. Endogenous endophthalmitis can be caused by bacteria, most commonly *Staphylococcus aureus*, or fungi, especially *Candida* genus (Schiedler et al. 2003). In those using intravenous drugs, *Candida albicans* is the most frequently infectious agent. The ocular localization of a candidiasis is due to direct penetration of the micelles into the bloodstream by injection of the substance. Lack of asepsis during preparation and inoculation or contamination with *Candida* of the drug itself through the diluent (lemon juice) or with infected water or saliva are factors that favour endophthalmitis (Connell et al. 2010).

Amongst drug users, the central nervous system may be secondary to infections that result from foci in other location, such as endocarditis and abscesses, or be associated with HIV infection. Neurological complications to the central nervous system may be directly related to retroviruses or secondary to unusual opportunistic infections before AIDS. Drugs can interact with the pathogenesis of HIV-related central nervous system damage through different routes that act on HIV replication, on the blood–brain barrier, and on neuroglia function. The major drug-related pathologies associated with drug use are progressive multifocal leucoencephalopathy, cryptococcal meningitis, toxoplasmosis, and cytomegalovirus disease (Ferrari et al. 2006).

The association between drug use, sexual behaviour, and sexually transmitted diseases has long been known because drugs can have significant effects on sexual behaviour. Sexually transmitted diseases (STDs) are a heterogeneous group of infections caused by a wide range of pathogens that are only or preferentially transmitted through sexual intercourse. These microorganisms can infect the same subject at the same time, resulting in several clinical pictures in the same individual. This is possible because some of the pathogens seem to have synergistic action in the transmission mechanism in the pathogenesis and clinical course of infectious diseases. All STDs (except hepatitis B virus infections) do not confer immunity. A summary of the many sexually transmitted diseases related to drug use is given in Table 24.4 (Leone and Girolomoni 2012).

24.5.4 Criminal behaviour

There is scientific evidence in support of the hypothesis that drug use is associated with criminal and violent behaviours amongst consumers. A study by Benson and colleagues, in 1984, highlighted that in a nine-year follow-up period, those who reported using drugs in the first interview (cannabis was the predominant substance, followed by opiates) had accumulated over time twice as many convictions as those who had not declared any use (Benson and Holmberg 1984).

A statistical association between the use of drugs and violent behaviour has been well documented in studies carried out amongst drug users as well as in community samples (Steinman and Zimmerman 2003; Loh et al. 2010). The use of cannabis seems to play a particular role in violent behaviour. Indeed, some longitudinal studies have shown that the use of cannabis at a young age is a predictor of antisocial behaviours, including the use of weapons, in adulthood (Loh et al. 2010; Brook et al. 2014).

More recently, it has been shown that violent and criminal behaviour can be considered to be a result of the severity of drug addiction, psychological, social and neurobiological characteristics, situational factors, and the psycho-pharmacological effects of certain substances (Lammers et al. 2014). This data is confirmed by a study of a subset of drug users, based on the episodes of violence committed, in which the most violent group was the one that also reported the heaviset consumption of cannabis and crack (Golder and Logan 2014).

Finally, it has emerged from scientific studies that more than 85% of minors with a history of drug use end up under investigation for several crimes. In these cases, tobacco and cannabis are the most consumed substances, in addition to other drugs. The consumption of psycho-drugs, though relatively minor, seems to be linked to serious offences such as rape, murder, attempted murder, and burglary. The use of cannabis appears to be related to homicides, the use of inhalants with rape, and the use of opioids with muggings and snatching-related crime (Sharma and Barkataki 2016).

24.5.5 Drugs and driving

The effect of driving under the influence of drugs is demonstrated by the severity of the consequences that result from accidents, injuries, avoidable deaths, and social costs. The adverse role of drugs on driving skill and road accidents has been analysed using different methodological approaches: experimental studies carried out through laboratory tests, driving simulations or

Table 24.4 Sexually transmitted diseases.

Pathogenic agent	Disease or associated syndrome
Bacteria	
Neisseria gonorrhoeae	Urethritis, cervicitis, bartolinitis, proctitis, pharyngitis,
Chlamydia tracomatis	salpingitis, epididymitis, amniositis
• Serotype L1,L2,L3	Venous lymph natal membrane
• Serotype D-K	Urethritis, cervicalitis, statitis, with alpiperite
Ureaplasma uralyticum	Urethritis, cervicitis, salpingitis
Ureaplasma parvum	Syphilis
Mycoplasma genitalium	Bacterial vaginosis
Mycoplasma hominis	Venereal ulcer
Treponema pallidum	Donovanosi (inguinal granuloma)
Gardnerella vaginalis	Shigellosis (anal intercourses)
Mobilunculus curtisii	Enteritis, proctocolitis (anal intercourses)
Mobilunculus muliebri	Proctocolite, bacteremia (in AIDS)
Haemophilus ducrey	
Calymmtobacterium granulomatis	
Shigella spp.	
Campylobacter spp.	
Helycobacter cinaedi	
Helycobacter fenneliae	
Virus	
Human immunodeficiency virus (HIV)	HIV disease, AIDS
Herpes simplex virus 1 and 2 (HSV 1,2)	Herpes simplex genitalis
Papillomavirus (HPV)	Condylomas, carcinomas
Hepatitis viruses (HAV, HBV, HCV, HDV)	Hepatitis
Citomegalovirus (CMV)	Symymonucleonucleosis syndrome
Epstain–Barr virus (EBV)	Infections from EBV
Poxvirus	Contagious mollusc
HTLV-1	Adult T cell leukaemia or lymphoma, paraparezes
HHV-8	tropical spastic
	Kaposi's sarcoma, lymphoma, multicentric Castelman disease
Protozoa	
Trichomonas vaginalis	Vaginitis, urethritis, balanitis
Entamoeba histolytica	Amebias (anal intercourses)
Giardia lamblia	Giardiasi (anal intercourses)
Fungi	
Candida albicans	Vulvovaginitis, balanitis, urethritis
Epidermophyton, trichophyton	Dermatomicosis
Parasites	
Phtirius pubis	Pubic pediculosis
Sarcoptes scabiei hominis	Human scabies
Enterobius vermicularis	Proctitis

roadside guidance, and epidemiological investigations that explore the prevalence of drug use in different populations through street surveys, prevalence studies in subgroups of drivers, accident risk studies, and analysis of responsibilities in causing accidents. In general, studies have shown that the use of any psychotropic substance can reduce the ability to drive a motor vehicle safely and is associated with a reduction in cognitive and/or psychomotor skills, a decrease in driver performance, and an increased risk of road accidents (Sexton et al. 2002; Ferrara et al. 2006; Ramaekers et al. 2006a; Solowij and Battisti 2008).

According to the European Monitoring Centre for Drugs and Drug Addiction, statistics show that in Europe more than 30 000 people die in road traffic collisions every year and about 1.7 million are injured. It is reported that about 425 000 deaths on the road are caused by drink-driving. At international level, in Europe, the United States, Australia, and Canada about 7% of drivers stopped during roadside surveys tested positive for drugs or alcohol in blood or saliva (EMCDDA 2017a).

Since 2007, several prevalence studies have been published on drug and alcohol driving in Europe. One of the most meaningful is the DRUID study showing that amongst EU drivers, 7.43% tested positive for alcohol or drugs in blood or saliva (EMCDDA 2014). Of those who tested positive for drugs, 1.9% tested positive for illicit drugs (mainly cannabis), 1.4% for prescription drugs, 0.37% for both alcohol and drugs, and 0.39% for other classes of drugs. Amongst severely injured drivers, about 50% tested positive for one psychoactive substance (alcohol, illicit drugs or both) and about 10% tested positive for illicit drugs only (EMCDDA 2012). Other EU studies showed that amongst drivers killed in road accidents, about 50% tested positive for at least one psychoactive substance. Moreover, cannabis was the most detected drug, with the highest percentage (35%) found in the UK (Wong et al. 2010; De Boni et al. 2011; Drummer et al. 2012).

In general, the effects of drugs on driving performance vary in relation to the dose of active substance consumed, the route of administration, the prior experience of the user, individual vulnerability, and the context of consumption. The main effects that illicit drugs have on driving performance according to the type of substance are described in the following sections.

24.5.5.1 Cannabis Both experimental and epidemiological studies that analyse the effects of drugs on psychomotor performance have shown dose-related impairment of the various functions necessary for driving (Ramaekers et al. 2004; Ménétrey et al. 2005; Khiabani et al. 2006). For cannabis, the effects, already evident even after small doses (5–10 mg of THC), can last up to 4–8 hours after the intake and are distinguished by their acute and chronic effects. Effects are amplified when cannabis is associated with alcohol or other psychoactive substances. They particularly affect speed and deviation from the normal driving position of the vehicle (Sexton et al. 2002; Ferrara et al. 2006). In summary, the effects of cannabis on driving performance are slow reaction times, reduced perception of peripheral light stimuli, reduced ocular motor control, spatial–temporal distortion, coordination difficulties, poor speed control, braking and acceleration errors, poorer judgement skills, risky overtaking manoeuvres, reduced attention, and reduction in short-term memory. The effects of simultaneous intake of cannabis and alcohol, one of the most commonly encountered associations amongst drivers, may be additive and multiply the adverse effects on driving (Chipman et al. 2003; Ramaekers et al. 2006b). The effects of the combined use of alcohol and cannabis are thus more severe than those resulting from the use of these substances taken individually (Liguori et al. 2002; O'Kane et al. 2002).

24.5.5.2 Cocaine The results of the few studies available report that effects of cocaine can be influenced by the induction of hypercortisolaemia, leading to symptoms such as mania, depression, poor concentration, hyperactivity, and impaired vigilance attention (Rush et al. 1999; Hopper et al. 2004). Snorted cocaine provokes effects immediately after consumption which can last up to two hours (and several days when cocaine is consumed in a binge). Studies have demonstrated that the probability of being involved in a road accident when on cocaine is higher when cocaine is consumed in association with other psychoactive substances (Dussault et al. 2002; Stoduto et al. 2012). Combined with alcohol, cocaine can partially oppose some effects of alcohol while it can reinforce the effects of other illicit drugs, such as cannabis (Farré et al. 1993; Foltin et al. 1993). Chronic use of cocaine amongst drivers can lead to difficulties in processing cognitive tasks regarding attention, memory, visuospatial perception, perceptual–motor speed, cognitive flexibility, problem-solving, abstraction, and executive functioning (Di Sclafani et al. 2002; Goldstein et al. 2004; Kelley et al. 2005), resulting in cognitive defects, impaired psychomotor performance, and impulsive behaviour.

24.5.5.3 Opioids

Studies have shown that opioids can cause cognitive and psychomotor impairment, whose intensity depends on the type of opioid and the administered dose. Effects of morphine consumption have been recorded above 5 mg dosage and have been shown to impair driving abilities (Walker et al. 2001). Fentanyl administered for hospital surgery can cause significant cognitive impairment, but this does not last more than four hours (Schneider et al. 1999). Methadone has resulted in driving impairment in naive subjects, but less in habitual consumers (Strand et al. 2011). Codeine has been associated with a greater chance of being involved in road accidents, even though it is unclear what type of driving impairment it causes (Bachs et al. 2009). Fentanyl causes a psychomotor function impairment up to two hours after intake, while the same effects caused by heroin consumption may last up to six hours. Impairment of psychomotor skills and of the cognitive functions involved in driving performance are the most frequently detected effects in the chronic use of opioids (Larsen et al. 1999; Strumpf et al. 2005).

24.5.5.4 Amphetamine/Methamphetamine

Studies have shown that amphetamine and methamphetamine can stimulate cognitive and psychomotor functions, especially in fatigued or sleep-deprived persons. However, they can also reduce driving capacity and impair cognitive functions (i.e. working memory, movement perception) (McKetin et al. 1999; Barch and Carter 2005). People who take stimulants alone at medicinal dosage are usually fit to drive, but are less fit when stimulants are taken in combination with sleep loss or alcohol intoxication, as often happens with drug users. Experimental studies of MDMA effects on driving performance have also found both negative (increased speed and increased speed variance, decreased ability to follow a car) and positive effects (decreased standard deviation of lateral position and increased psychomotor speed) (Ramaekers et al. 2012). The effects on psychomotor performance can last over five hours, in some cases for several days.

24.5.5.5 Benzodiazepines and other medicines

Benzodiazepines and Z-hypnotics can have different effects on driving performance. Some benzodiazepines and benzodiazepine-like drugs have little or no effect, while others, such as intermediate-acting benzodiazepines, result in greater impairment, especially lorazepam and alprazolam. A few studies carried out on long-acting benzodiazepines reported important impairment (clonazepam and diazepam). The most common negative effects were cognitive impairment, reduced memory, reduced psychomotor performance, impaired standard deviation of lateral position, and impaired driving (Stillwell 2003; Leufkens et al. 2007). The effects caused by the consumption of benzodiazepines and Z-hypnotics do not usually last longer than 8–10 hours, leaving no or low effects after night-time. However, this will vary according to the substance and the dosage administered (Berghaus et al. 2010). When taken in combination with alcohol, benzodiazepines cause clear impairment and the risk of being involved in or responsible for an accident increases when other psychoactive substances are taken. When benzodiazepines are consumed chronically, tolerance may develop, showing that effects on day time performance, including driving, may diminish.

24.5.5.6 Drug use in the workplace The extent of the spread of illicit drug consumption in industrialised countries leads to the impact that this type of consumption may have on the active and productive population of working age (Mollica and Serpelloni 2011). As a result, over time a great deal of attention has been paid to the use of drugs as a risk factor for accidents at work (Alleyne et al. 1991; Lehman and Simpson 1992; National Research Council 1994). In Europe, around 30 million people use drugs and many of them are adults, with working skills and/or employed. Moreover, more than 40% of people in drug rehabilitation have a job occupation. In the UK, about 10–13% of workers reported drug use in the last year (7% in the last month) and about 30% of cannabis users are employed (Vermeeren and Coenen 2011).

The intake of psychotropic substances while performing works at risk increases the probability of unfavourable and unexpected events (accidents) occurring (Holcom et al. 1993). Moreover, since the 1990s, numerous studies have documented a clear link between the risk of accidents at work and the use of substances. This risk increases from 50 to 100% depending on the substance used (alcohol, cannabis, other substances), the dose consumed, and the frequency of drugs intake (Hingson et al. 1985; Zwerling and Orav 1990; Gutierrez-Fisac et al. 1992).

In addition to the risk of work-related injuries related to drug use, the use of substances may also have other consequences at work, including absenteeism, increased turnover, and the provision of disciplinary actions (SAMHSA 1999; Bush and Autry 2002; Phillips et al. 2015).

Numerous studies have been carried out using driving simulators, road tests, and psychometric tests to evaluate the alteration of driving skills of motor vehicles in the workplace. These studies have found that driving and cognitive abilities are altered in a dose-dependent manner related to the amount of drugs in the blood. Furthermore, these studies have shown that the use of drugs, especially cannabis, can negatively influence a worker's attention to driving vehicles, his/her perception of time and speed, and his/her ability to learn from experience. Other studies carried out on workers have confirmed that individuals show impaired motor activity and decreased coordination ability in divided attention tasks as a result of drug use (Ramaekers et al. 2006b).

In the workplace, the most common consequences of drug use, particularly cannabis use, are delayed decision making, incorrect cognitive function, diminished concentration, time distortion, impaired memory, paranoia, and drowsiness (Dougherty 2016).

To counteract the use of drugs in the workplace, a form of control and prevention has been introduced: workplace drug testing. This involves carrying out toxicological tests on workers who perform risk-based tasks to assess their possible use of drugs, the effects that such use may have on their work performance, and any addiction that the worker may have developed. Europe, the United States, and Canada implement this control and prevention in different ways (some countries perform tests only on saliva, others on saliva and blood, some countries perform controls without notice, others with notice, etc.). However, in general, most countries have developed guidelines and/or rules regulating this activity and giving indication on how to handle any workers tested positive. According to scientific literature, workplace drug testing represents a valid safety strategy (Miller et al. 2007; Pidd and Roche 2014). In a general analysis of drug testing carried out in various European countries, the percentage of workers who tested positive ranged from 1 to 20% and pre-employment drug testing performed in several companies recorded 5% positivity (Brunt et al. 2017). In the United States, over 8% of full-time workers aged 18–64 years tested positive (Alleyne et al. 1991; Lehman and Simpson 1992; Gust and Walsh 1989).

References

Advokat, C., Comaty, J., and Julien, R. (2014). *Julien's Primer of Drug Action*, 13e. New York: Worth Publishers

Alleyne, B.C., Stuart, P., and Copes, R. (1991). Alcohol and other drug use in occupational facilities. *J. Occup. Med.* 33 (4): 496–500.

Arsenault, L., Cannon, M., Poulton, R. et al. (2002). Cannabis use in adolescence and risk for adult psychosis: longitudinal prospective study. *BMJ* 325 (7374): 1212–1213.

Bachs, L.C., Engeland, A., Morland, J.G., and Skurtveit, S. (2009). The risk of motor vehicle accidents involving drivers with prescriptions for codeine or tramadol. *Clin. Pharmacol. Ther.* 85: 596–599.

Balster, R.L. (1998). Neural basis of inhalant abuse. *Drug Alcohol Depend.* 51 (1–2): 207–214.

Barch, D.M. and Carter, C.S. (2005). Amphetamine improves cognitive function in medicated individuals with schizophrenia and in healthy volunteers. *Schizophr. Res.* 77: 43–58.

Baumann, M.H., Partilla, J.S., Lehner, K.R. et al. (2013). Powerful cocaine-like actions of 3,4-methylenedioxypyrovalerone (MDPV), a principal constituent of psychoactive 'bath salts' products. *Neuropsychopharmacology* 38 (4): 552–562.

Bell, C., Slim, J., Flaten, H.K. et al. (2015). Butane hash oil burns associated with marijuana liberalization in Colorado. *J. Med. Toxicol.* 11 (4): 422–425.

Benson, G. and Holmberg, M.B. (1984). Drug-related criminality among young people. *Acta Psychiatr. Scand.* 70 (5): 487–502.

Berghaus, G., Sticht, G., Grellner, W., et al. (2010), Meta-analysis of empirical studies concerning the effects of medicines and illegal drugs including pharmacokinetics on safe driving, DRUID Deliverable 1.1.2b, Bundesanstalt für Strassenwesen, European Commission under the Transport RTD Programme of the 6th Framework Programme, UWURZ, Cologne.

Bossong, M.G., van Berckel, B.N., Boellaard, R. et al. (2008). Delta 9-tetrahydrocannabinol induces dopamine release in the human striatum. *Neuropsychopharmacology* 34 (3): 759–766.

Brenneisen, R. (2007). Chemistry and analysis of phytocannabinoids and other cannabis constituents. In: *Marijuana and the Cannabinoids, Forensic Science and Medicine* (ed. M.A. Elsohly), 17–49. Humana Press.

Brook, J.S., Lee, J.Y., Finch, S.J., and Brook, D.W. (2014). Developmental trajectories of marijuana use from adolescence to adulthood: relationship with using weapons including guns. *Aggress. Behav.* 40 (3): 229–237.

Brunt, T.M., Nagy, C., Bücheli, A., et al. (2017). Drug testing in Europe: monitoring results of the Trans European Drug Information (TEDI) project. *Drug Test Anal.* 9 (2): 188–198.

Budney, A.J. and Hughes, J.R. (2006). The cannabis withdrawal syndrome. *Curr. Opin. Psychiatry* 19 (3): 233–238.

Bush, D.M. and Autry, J.H. (2002). Substance abuse in the workplace: epidemiology, effects, and industry response. *Occupa. Med. State Art Rev.* 17: 13–25.

Bussi, M., Trimarchi, M., Serpelloni, G., and Rimondo, C. (2011). *Linee di indirizzo – Uso di cocaina e lesioni distruttive facciali: linee di indirizzo per gli specialisti otorinolaringoiatri*. Rome: Dipartimento Politiche Antidroga, Presidenza del Consiglio dei Ministri.

Büttner, A. (2012). Neuropathological alterations in cocaine abuse. *Curr. Med. Chem.* 19 (33): 5597–5600.

Calafat, A., Fernández, C., Juan, M. et al. (2001). *Risk and Control in the Recreational Drug Culture. Sonar Project*. Palma de Mallorca: Irefrea.

Calatayud, J. and González, A. (2003). History of the development and evolution of local anesthesia since the coca leaf. *Anesthesiology* 98 (6): 1503–1508.

CDC (2014). *Behavioral Risk Factor Surveillance System (BRFSS)*. Atlanta: Centers for Disease Control and Prevention.

Center for the Study of Health and Risk Behaviors (2015). *Young Adult Health Survey (YAHS)*. Washinghton: University of Washington.

CESAR, Cocain (Powder). Available at: http://www.cesar.umd.edu/ccsar/drugs/cocaine.asp [Accessed 6 October 2018].

CHA (2016). Monitoring Health Concerns related to Marijuana in Colorado 2000-Jun 2015. Colorado Hospital Association, US Department of Public Health and Environment, Colorado.

Chan, G.C.K., Hall, W., Freeman, T.P. et al. (2017). User characteristics and effect profile of butane hash oil: an extremely high-potency cannabis concentrate. *Drug Alcohol Depend.* 178: 32–38.

Chang, L., Ernst, T., Speck, O., and Grob, C.S. (2005). Additive effects of HIV and chronic methamphetamine use on brain metabolite abnormalities. *Am. J. Psychiatry* 162 (2): 361–369.

Chen, C.Y., Wagner, F.A., and Anthony, J.C. (2002). Marijuana use and the risk of major depressive episode: epidemiological evidence from the United States National Comorbidity Survey. *Soc. Psychiatry Psychiatr. Epidemiol.* 37 (5): 199–206.

Chipman, M.L., Macdonald, S., and Mann, R.E. (2003). Being 'at fault' in traffic crashes: does alcohol, cannabis, cocaine, or polydrug abuse make a difference? *Inj. Prev.* 9 (4): 343–348.

Colorado Department of Public Health and Environment (2016). Colorado Violent Death Reporting System, Colorado: US Department of Public Health and Environment.

Colorado Department of Transportation (2015). Fatality Analysis Reporting System, Washington: US Department of Transportation.

Connell, P.P., O'Neill, E.C., Amirul Islam, F.M. et al. (2010). Endogenous endophthalmitis associated with intravenous drug abuse: seven-year experience at a tertiary referral center. *Retina* 30 (10): 1721 1725.

Cunningham, N. (2008). Hallucinogenic plants of abuse. *Emerg. Med. Australas.* 20 (2): 167–174.

Curtin, K., Fleckenstein, A.E., Robison, R.J. et al. (2015). Methamphetamine/amphetamine abuse and risk of Parkinson's disease in Utah: a population-based assessment. *Drug Alcohol Depend.* 146: 30–38.

Davidson, C., Opacka-Juffry, J., Arevalo-Martin, A. et al. (2017). Spicing up pharmacology: a review of synthetic cannabinoids from structure to adverse events. *Adv. Pharmacol.* 80: 135–168.

De Boni, R., Bozzetti, M.C., Hilgert, J. et al. (2011). Factors associated with alcohol and drug use among traffic crash victims in southern Brazil. *Accid. Anal. Prev.* 43 (4): 1408–1413.

De Gregorio, D., Comai, S., Posa, L., and Gobbi, G. (2016). d-lysergic acid diethylamide (LSD) as a model of psychosis: mechanism of action and pharmacology. *Int. J. Mol. Sci.* 17 (11): pii: E1953.

Degenhardt, L., Hall, W., and Lynskey, M. (2003). Exploring the association between cannabis use and depression. *Addiction* 98 (11): 1493–1504.

Degenhardt, L., Hall, W., Warner-Smith, M., and Lynskey, M. (2004). Illicit drug use. In: *Comparative Quantification of Health Risks: Global and Regional Burden of Disease Attributable to Selected Major Risk Factors* (ed. M. Ezzati et al.), 1109–1176. Geneva: World Health Organization.

Di Sclafani, V., Tolou-Shams, M., Price, L.J., and Fein, G. (2002). Neuropsychological performance of individuals dependent on crack-cocaine, or crack-cocaine and alcohol, at 6 weeks and 6 months of abstinence. *Drug Alcohol Depend.* 66: 161–171.

Diana, M., Melis, M., Muntoni, A.L., and Gessa, G.L. (1998). Mesolimbic dopaminergic decline after cannabinoid withdrawal. *Proc. Natl. Acad. Sci.* 95 (17): 10269–10273.

Dipartimento Politiche Antidroga (2009a). Anfetamine & metanfetamina? Informazioni per i giovani. Dipartimento Politiche Antidroga, Presidenza del Consiglio dei Ministri. Available at: http://www.droganograzie.it/schede_sostanze.html [Accessed 6 October 2018].

Dipartimento Politiche Antidroga (2009b). Eroina? Informazioni per i giovani. Dipartimento Politiche Antidroga, Presidenza del Consiglio dei Ministri. Available at: http://www.droganograzie.it/schede_sostanze.html [Accessed 6 October 2018].

Dipartimento Politiche Antidroga (2009c), LSD *Informazioni per i giovani.* Dipartimento Politiche Antidroga, Presidenza del Consiglio dei Ministri. Available at http://www.droganograzie.it/schede_sostanze.html [Accessed 6 October 2018].

Dougherty, T.L. (2016). Marijuana use and its impact on workplace safety and productivity. *Occup. Health Saf.* 85 (2): 38–40.

Drent, M., Wijnen, P., and Bast, A. (2012). Interstitial lung damage due to cocaine abuse: pathogenesis, pharmacogenomics and therapy. *Curr. Med. Chem.* 19 (33): 5607–5611.

Drummer, O.H., Kourtis, I., Beyer, J. et al. (2012). The prevalence of drugs in injured drivers. *Forensic Sci. Int.* 215 (1–3): 14–17.

Drummond, D.C. (2001). Theories of drug craving, ancient and modern. *Addiction* 96 (1): 33–46.

Dussault, C., Brault, M., Bouchard, J., and Lemire, A.M. (2002). The contribution of alcohol and other drugs among fatally injured drivers in Québec: some preliminary results. In: *Proceedings of the 16th International Conference on Alcohol, Drugs and Traffic Safety (Montréal), La Société de l'Assurance Automobile du Québec* (ed. D. Mayhew and C. Dussault). Canada: Montréal.

Ellenhorn, M.J., Schonwald, S., Ordog, G., and Wasserberger, J. (1997). *Ellenhorn's Medical Toxicology: Diagnosis and Treatment of Human Poisoning*, 2e, 394. Baltimore, MD: Williams and Wilkins.

ElSohly, M.A. and Slade, D. (2005). Chemical constituents of marijuana: the complex mixture of natural cannabinoids. *Life Sci.* 78 (5): 539–548.

EMCDDA (2002). Drugs in Focus, Recreational drug use – a key EU challenge. Lisbon, EMCDDA. ISSN 1681-5157.

EMCDDA (2012), Driving Under the Influence of Drugs, Alcohol and Medicines in Europe – findings from the DRUID project, Lisbon: EMCDDA.

EMCDDA (2014). *Drug Use, Impaired Driving and Traffic Accidents*, 2e. Lisbon: EMCDDA.

EMCDDA (2015a). New psychoactive substances in Europe. An update from the EU Early Warning System. Lisbon: EMCDDA.

EMCDDA (2015b). The EU drugs strategy (2013–20) and its action plan (2013–16) (updated 15.5.2015). Lisbon: EMCDDA.

EMCDDA (2016). The Internet and Drug Markets, Insights Series No. 21, Luxembourg: Publications Office of the European Union.

EMCDDA (2017a). *Drugs and Driving*. Lisbon: EMCDDA.

EMCDDA (2017b), EU Drug Markets Report. Poster, Lisbon: EMCDDA.

EMCDDA–Europol (2009). *Methamphetamine: A European Union Perspective in the Global Context*. Lisbon: EMCDDA–Europol.

EMCDDA.europa.eu (2018). EMCDDA's oficial website. [online] Available at: http://www.emcdda.europa.eu/stats07/PDU/methods [Accessed 06 October 2018].

EU Council Framework Decision 2004/757/JHA of 25 October 2004 laying down minimum provisions on the constituent elements of criminal acts and penalties in the field of illicit drug trafficking. Available at: https://eur-lex.europa.eu/legal-content/GA/TXT/?uri=CELEX:32004F0757

EU Council Recommendations, EU Drug strategy 2013–2020, Official Journal of the European Union, 29.12.2012, 402/01.

Farré, M., Delatorre, R., Llorente, M. et al. (1993). Alcohol and cocaine interactions in humans. *J. Pharmacol. Exp. Ther.* 266: 1364–1373.

Ferrara, S.D., Snenghi, R., and Boscolo, M. (2006). *Idoneità alla guida e sostanze psicoattive*. Padova: Piccin Nuova Libraria.

Ferrari, S., Vento, S., Monaco, S. et al. (2006). Human immunodeficiency virus-associated peripheral neuropathies. *Mayo Clin. Proc.* 81: 213–219.

Foltin, R.W., Fischman, M.W., Pippen, P.A., and Kelly, T.H. (1993). Behavioral effects of cocaine alone and in combination with ethanol or marijuana in humans. *Drug Alcohol Depend.* 32: 93–106.

Fonseca, A.C. and Ferro, J.M. (2013). Drug abuse and stroke. *Curr. Neurol. Neurosci. Rep.* 13 (2): 325.

Franz, C.A. and Frishman, W.H. (2016). Marijuana use and cardiovascular disease. *Cardiol. Rev.* 24 (4): 158–162.

Friedman, H., Newton, C., and Klein, T.W. (2003). Microbial infections, immunomodulation, and drugs of abuse. *Clin. Microbiol. Rev.* 16 (2): 209–219.

Gessa, G.L., Melis, M., Muntoni, A.L., and Diana, M. (1998). Cannabinoids activate mesolimbic dopamine neurons by an action on cannabinoid CB1 receptors. *Eur. J. Pharmacol.* 341 (1): 39–44.

Godfrey, C., Stewart, S., and Gossop, M. (2004). National treatment outcome research study: economic analysis of the two-year outcome data: report to the Department of Health. *Addiction* 99 (6): 697–707.

Golder, S. and Logan, T.K. (2014). Violence, victimization, criminal justice involvement, and sub-stance use among drug-involved men. *Violence Vict.* 29 (1): 53–72.

Goldstein, R.Z., Leskovjan, A.C., Hoff, A.L. et al. (2004). Severity of neuropsychological impairment in cocaine and alcohol addiction: association with metabolism in the prefrontal cortex. *Neuropsychologia* 42: 1447–1458.

Goldstein, R.A., DesLauriers, C., and Burda, A.M. (2009). Cocaine: history, social implications, and toxicity–a review. *Semin. Diagn. Pathol.* 55 (1): 6–38.

Gottschalk, L., Aronow, W., and Prakash, R. (1997). Effect of cannabis and placebo-cannabis smoking on psychological state and on psychophysiological and cardiovascular functioning in angina patients. *Biol. Psychiatry* 12 (2): 255–266.

UK Government. Drugs penalties. Available at: https://www.gov.uk/penalties-drug-possession-dealing [Accessed 6 October 2018].

Grant, I., Gonzalez, R., Carey, C.L. et al. (2003). Non-acute (residual) neurocognitive effects of cannabis use: a meta-analytic study. *J. Int. Neuropsychol. Soc.* 9 (5): 679–689.

Grella, C.E. (2008). From generic to gender-responsive treatment: changes in social policies, treatment services, and outcomes of women in substance abuse treatment. *J. Psychoactive Drugs* 40 (5): 327–343.

Gust, S.W. and Walsh, J.M. (1989). *Drugs in the Workplace: Research and Evaluation Data.* Washington DC: National Institute on Drug Abuse.

Gutierrez-Fisac, J.L., Regidor, E., and Ronda, E. (1992). Occupational accidents and alcohol consumption in Spain. *Int. J. Epidemiol.* 21 (6): 1114–1120.

Hackam, D.G. (2015). Cannabis and stroke: systematic appraisal of case reports. *Stroke* 46 (3): 852–856.

Hall, W. and Degenhardt, L. (2009). Adverse health effects of non-medical cannabis use. *Lancet* 374 (9698): 1383–1391.

Harvey, M.A., Sellman, J.D., Porter, R.J., and Frampton, C.M. (2007). The relationship between non-acute adolescent cannabis use and cognition. *Drug Alcohol. Rev.* 26 (3): 309–319.

Hayatbakhsh, M.R., Najman, J.M., Jamrozik, K. et al. (2007). Cannabis and anxiety and depression in young adults: a large prospective study. *J. Am. Acad. Child Adolesc. Psychiatry* 46 (3): 408–417.

Heal, D.J., Smith, S.L., Gosden, J., and Nutt, D.J. (2013). Amphetamine, past and present – a pharmacological and clinical perspective. *J. Psychopharmacol.* 27 (6): 479–496.

Henquet, C., Krabbendam, L., de Graaf, R. et al. (2006). Cannabis use and expression of mania in the general population. *J. Affect. Disord.* 95 (1–3): 103–110.

Hind, C.R. (1990). Pulmonary complications of intravenous drug misuse: infective and HIV related complications. *Thorax* 45 (12): 957–961.

Hingson, R.W., Lederman, R.I., and Walsh, D.C. (1985). Employee drinking patterns and accidental injury: a study of four New England states. *J. Stud. Alcohol* 46 (4): 298–303.

Holcom, M.L., Lehman, W.E.K., and Simpson, D.D. (1993). Employee accidents: influences of personal characteristics, job characteristics, and substance use in jobs differing in accident potential. *J. Safety Res.* 24 (4): 205–221.

Hollister, L.E. (1992). Marijuana and immunity. *J. Psychoactive Drugs* 24 (2): 159–164.

Hopper, J.W., Karlsgodt, K.H., Adler, C.M. et al. (2004). Effects of acute cortisol and cocaine administration on attention, recall and recognition task performance in individuals with cocaine dependence. *Hum. Psychopharmacolo. Clin. Exp.* 19: 511–516.

John, W.S. and Wu, L.T. (2017). Trends and correlates of cocaine use and cocaine use disorder in the United States from 2011 to 2015. *Drug Alcohol Depend.* 180: 376–384.

Johns, A. (2001). Psychiatric effects of cannabis. *Br. J. Psychiatry* 178 (2): 116–122.

Johnston, L.D., O'Malley, P.M., Miech, R.A. et al. (2016). *Monitoring the Future National Survey Results on Drug Use, 1975–2015: Overview, Key Findings on Adolescent Drug Use.* Ann Arbor: Institute for Social Research, University of Michigan.

Kelley, B.J., Yeager, K.R., Pepper, T.H., and Beversdorf, D.Q. (2005). Cognitive impairment in acute cocaine withdrawal. *Cogn. Behav. Neurol.* 18: 108–112.

Kern, A.M., Akerman, S.C., and Nordstrom, B.R. (2014). Opiate dependence in schizophrenia: case presentation and literature review. *J. Dual Diagn.* 10 (1): 52–57.

Khiabani, H.Z., Bramness, J.G., Bjørneboe, A., and Mørland, J. (2006). Relationship between THC concentration in blood and impairment in apprehended drivers. *Traffic Inj. Prev.* 7: 111–116.

Koob, G.F. and Le Moal, M. (2001). Drug addiction, dysregulation of reward, and allostasis. Review. *Neuropsychopharmacology* 24 (2): 97–129.

Kreek, M.J., Ragunath, J., Plevy, S. et al. (1984). ACTH, cortisol and beta-endorphin response to metyrapone testing during chronic methadone maintenance treatment in humans. *Neuropeptides* 5 (1–3): 277–278.

Kreek, M.J., Levran, O., Reed, B. et al. (2012). Opiate addiction and cocaine addiction: underlying molecular neurobiology and genetics. *J. Clin. Invest.* 122 (10): 3387–3393.

Kyzar, E.J., Nichols, C.D., Gainetdinov, R.R. et al. (2017). Psychedelic drugs in biomedicine. *Trends Pharmacol. Sci.* 38 (11): 992–1005.

van Laar, M., van Dorsselaer, S., Monshouwer, K., and de Graaf, R. (2007). Does cannabis use predict the first incidence of mood and anxiety disorders in the adult population? *Addiction* 102 (8): 1251–1260.

Laing, R. (ed.) (2003). *Hallucinogens: A Forensic Drug Handbook*, 1e. Academic Press.

Lammers, S.M., Soe-Agnie, S.E., de Haan, H.A. et al. (2014). Substance use and criminality: a review. *Tijdschr. Psychiatr.* 56 (1): 32–39.

Larrimore, A. and Powell, E. (2015). Dangerous inhalants. *Journal of Emergency Medical Services* 40 (11): 22–23.

Larsen, B., Otto, H., Dorscheid, E., and Larsen, R. (1999). Effects of long-term opioid therapy on psychomotor function in patients with cancer pain or non-malignant pain. *Anaesthesist* 48: 613–624.

Le Moing, V., Rabaud, C., Journot, V. et al. (2006). Incidence and risk factors of bacterial pneumonia requiring hospitalization in HIV infected patients started on a protease inhibitor-containing regimen. *HIV Med.* 7 (4): 261–267.

Lehman, W. and Simpson, D. (1992). Employee substance use and on-the-job behaviors. *J. Appl. Psychol.* 77 (3): 309–321.

Leone, L. and Girolomoni, G. (2012). Infezioni a trasmissione sessuale. In: *Uso di sostanze stupefacenti e patologie infettive correlate* (ed. G. Serpelloni and M. Cruciani). Rome: Dipartimento Politiche Antidroga.

Leufkens, T.R., Vermeeren, A., Smink, B.E. et al. (2007). Cognitive, psychomotor and actual driving performance in healthy volunteers after immediate and extended release formulations of alprazolam 1 mg. *Psychopharmacology (Berlin)* 191: 951–959.

LeVert, S. (2006). *The Facts about Heroin.* New York: Marshall Cavendish Benchmark.

Li, W., Li, Q., Zhu, J. et al. (2013). White matter impairment in chronic heroin dependence: a quantitative DTI study. *Brain Res.* 1531: 58–64.

Liguori, A., Gatto, C.P., and Jarrett, D.B. (2002). Separate and combined effects of marijuana and alcohol on mood, equilibrium and simulated driving. *Psychopharmacology (Berlin)* 163 (3–4): 399–405.

Loh, K., Walton, M.A., Harrison, S.R. et al. (2010). Prevalence and correlates of handgun access among adolescents seeking care in an urban emergency department. *Accid. Anal. Prev.* 42 (2): 347–353.

Lutchmansingh, D., Pawar, L., and Savici, D. (2014). Legalizing cannabis: a physician's primer on the pulmonary effects of marijuana. *Curr. Respir. Care Rep.* 3 (4): 200–205.

Lynskey, M. and Hall, W. (2000). The effects of adolescent cannabis use on educational attainment: a review. *Addiction* 95 (11): 1621–1630.

Maraj, S., Figueredo, V.M., and Lynn Morris, D. (2010). Cocaine and the heart. *Clin. Cardiol.* 33 (5): 264–269.

McGlothlin, W.H. and West, L.J. (1968). The marihuana problem: an overview. *Am. J. Psychiatry* 125 (3): 126–134.

McGuinness, T.M. (2009). Update on cannabis. *J. Psychosoc. Nurs. Ment. Health Serv.* 47 (10): 19–22.

McKetin, R., Ward, P.B., Catts, S.V. et al. (1999). Changes in auditory selective attention and event-related potentials following oral administration of d-amphetamine in humans. *Neuropsychopharmacology* 21: 380–390.

Medina, K.L., Hanson, K.L., Schweinsburg, A.D. et al. (2007). Neuropsychological functioning in adolescent marijuana users: subtle deficits detectable after a month of abstinence. *J. Int. Neuropsychol. Soc.* 13 (5): 807–820.

Meier, M.H., Caspi, A., Ambler, A. et al. (2012). Persistent cannabis users show neuropsychological decline from childhood to midlife. *Proc. Natl. Acad. Sci.* 109 (40): 2657–2664.

Ménétrey, A., Augsburger, M., and Favrat, B. (2005). Assessment of driving capability through the use of clinical and psychomotor tests in relation to blood cannabinoids levels. *J. Anal. Toxicol.* 29: 327–338.

Mengoli, C. (2012). Infezioni della cute e dei tessuti molli nel tossicodipendente con uso parenterale delle sostanze. In: *Uso di sostanze stupefacenti e patologie infettive correlate* (ed. G. Serpelloni and M. Cruciani). Rome: Dipartimento Politiche Antidroga, Presidenza del Consiglio dei Ministri.

Miller, N.S., Dackis, C.A., and Gold, M.S. (1987). The relationship of addiction, tolerance, and dependence to alcohol and drugs: a neurochemical approach. *J. Subst. Abuse Treat.* 4 (3–4): 197–207.

Miller, T.R., Zaloshnja, E., and Spicer, R.S. (2007). Effectiveness and benefit-cost of peer-based workplace substance abuse prevention coupled with random testing. *Accid. Anal. Prev.* 39 (3): 565–573.

Mittleman, M.A., Lewis, R.A., Maclure, M. et al. (2001). Triggering myocardial infarction by cannabis. *Circulation* 103 (23): 2805–2809.

Moffitt, T.E., Meier, M.H., Caspi, A., and Poulton, R. (2013). Reply to Rogeberg and Daly: no evidence that socio-economic status or personality differences confound the association between cannabis use and IQ decline. *Proc. Natl. Acad. Sci.* 110 (11): 980–982.

Mollica, R. and Serpelloni, G. (2011). e gruppo di lavoro Progetto DTLR, Cannabis e mondo del lavoro: lavoratori con mansioni a rischio. In: *Cannabis e danni alla salute* (ed. G. Serpelloni, M. Diana, M. Gomma and C. Rimondo). Rome: Dipartimento Politiche Antidroga.

Morris, B.J., Cochran, S.M., and Pratt, J.A. (2005). PCP: from pharmacology to modelling schizophrenia. *Curr. Opin. Pharmacol.* 5 (1): 101–116.

Murpy, L. (2001). Endokrinum. In: *Cannabis Und Cannabinoide. Pharmakologie, Toxikologie Und Therapeutisches Potential* (ed. F. Grotenhermen). Bern: Huber.

Murray, M.R., Morrison, P.D., Henquet, C., and Di Forti, M. (2008). Cannabis, the mind and society: the hash realities. *Nat. Rev. Neurosci.* 8 (11): 885–895.

National Collaborating Centre for Mental Health (2008). Drug misuse: psychosocial interventions, National Clinical Practice Guideline Number 51, Leicester British: Psychological Society.

National Research Council (1994). *Under the Influence? Drugs and the American Work Force.* Washington, DC: National Academy Press.

NIDA (2007). Neurobiology of Drug Addiction. Definition of Tolerance. National Institute on Drug Abuse. Available at https://www.drugabuse.gov/publications/teaching-packets/neurobiology-drug-addiction/section-iii-action-heroin-morphine/6-definition-tolerance [Accessed 6 October 2018].

NIDA (2016). The Science of Drug Use and Addiction: The Basics. National Institute on Drug Abuse. Available at https://www.drugabuse.gov/publications/media-guide/science-drug-use-addiction-basics [Accessed 6 October 2018].

NIDA (2016a). Cocaine. Research report series. National Institute on Drug Abuse. Available at: https://d14rmgtrwzf5a.cloudfront.net/sites/default/files/1141-cocaine.pdf [Accessed 6 October 2018].

NIDA (2016b). Drug Facts, MDMA (Ecstasy/Molly)? National Institute on Drug Abuse. Available at https://www.drugabuse.gov/publications/drugfacts/mdma-ecstasymolly [Accessed 6 October 2018].

NIDA (2016c). Drug Facts, Hallucinogens. National Institute on Drug Abuse. Available at: https://www.drugabuse.gov/publications/drugfacts/hallucinogens [Accessed 6 October 2018].

NIDA. (2016d). Drug Facts, Cocaine. National Institute on Drug Abuse. Available at https://www.drugabuse.gov/publications/research-reports/cocaine/what-cocaine [Accesses 6 Oct. 2018].

NIDA (2017a). Drug Facts, Heroin. National Institute on Drug Abuse. Available at: https://www.drugabuse.gov/publications/drugfacts/heroin [Accessed 6 October 2018].

NIDA (2017b). Drug Facts, Inhalants. National Institute on Drug Abuse. Available at: https://www.drugabuse.gov/publications/drugfacts/inhalants [Accessed 6 October 2018].

NIDA (2018a). Drug Facts, Synthetic Cannabinoids (K2/Spice). National Institute on Drug Abuse. Available at: https://www.drugabuse.gov/publications/drugfacts/synthetic-cannabinoids-k2spice [Accessed 6 October 2018].

NIDA (2018b). Drug Facts, Synthetic cathinones ("Bath Salts"). National Institute on Drug Abuse. Available at: https://www.drugabuse.gov/publications/drugfacts/synthetic-cathinones-bath-salts [Accessed 6 October 2018].

NIDA (2018c). Drug Facts, Methamphetamine. National Institute on Drug Abuse. Available at: https://www.drugabuse.gov/publications/drugfacts/methamphetamine [Accessed 6 October 2018].

NIDA (2018d). DrugFacts, Drug Use and Viral Infections (HIV, Hepatitis). National Institute on Drug Abuse. Available at: https://www.drugabuse.gov/publications/drugfacts/drug-use-viral-infections-hiv-hepatitis [Accessed 6 October 2018].

O'Kane, C.J., Tutt, D.C., and Bauer, L.A. (2002). Cannabis and driving: a new perspective. *Emerg. Med. (Fremantle)* 14 (3): 296–303.

Phillips, J.A., Holland, M.G., Baldwin, C.C. et al. (2015). Marijuana in the workplace: guidance for occupational health professionals and employers. *Workplace Health Saf.* 63 (4): 139–164.

Pidd, K. and Roche, A.M. (2014). How effective is drug testing as a workplace safety strategy? A systematic review of the evidence. *Accid. Anal. Prev.* 71: 154–165.

Platt, J. (2000). *Cocaine Addiction: Theory, Research, and Treatment*, 52. Cambridge: Harvard University Press.

Platt, L., Easterbrook, P., Gower, E. et al. (2016). Prevalence and burden of HCV co-infection in people living with HIV: a global systematic review and meta-analysis. *Lancet Infect. Dis.* 16 (7): 797–808.

Puighermanal, E., Marsicano, G., Busquets-Garcia, A. et al. (2009). Cannabinoid modulation of hippocampal long-term memory is mediated by mTOR signalling. *Nat. Neurosci.* 12 (9): 1152–1158.

Qiu, Y., Jiang, G., Su, H. et al. (2013). Progressive white matter microstructure damage in male chronic heroin dependent individuals: a DTI and TBSS study. *PLoS One* 8 (5): 63212.

Quest Diagnostics (2018) Drug Positivity in US Workforce Rises to Highest Level in a Decade, Available at http://newsroom.questdiagnostics.com/2016-09-15-Drug-Positivity-in-U-S-Workforce-Rises-to-Nearly-Highest-Level-in-a-Decade-Quest-Diagnostics-Analysis-Finds [Accessed 6 October 2018].

Quickfall, J. and Crockford, D. (2006). Brain neuroimaging in cannabis use: a review. *J. Neuropsychiatry Clin. Neurosci.* 18 (3): 318–332.

Ramaekers, J.G., Berghaus, G., van Laar, M., and Drummer, O.H. (2004). Dose related risk of motor vehicle crashes after cannabis use. *Drug Alcohol Depend.* 73 (2): 109–119.

Ramaekers, J.G., Kauert, G., van Ruitenbeek, P. et al. (2006a). High-potency marijuana impairs executive function and inhibitory motor control. *Neuropsychopharmacology* 31: 2296–2303.

Ramaekers, J.G., Moeller, M.R., van Ruitenbeek, P. et al. (2006b). Cognition and motor control as a function of Delta(9)-THC concentration in serum and oral fluid: limits of impairment. *Drug Alcohol Depend.* 85: 114–122.

Ramaekers, J.G., Kuypers, K.P., Bosker, W.M. et al. (2012). Effects of stimulant drugs on actual and simulated driving: perspectives from four experimental studies conducted as part of the DRUID research consortium. *Psychopharmacology (Berlin)* 222: 413–418.

Ranganathan, M. and D'Souza, D.C. (2006). The acute effects of cannabinoids on memory in humans: a review. *Psychopharmacology* 188 (4): 425–444.

Reece, A.S. (2009). Chronic toxicology of cannabis. *Clin. Toxicol. (Phila).* 47 (6): 517–524.

Riezzo, I., Fiore, C., De Carlo, D. et al. (2012). Side effects of cocaine abuse: multiorgan toxicity and pathological consequences. *Curr. Med. Chem.* 19 (33): 5624–5646.

Romanowski, K.S., Barsun, A., Kwan, P. et al. (2017). Butane hash oil burns: a 7-year perspective on a growing problem. *J. Burn Care Res.* 38 (1): 165–171.

Rush, C.R., Baker, R.W., and Wright, K. (1999). Acute physiological and behavioral effects of oral cocaine in humans: a dose–response analysis. *Drug Alcohol Depend.* 55: 1–12.

Russo, G. and Rezza, G. (2012). Sepsi ed endocarditi infettive nel tossicodipendente. In: *Uso di sostanze stupefacenti e patologie infettive correlate* (ed. G. Serpelloni and M. Cruciani). Rome: Dipartimento Politiche Antidroga, Presidenza del Consiglio dei Ministri.

SAM (2016). Lessons Learned after four years of Marijuana Legalization, Smart Approaches to Marijuana, Virginia.

SAMHSA (1999). Worker Drug Use and Workplace Policies and Programs: Results from the 1994 and 1997 Household Survey, DHHS Publication no. (SMA) 99–3252. Rockville, MD.

Schiedler, V., Scott, I.U., Flynn, H.W.j. et al. (2003). Culture-proven endogenous Endophthalmitis: clinical features and visual acuity outcomes. *Am. J. Ophthalmol.* 137 (4): 725–731.

Schneider, U., Bevilacqua, C., Jacobs, R. et al. (1999). Effects of fentanyl and low doses of alcohol on neuropsychological performance in healthy subjects. *Neuropsychobiology* 39: 38–43.

Schweinsburg, A.D., Nagel, B.J., Schweinsburg, B.C. et al. (2008). Abstinent adolescent marijuana users show altered fMRI response during spatial working memory. *Psychiatry Res. Neuroimaging* 163: 40–51.

Serpelloni, G. (2013). *New Drugs: Update e Piano di Azione Nazionale per la prevenzione della diffusione delle Nuove sostanze Psicoattive (NSP) e dell'offerta in internet.* Rome: Dipartimento Politiche Antidroga, Presidenza del Consiglio dei Ministri. Available at: http://www.en.npsalert.it/modules/pubbdetails/695/New+Drugs+2014+.html?ln=en Accessed 6 October 2018.

Serpelloni, G., Rimondo, C., Macchia, T. et al. (2013). *New Drugs: Update e Piano di Azione Nazionale per la prevenzione della diffusione delle Nuove sostanze Psicoattive (NSP) e dell'offerta in internet.* Rome: Dipartimento Politiche Antidroga, Presidenza del Consiglio dei Ministri.

Sexton, B.F., Tunbridge, R.J., Board, A., Jackson, P.G. (2002). The influence of cannabis and alcohol on driving, Summary of TRL Report TRL. Available at: http://www.grotenhermen.com/driving/trl2.pdf [Accessed 6 October 2018].

Sharma, S. and Barkataki, B. (2016). Substance use and criminality among juveniles-under-enquiry in New Delhi. *Indian J. Psychiatry* 58 (2): 178–182.

Sherry, C.J. (2001). *Inhalants.* New York: The Rosen Publishing Group Inc.

Sidney, S., Quesenberry, C.P. Jr., Friedman, G.D., and Tekawa, I.S. (1997). Marijuana use and cancer incidence (California, United States). *Cancer Causes Control* 8 (5): 722–728.

Sinha, R. (2013). The clinical neurobiology of drug craving. *Curr. Opin. Neurobiol.* 23 (4): 649–654.

Skowronska, M., McDonald, M., Velichkovska, M. et al. (2018). Methamphetamine increases HIV infectivity in neural progenitor cells. *J. Biol. Chem.* 293 (1): 296–311.

Solowij, N. and Battisti, R. (2008). The chronic effects of cannabis on memory in humans: a review. *Curr. Drug Abuse Rev.* 1 (1): 81–98.

Solowij, N. and Pesa, N. (2012). Cannabis and cognition: short and long term effects. In: *Marijuana and Madness*, 2nde (ed. D.M.R. Castle and D.C. D'Souza), 91–102. New York: Cambridge University Press.

Spronk, D.B., van Wel, J.H.P., Ramaekers, J.G., and Verkes, R.J. (2013). Characterizing the cognitive effects of cocaine: a comprehensive review. *Neurosci. Biobehav. Rev.* 37 (8): 1838–1859.

Steinman, K.J. and Zimmerman, M.A. (2003). Episodic and persistent gun-carrying among urban African-American adolescents. *J. Adolesc. Health.* 32 (5): 356–364.

Stillwell, M.E. (2003). Zaleplon and driving impairment. *J. Forensic Sci.* 48: 677–679.

Stoduto, G., Mann, R.E., Ialomiteanu, A. et al. (2012). Examining the link between collision involvement and cocaine use. *Drug Alcohol Depend.* 123: 260–263.

Strand, M. C., Fjeld, B., Marianne, A., Morland, J. (2011), Psychomotor relevant performance: 1. After single dose administration of opioids, narcoanalgesics and hallucinogens to drug naïve subjects, 2. In patients treated chronically with morphine or methadone/buprenorphine, DRUID Deliverable 1.1.2c, Bundesanstalt für Strassenwesen, Bergisch-Gladbach.

Strumpf, M., Willweber-Strumpf, A., Herberg, K.W., and Zenz, M. (2005). Safety-relevant performance of patients on chronic opioid therapy. *Der Schmerz* 19: 426 433.

Tapert, S.F., Granholm, E., Leedy, N.G., and Brown, S.A. (2002). Substance use and withdrawal: neuro-psychological functioning over 8 years in youth. *J. Int. Neuropsychol. Soc.* 8 (7): 873–883.

Tiffany, S.T., Warthen, M.W., and Goedeker, K.C. (2008). The functional significance of craving in nicotine dependence. In: *The Motivational Impact of Nicotine and its Role in Tobacco Use* (ed. R. Devino and A. Caggiula), 171 197. Lincoln, NE: University of Nebraska Press.

US Drug Enforcement Administration (2015). Special report: opiates and related drugs reported in NFLIS, 2009–2014. Springfield, VA: US Drug Enforcement Administration.

US Drug Enforcement Administration (2016). 2015 Annual Report. Springfield, VA: Diversion Control Division, National Forensic Laboratory Information System, US Drug Enforcement Administration.

UNDCP (2000). Global illicit drug trends 2000. Vienna: United Nations International Drug Control Programme.

UNODC (2003a). *Terminology and Information on Drugs*, 2e. New York: United Nations.

UNODC (2003b). *Terminology and Information on Drugs*, 2e. Vienna: United Nations.

UNODC (2009). *World Drug Report.* Vienna: United Nations.

UNODC (2013a). *The Challenge of New Psychoactive Substances.* Vienna: United Nations.

UNODC (2013b). *The international drug control conventions.* New York: United Nations.

UNODC (2016). *Terminology and information on drugs*, 3rde. New York: United Nations.

UNODC (2017). *World Drug Report.* Vienna: United Nations.

Van Etten, M.L. and Anthony, J.C. (2001). Male–female differences in transitions from first drug opportunity to first use: searching for subgroup variation by age, race, region, and urban status. *J. Women Health Gend. Based Med.* 10 (8): 797 804.

Vermeeren, A. and Coenen, A.M. (2011). Effects of the use of hypnotics on cognition. *Prog. Brain Res.* 190: 89–103.

Verstraete, A.G. (ed.) (2011). *Workplace Drug Testing.* London, Chicago: Pharmaceutical Press.

Volkow, N.D., Chang, L., Wang, G.J. et al. (2001). Association of dopamine transporter reduction with psychomotor impairment in methamphetamine abusers. *Am. J. Psychiatry* 158 (3): 377–382.

Volkow, N.D., Swanson, J.M., Evins, A.E. et al. (2016). Effects of cannabis use on human behavior, including cognition, motivation, and psychosis: a review. *JAMA Psychiatry* 73 (3): 292–297.

Walker, D.J., Zacny, J.P., Galva, K.E., and Lichtor, J.L. (2001). Subjective, psychomotor, and physiological effects of cumulative doses of mixed-action opioids in healthy volunteers. *Psychopharmacology* 155: 362–371.

Wang, G.J., Volkow, N.D., Chang, L. et al. (2004). Partial recovery of brain metabolism in methamphetamine abusers after protracted abstinence. *Am. J. Psychiatry* 161 (2): 242–248.

Wang, X., Li, B., Zhou, X. et al. (2012). Changes in brain gray matter in abstinent heroin addicts. *Drug Alcohol Depend.* 126 (3): 304–308.

Wayman, W.N. and Woodward, J.J. (2017). Exposure to the abused inhalant toluene alters medial prefrontal cortex physiology. *Neuropsychopharmacology* 43 (4): 912–924.

WHO (1992). *The ICD-10 Classification of Mental and Behavioural Disorders: Clinical Descriptions and Diagnostic Guidelines.* Geneva: WHO Press.

WHO (2018). Substance abuse. Available at: http://www.who.int/topics/substance_abuse/en [Accessed 20 October 2018].

Wilson, M.L. and Winn, W. (2008). Laboratory diagnosis of bone, joint, soft tissue and skin infections. *CID* 46 (3): 453–457.

Winstock, A., Barratt, M., Ferris, J., Maier, L. (2017), Global Drug Survey 2017, National Drug and Alcohol Research Centre, Australia.

Wolf, M.E. (2010). The Bermuda triangle of cocaine-induced neuroadaptations. *Trends Neurosci.* 33 (9): 391–398.

Wong, O.F., Tsui, K.L., Lam, T.S. et al. (2010). Prevalence of drugged drivers among non-fatal driver casualties presenting to a trauma centre in Hong Kong. *Hong Kong Med. J.* 16 (4): 246–251.

Zhang, Z.F., Morgenstern, H., Spitz, M.R. et al. (1999). Marijuana use and increased risk of squamous cell carcinoma of the head and neck. *Cancer Epidemiol. Biomarkers Prev.* 8 (12): 1071–1078.

Zwerling, C.J.R. and Orav, J.E. (1990). The efficacy of preemployment drug screening for marijuana and cocaine in predicting employment outcome. *JAMA* 264 (20): 2639–2243.

Index

Essential Forensic Medicine, First Edition. Edited by Peter Vanezis.
© 2020 John Wiley & Sons Ltd. Published 2020 by John Wiley & Sons Ltd.